BASIC IMMUNOLOGY

BASIC IMMUNOLOGY

Functions and Disorders of the Immune System

Second Edition

Abul K. Abbas, MBBS

Professor and Chair
Department of Pathology
University of California, San Francisco, School of Medicine
San Francisco, California

Andrew H. Lichtman, MD, PhD

Associate Professor of Pathology
Harvard Medical School
Brigham and Women's Hospital
Boston, Massachusetts

Illustrated by David L. Baker, MA, and Alexandra Baker, MS, CMI

SAUNDERS

An Imprint of Elsevier

SAUNDERS
An Imprint of Elsevier

The Curtis Center
Independence Square West
Philadelphia, PA 19106-3399

ISBN: 0-7216-0241-X

BASIC IMMUNOLOGY: FUNCTIONS AND DISORDERS OF THE IMMUNE SYSTEM

NOTICE

Immunology is an ever-changing field. Standard safety precautions must be followed, but as new research and clinical experience broaden our knowledge, changes in treatment and drug therapy may become necessary or appropriate. Readers are advised to check the most current product information provided by the manufacturer of each drug to be administered to verify the recommended dose, the method and duration of administration, and contraindications. It is the responsibility of the treating physician, relying on experience and knowledge of the patient, to determine dosages and the best treatment for each individual patient. Neither the publisher nor the editor assume any liability for any injury and/or damage to persons or property arising from this publication.

The Publisher

First Edition 2001. Second Edition 2004.

Library of Congress Cataloging-in-Publication Data

Abbas, Abul K.
   Basic immunology: functions and disorders of the immune system / Abul K. Abbas, Andrew H. Lichtman; illustrated by David L. Baker and Alexandra Baker. – 2nd ed.
      p. ; cm.
   Includes index.
   ISBN 0-7216-0241-X
   1. Immunology. 2. Immunity. 3. Immunologic diseases. I. Lichtman, Andrew H. II. Title.
   [DNLM: 1. Immunity. 2. Hypersensitivity. 3. Immune System–physiology. 4. Immunologic Deficiency Syndromes. QW 504 A122b 2004]
   QR181.A28 2004
   616.07'9 – dc21
      2003050607

Acquisitions Editor: Jason Malley
Project Manager: Linda Lewis Grigg
Designer: Gene Harris

BS / CTP
Printed in China.

Last digit is the print number: 9 8 7 6 5 4 3 2 1

To
Ann, Jonathan, Rehana
Sheila, Eben, Ariella, Amos, Ezra

Preface

The second edition of *Basic Immunology* has been revised to reflect new advances in our understanding of the immune system and to improve on the presentation of information in ways most useful to students and teachers. We have been extremely gratified by how well the first edition of *Basic Immunology* has been received by students in the courses that we teach, and the guiding principles on which the book is based have not changed from the first edition. As teachers of immunology, we are becoming increasingly aware that assimilating detailed information and experimental approaches is difficult in many medical school and undergraduate courses. The problem of how much detail is appropriate has become a pressing one because of the continuous and rapid increase in the amount of information in all the biomedical sciences. This problem is compounded by the development of integrated curricula in many medical schools, with reduced time for didactic teaching and an increasing emphasis on social and behavioral sciences and primary health care. For all these reasons, we have realized the value for many medical students of presenting the principles of immunology in a concise and clear manner.

It is our view that several developments have come together to make the goal of a concise and modern consideration of immunology a realistic one. Most important, immunology has matured as a discipline, so that it has now reached the stage when the essential components of the immune system, and how they interact in immune responses, are understood quite well. There are, of course, many details to be filled in, and the longstanding challenge of applying basic principles to human diseases remains a difficult task.

Nevertheless, we can now teach our students, with reasonable confidence, how the immune system works. The second important development has been an increasing emphasis on the roots of immunology, which lie in its role in defense against infections. As a result, we are better able to relate experimental results, using simple models, to the more complex, but physiologically relevant, issue of host defense against infectious pathogens.

This book has been written to address the perceived needs of both medical school and undergraduate curricula and to take advantage of the new understanding of immunology. We have tried to achieve several goals. First, we have presented the most important principles governing the function of the immune system. Our fundamental objective has been to synthesize the key concepts from the vast amount of experimental data that emerge in the rapidly advancing field of immunology. The choice of what is most important is based largely on what is most clearly established by experimentation, what our students find puzzling, and what explains the wonderful efficiency and economy of the immune system. Inevitably, however, such a choice will have an element of bias, and our bias is toward emphasizing the cellular interactions in immune responses and limiting the description of many of the underlying biochemical and molecular mechanisms to the essential facts. Second, we have focused on immune responses against infectious microbes, and all our discussions of the immune system are in this context. Third, we have emphasized immune responses in humans (rather than experimental animals), drawing on parallels with experimental situations whenever necessary. Fourth, we have made liberal use of illustrations to highlight important principles but have reduced factual details that may be found in more comprehensive textbooks. Fifth, we have discussed immunologic diseases also from the perspective of principles, emphasizing their relation to normal immune responses and avoiding details of clinical syndromes and treatments. We have added selected clinical cases in the Appendix, to illustrate how the concepts of immunology may be applied to common human diseases. Finally, we have realized that in any concise discussion of complex phenomena, it is inevitable that exceptions and caveats will fall by the wayside. We have avoided exceptions and caveats without hesitation, but with a willingness to modify our conclusions as new information continues to emerge.

It is our hope that students will find this book clear, cogent, and manageable. Most important, we hope the book will convey our sense of wonder about the immune system and excitement about how the field has evolved and how it continues to be relevant to human health and disease. Finally, although we were spurred to tackle this project because of our associations with medical school courses, we hope the book will be valued more widely by students of allied health and biology as well. We will have succeeded if the book can answer many of the questions these students have about the immune system and, at the same time, encourage them to delve even more deeply into immunology.

Several individuals played key roles in the writing of this book. Our editor, Jason Malley, has been a skilled and helpful colleague throughout. We have been fortunate to again work with David and Alexandra Baker of DNA Illustrations, who have translated ideas into pictures that are informative and aesthetically pleasing. Our project manager, Linda Grigg, kept the project organized and on track despite pressures of time and logistics. To all of them we owe our many thanks.

Abul K. Abbas
Andrew H. Lichtman

Contents

ix

Introduction to the Immune System

The Nomenclature, General Properties, and Components of the Immune System

Immunity is defined as resistance to disease, specifically infectious disease. The collection of cells, tissues, and molecules that mediate resistance to infections is called the *immune system*, and the coordinated reaction of these cells and molecules to infectious microbes is the *immune response*. Immunology is the study of the immune system and its responses to invading pathogens. **The physiologic function of the immune system is to prevent infections and to eradicate established infections,** and this is the principal context in which immune responses are discussed throughout this book.

The importance of the immune system for health is dramatically illustrated by the frequent observation that individuals with defective immune responses are susceptible to serious, often life-threatening infections (Fig. 1-1). Conversely, stimulating immune responses against microbes by the process of vaccination is the most effective method for protecting individuals against infections and is, for example, the approach that has led to the worldwide eradication of smallpox (Fig. 1-2). The emergence of the acquired immunodeficiency syndrome (AIDS) since the 1980s has tragically emphasized the importance of the immune system for defending individuals against infections. But the impact of immunology goes beyond infectious disease (see Fig. 1-1). The immune response is the major barrier to successful organ transplantation, an increasingly used therapy for organ

Role of the immune system	Implications
Defense against infections	Deficient immunity results in increased susceptibility to infections; exemplified by AIDS Vaccination boosts immune defenses and protects against infections
The immune system recognizes and responds to tissue grafts and newly introduced proteins	Immune responses are important barriers to transplantation and gene therapy
Defense against tumors	Potential for immunotherapy of cancer
Antibodies are highly specific reagents for detecting any class of molecules	Immunologic approaches for laboratory testing are widely used in clinical medicine and research

Figure 1–1   The importance of the immune system. Some of the functions and features of the immune system, and their importance in health and disease, are summarized.

Disease	Max. number of cases	Number of cases in 2000	Percent change
Diphtheria	206,939 (1921)	2	-99.99
Measles	894,134 (1941)	63	-99.99
Mumps	152,209 (1968)	315	-99.80
Pertussis	265,269 (1934)	6,755	-97.73
Polio (paralytic)	21,269 (1952)	0	-100.0
Rubella	57,686 (1969)	152	-99.84
Tetanus	1,560 (1923)	26	-98.44
Haemophilus influenzae type B	~20,000 (1984)	1,212	-93.14
Hepatitis B	26,611 (1985)	6,646	-75.03

Figure 1–2   The effectiveness of vaccination for some common infectious diseases. There is a striking decrease in the incidence of selected infectious diseases for which effective vaccines have been developed. In some cases, such as with hepatitis B, a vaccine has become available and the incidence of the disease is continuing to decrease. (Adapted from Orenstein WA, AR Hinman, KJ Bart, and SC Hadler. Immunization. *In* GL Mandell, JE Bennett, and R Dolin [eds]. Principles and Practices of Infectious Diseases, 4th ed. Churchill Livingstone, New York, 1995, and Morbidity and Mortality Weekly Reports, Centers for Disease Control 49:1159-1201, 2001.)

failure. Attempts to treat cancers by stimulating immune responses against cancer cells are being tried for many human malignancies. Furthermore, abnormal immune responses are the causes of many diseases with serious morbidity and mortality. For all these reasons, the field of immunology has captured the attention of clinicians, scientists, and the lay public.

In this opening chapter of the book, the topics introduced are the nomenclature of immunology, some of the important general properties of all immune responses, and the cells and tissues that are the principal components of the immune system. In particular, the following questions are addressed:

- What types of immune responses protect individuals from infections?

- What are the important characteristics of immunity, and what mechanisms are responsible for these characteristics?

- How are the cells and tissues of the immune system organized so they are able to find microbes and respond to them in ways that lead to their elimination?

Basic principles are introduced in this chapter that set the stage for much more detailed discussions of immune responses in the remainder of this book.

Innate and Adaptive Immunity

Host defense mechanisms consist of innate immunity, which mediates the initial protection against infections, and adaptive immunity, which develops more slowly and mediates the later, even more effective, defense against infections (Fig. 1-3). The term *innate immunity* (also called natural or native immunity) refers to the fact that this type of host defense is always present in healthy individuals, prepared to block the entry of microbes and to rapidly eliminate microbes that do succeed in entering host tissues. *Adaptive immunity* (also called specific or acquired immunity) is the type of host defense that is stimulated by microbes that invade tissues, that is, it adapts to the presence of microbial invaders.

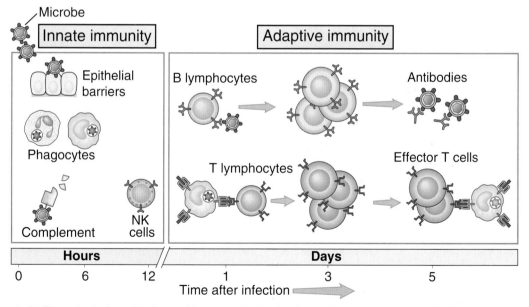

Figure 1–3   The principal mechanisms of innate and adaptive immunity. The mechanisms of innate immunity provide the initial defense against infections. Some of the mechanisms prevent infections (e.g., epithelial barriers) and others eliminate microbes (e.g., phagocytes, NK cells, and the complement system). Adaptive immune responses develop later and are mediated by lymphocytes and their products. Antibodies block infections and eliminate microbes, and T lymphocytes eradicate intracellular microbes. The kinetics of the innate and adaptive immune responses are approximations and may vary in different infections.

The first line of defense in innate immunity is provided by epithelial barriers and by specialized cells and natural antibiotics present in epithelia, all of which function to block the entry of microbes. If microbes do breach epithelia and enter the tissues or circulation, they are attacked by phagocytes, specialized lymphocytes called natural killer (NK) cells, and several plasma proteins, including the proteins of the complement system. All these mechanisms of innate immunity specifically recognize and react against microbes but do not react against noninfectious foreign substances. Different mechanisms of innate immunity may be specific for molecules produced by different classes of microbes. In addition to providing early defense against infections, innate immune responses enhance adaptive immune responses against the infectious agents. The components and mechanisms of innate immunity are discussed in detail in Chapter 2.

Although innate immunity can effectively combat many infections, microbes that are pathogenic for humans (i.e., capable of causing disease) have evolved to resist innate immunity. Defense against these infectious agents is the task of the adaptive immune response, and this is why defects in the adaptive immune system result in increased susceptibility to infections. The adaptive immune system consists of lymphocytes and their products, such as antibodies. Whereas the mechanisms of innate immunity recognize structures shared by classes of microbes, the cells of adaptive immunity, namely, lymphocytes, express receptors that specifically recognize different substances produced by microbes as well as noninfectious molecules. These substances are called **antigens.** Adaptive immune responses are only triggered if microbes or their antigens pass through epithelial barriers and are delivered to lymphoid organs where they can be recognized by lymphocytes. Adaptive immune responses generate mechanisms that are specialized to combat different types of infections. For example, antibodies function to eliminate microbes in extracellular fluids, and activated T lymphocytes eliminate microbes living inside cells. These specialized mechanisms of adaptive immunity are described throughout the book. Adaptive immune responses often use the cells and molecules of the innate immune system to eliminate microbes, and adaptive immunity functions to greatly enhance these antimicrobial mechanisms of innate immunity. For instance, antibodies (a component of adaptive immunity) bind to microbes, and these coated microbes avidly bind to and activate phagocytes (a component of innate immunity), which ingest and destroy the microbes. There are many similar examples of the cooperation between innate and adaptive immunity that are referred to in later chapters. By convention the terms *immune system* and *immune response* refer to adaptive immunity, unless stated otherwise.

Types of Adaptive Immunity

There are two types of adaptive immunity, called *humoral immunity* and *cell-mediated immunity,* that are mediated by different cells and molecules and are designed to provide defense against extracellular microbes and intracellular microbes, respectively (Fig. 1-4). Humoral immunity is mediated by proteins called **antibodies,** which are produced by cells called **B lymphocytes.** Antibodies are secreted into the circulation and mucosal fluids, and they neutralize and eliminate microbes and microbial toxins that are present in the blood and in the lumens of mucosal organs, such as the gastrointestinal and respiratory tracts. One of the most important functions of antibodies is to stop microbes that are present at mucosal surfaces and in the blood from gaining access to and colonizing host cells and connective tissues. In this way, antibodies prevent infections from ever getting established. Antibodies do not have access to microbes that live and divide inside infected cells. Defense against such intracellular microbes is called cell-mediated immunity because it is mediated by cells called **T lymphocytes.** Some T lymphocytes activate phagocytes to destroy microbes that have been ingested by the phagocytes into phagocytic vesicles. Other T lymphocytes kill any type of host cells that are harboring infectious microbes in the cytoplasm. As is discussed in Chapter 3 and later chapters, the antibodies produced by B lymphocytes are designed to specifically recognize extracellular microbial antigens, whereas T lymphocytes recognize antigens produced by intracellular microbes. Another important difference between B and T lymphocytes is that most T cells recognize only microbial protein antigens, whereas antibodies are able to recognize many different types of

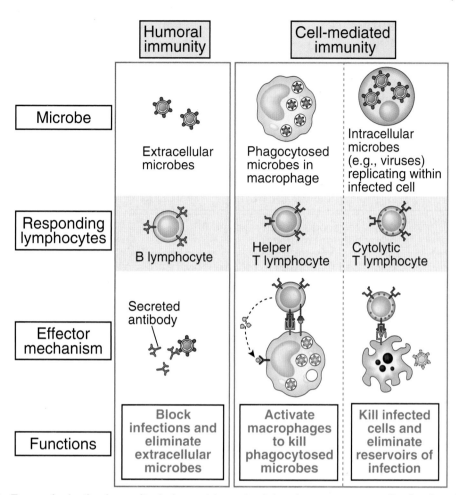

Figure 1–4 Types of adaptive immunity. In humoral immunity, B lymphocytes secrete antibodies that eliminate extracellular microbes. In cell-mediated immunity, T lymphocytes either activate macrophages to destroy phagocytosed microbes or kill infected cells.

microbial molecules, including proteins, carbohydrates, and lipids.

Immunity may be induced in an individual by infection or vaccination (active immunity) or conferred on an individual by transfer of antibodies or lymphocytes from an actively immunized individual (passive immunity). An individual who is exposed to the antigens of a microbe mounts an active response to eradicate the infection and develops resistance to later infection by that microbe. Such an individual is said to be "immune" to that microbe, in contrast to a "naive" individual who has not previously encountered that microbe's antigens. We will be concerned mainly with the mechanisms of active immunity. In passive immunity, a naive individual receives cells (e.g., lymphocytes) or molecules (e.g., antibodies) from another individual who is immune to an infection; for the limited lifetime of the transferred antibodies or cells, the recipient is able to combat the infection. Passive immunity is therefore useful for rapidly conferring immunity even before the individual is able to mount an active response, but it does not induce long-lived resistance to the infection. An excellent example of passive immunity is seen in newborns, whose immune systems are not mature enough to respond to many pathogens but who are protected against infections by acquiring antibodies from their mothers through the placenta and milk.

Properties of Adaptive Immune Responses

The most important properties of adaptive immunity, and the ones that distinguish it from innate immunity, are a fine specificity for structurally distinct antigens and memory of prior exposure to antigen (Fig. 1-5).

Specificity

The specificity of immune responses is illustrated by the observation that prior exposure to an antigen results in heightened responses to subsequent challenge with that antigen but not to challenge with other, even quite similar antigens (Fig. 1-6). The immune system has the potential for distinguishing

Property	Significance for immunity to microbes
Specificity	Ability to recognize and respond to many different microbes
Memory	Enhanced responses to recurrent or persistent infections
Specialization	Responses to distinct microbes are optimized for defense against these microbes
Nonreactivity to self antigens	Prevents injurious immune responses against host cells and tissues

Figure 1–5 Properties of adaptive immune responses. The important properties of adaptive immune responses, and how each feature contributes to host defense against microbes, are summarized.

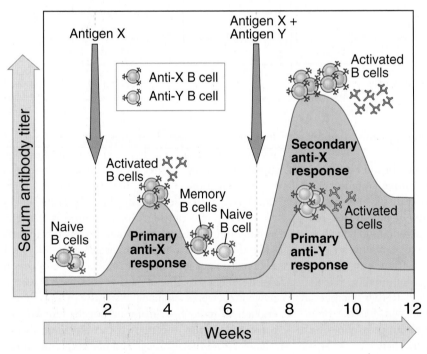

Figure 1–6 Specificity and memory in adaptive immunity, illustrated by primary and secondary immune responses. Antigens X and Y induce the production of different antibodies (specificity). The secondary response to antigen X is more rapid and larger than the primary response (memory) and is different from the primary response to antigen Y (again reflecting specificity). Antibody levels decline with time after each immunization.

among at least a billion different antigens or portions of antigens. Specificity for many different antigens implies that the total collection of lymphocyte specificities, sometimes called the lymphocyte repertoire, is extremely diverse. The basis of this remarkable specificity and diversity is that lymphocytes express clonally distributed receptors for antigens, meaning that the total population of lymphocytes consists of many different clones (each of which is made up of one cell and its progeny), and each clone expresses an antigen receptor that is different from the receptors of all other clones. The clonal selection hypothesis, formulated in the 1950s, correctly predicted that clones of lymphocytes specific for different antigens arise before encounter with these antigens, and each antigen elicits an immune response by selecting and activating the lymphocytes of a specific clone (Fig. 1-7). We now know how the specificity and diversity of lymphocytes are generated (see Chapter 4).

Memory

The immune system mounts larger and more effective responses to repeated exposures to the same antigen. The response to the first exposure to antigen, called the **primary immune response,** is mediated by lymphocytes, called **naive lymphocytes,** that are seeing antigen for the first time. The term *naive lymphocyte* refers to the fact that these cells are immunologically inexperienced, not having previously recognized and responded to antigens. Subsequent encounters with the same antigen lead to responses, called **secondary immune responses,** that are usually more rapid, larger, and better able to eliminate the antigen than are the primary responses (see Fig. 1-6). Secondary responses are the result of the activation of **memory lymphocytes,** which are long-lived cells that were induced during the primary immune response. Immunologic memory optimizes the ability of the immune system to

Figure 1–7 The clonal selection hypothesis. Mature lymphocytes with receptors for many antigens develop before encounter with these antigens. Each antigen (e.g., the examples X and Y) selects a preexisting clone of specific lymphocytes and stimulates the proliferation and differentiation of that clone. The diagram shows only B lymphocytes giving rise to antibody-secreting effector cells, but the same principle applies to T lymphocytes. The antigens shown are surface molecules of microbes, but the clonal selection hypothesis is also true for soluble antigens.

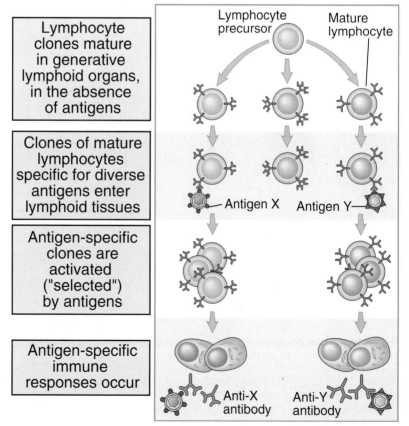

Lymphocyte clones mature in generative lymphoid organs, in the absence of antigens

Clones of mature lymphocytes specific for diverse antigens enter lymphoid tissues

Antigen-specific clones are activated ("selected") by antigens

Antigen-specific immune responses occur

Lymphocyte precursor

Mature lymphocyte

Antigen X   Antigen Y

Anti-X antibody   Anti-Y antibody

combat persistent and recurrent infections, because each encounter with a microbe generates more memory cells and activates previously generated memory cells. Memory is also one of the reasons why vaccines confer long-lasting protection against infections.

Immune responses have other characteristics that are important for their functions (see Fig. 1-5). Immune responses are specialized, and different responses are designed to best defend against different classes of microbes. The immune system is able to react against an enormous number and variety of microbes and other foreign antigens, but it normally does not react against the host's own potentially antigenic substances, so-called self antigens. All immune responses are self-limited and decline as the infection is eliminated, allowing the system to return to a resting state, prepared to respond to another infection. Much of the science of immunology is devoted to understanding the mechanisms underlying these characteristics of adaptive immune responses.

Phases of Immune Responses

Immune responses consist of sequential phases: antigen recognition, activation of lymphocytes, elimination of antigen, decline, and memory (Fig. 1-8). Each phase corresponds to particular reactions

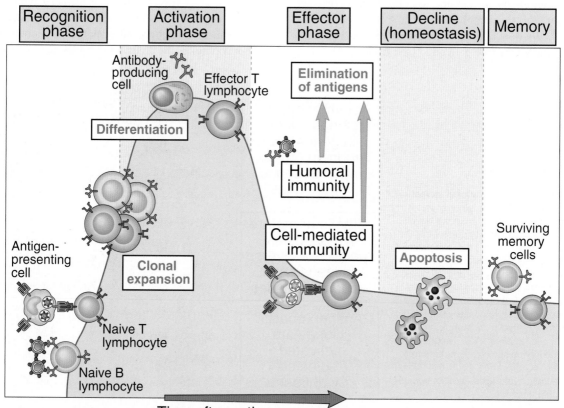

Figure 1-8 Phases of adaptive immune responses. Adaptive immune responses consist of sequential phases: recognition of antigen by specific lymphocytes, activation of lymphocytes (consisting of their proliferation and differentiation into effector cells), and the effector phase (elimination of antigen). The response declines as antigen is eliminated and most of the antigen-stimulated lymphocytes die by apoptosis. The antigen-specific cells that survive are responsible for memory. The duration of each phase may vary in different immune responses. The y-axis represents an arbitrary measure of the magnitude of the response. These principles apply to humoral immunity (mediated by B lymphocytes) and cell-mediated immunity (mediated by T lymphocytes).

of lymphocytes and other components of the immune system. During the recognition phase, naive antigen-specific lymphocytes locate and recognize the antigens of microbes. The subsequent activation of the lymphocytes requires at least two types of signals (Fig. 1-9). Antigen binding to the antigen receptors of lymphocytes (known as *signal 1*) is required to initiate all immune responses. In addition, other signals (collectively termed *signal 2*), which are provided by microbes and by innate immune responses to microbes, are needed for the activation of lymphocytes in primary immune responses. This requirement for microbe-induced second signals ensures that adaptive immune responses are elicited by microbes and not by harmless noninfectious antigens. The "two-signal" concept of lymphocyte activation is discussed

again in Chapter 2 and in later chapters. During the activation phase, the lymphocyte clones that have encountered antigens undergo rapid cell division, generating a large number of progeny; this process is called **clonal expansion.** Some of the lymphocytes differentiate from naive cells into cells, often called **effector lymphocytes,** that produce substances whose function is to eliminate antigens. For instance, B lymphocytes differentiate into effector cells that secrete antibodies, and some T lymphocytes differentiate into effector cells that kill infected host cells. The effector cells and their products eliminate the microbe, often with the help of components of innate immunity; this phase of antigen elimination is called the **effector phase** of the immune response. Once the infection is cleared, the stimulus for lymphocyte activation is eliminated. As a result, most of the cells that were activated by the antigens die by a regulated process of cell death, called **apoptosis,** and the dead cells are rapidly cleared by phagocytes without eliciting a harmful reaction. After the immune response subsides, the cells that remain are memory lymphocytes, which may survive in a state of rest for months or years, able to respond rapidly to a repeat encounter with the microbe.

Cells of the Immune System

The cells of the immune system consist of lymphocytes, specialized cells that capture and display microbial antigens, and effector cells that eliminate microbes (Fig. 1-10). In the following section the important functional properties of the major cell populations are discussed; the details of the morphology of these cells may be found in histology textbooks.

Lymphocytes

Lymphocytes are the only cells with specific receptors for antigens and are thus the key mediators of adaptive immunity. Although all lymphocytes are morphologically similar and rather unremarkable in appearance, they are extremely heterogeneous in lineage, function, and phenotype and are capable of complex biologic responses and activities (Fig. 1-11). In modern times these cells are often distinguished by surface proteins that may be identified by panels of monoclonal antibodies. The standard nomenclature

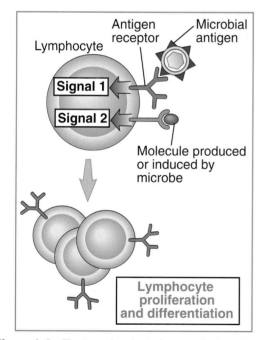

Figure 1-9 The two-signal requirement for lymphocyte activation. Antigen recognition by lymphocytes provides signal 1 for the activation of the lymphocytes, and components of microbes or substances produced during innate immune responses to microbes provide signal 2. In this illustration, the lymphocytes could be T cells or B cells. By convention, the major second signals for T cells are called "costimulators" because they function together with antigens to stimulate the cells. The nature of second signals for T and B lymphocytes is described in later chapters.

Cell type	Principal function(s)
Lymphocytes: B lymphocytes; T lymphocytes; natural killer cells 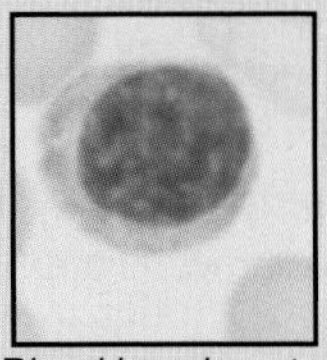 *Blood lymphocyte*	Specific recognition of antigens B lymphocytes: mediators of humoral immunity T lymphocytes: mediators of cell-mediated immunity Natural killer cells: cells of innate immunity
Antigen-presenting cells: dendritic cells; macrophages; follicular dendritic cells 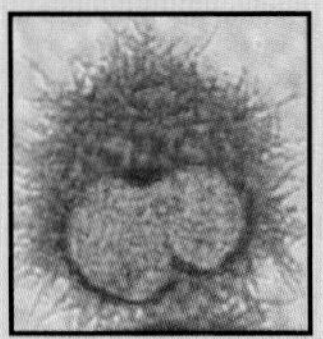 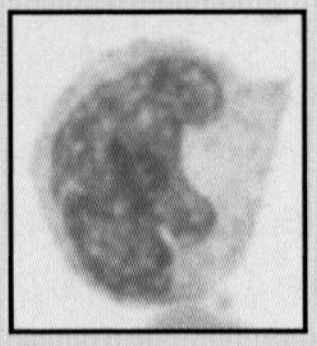 *Dendritic cell* *Blood monocyte*	Capture of antigens for display to lymphocytes: Dendritic cells: initiation of T cell responses Macrophages: initiation and effector phase of cell-mediated immunity Follicular dendritic cells: display of antigens to B lymphocytes in humoral immune responses
Effector cells: T lymphocytes; macrophages; granulocytes 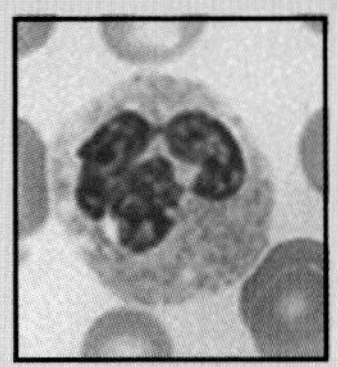 *Neutrophil*	Elimination of antigens: T lymphocytes: helper T cells and cytolytic T lymphocytes Macrophages and monocytes: cells of the mononuclear phagocyte system Granulocytes: neutrophils, eosinophils

Figure 1–10   The principal cells of the immune system. The major cell types involved in immune responses, and their functions, are shown. Micrographs in the left panels illustrate the morphology of some of the cells of each type.

for these proteins is the "CD" (cluster of differentiation) numerical designation, which is used to delineate surface proteins that define a particular cell type or stage of cell differentiation and are recognized by a cluster or group of antibodies. (A list of CD molecules is provided in Appendix I.)

As alluded to earlier, B lymphocytes are the only cells capable of producing antibodies; therefore, they are the cells that mediate humoral immunity. B cells express membrane forms of antibodies that serve as the receptors that recognize antigens and initiate the process of activation of the cells. Soluble antigens and antigens on the surface of microbes and other cells may bind to these B lymphocyte antigen receptors and elicit humoral immune responses. T lymphocytes are the cells of cell-mediated immunity. The antigen receptors of T lymphocytes only recognize peptide fragments of protein antigens that are bound to specialized peptide display molecules called major histocompatibility complex (MHC) molecules, on the surface of specialized cells called antigen-presenting cells (APCs) (see Chapter 3). Among T lymphocytes, CD4+ T cells are called **helper T cells** because they help B lymphocytes to produce antibodies and help

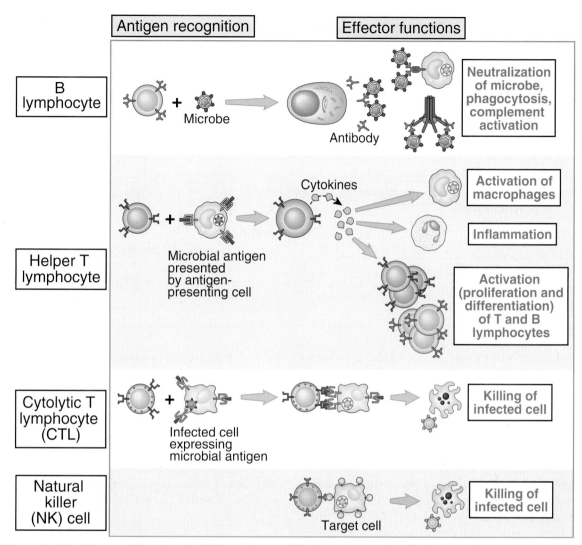

Figure 1–11 Classes of lymphocytes. Different classes of lymphocytes recognize distinct types of antigens and differentiate into effector cells whose function is to eliminate the antigens. B lymphocytes recognize soluble or cell surface antigens and differentiate into antibody-secreting cells. Helper T lymphocytes recognize antigens on the surfaces of antigen-presenting cells and secrete cytokines, which stimulate different mechanisms of immunity and inflammation. Cytolytic T lymphocytes recognize antigens on infected cells and kill these cells. (Note that T lymphocytes recognize peptides that are displayed by MHC molecules; this process is discussed in much more detail in Chapter 3.) Natural killer cells recognize changes on the surface of infected cells and kill these cells.

phagocytes to destroy ingested microbes. CD8+ T lymphocytes are called **cytolytic,** or **cytotoxic, T lymphocytes (CTLs)** because they kill cells harboring intracellular microbes, that is, they lyse other cells. A third class of lymphocytes is called natural killer (NK) cells; these cells are mediators of innate immunity and

do not express the kinds of clonally distributed antigen receptors that B cells and T cells do.

All lymphocytes arise from stem cells in the bone marrow (Fig. 1-12). B lymphocytes mature in the bone marrow, and T lymphocytes mature in an organ called the thymus; these sites in which mature

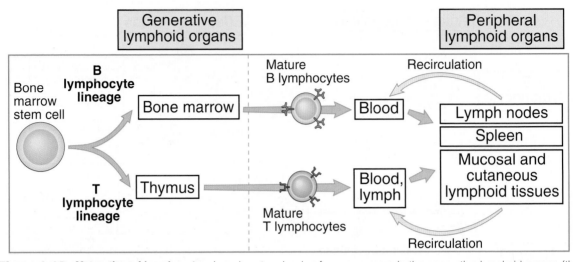

Figure 1-12 Maturation of lymphocytes. Lymphocytes develop from precursors in the generative lymphoid organs (the bone marrow and thymus). Mature lymphocytes enter the peripheral lymphoid organs, where they respond to foreign antigens and from where they recirculate in the blood and lymph.

lymphocytes are produced are called the generative lymphoid organs. Mature lymphocytes leave the generative lymphoid organs and enter the circulation and the peripheral lymphoid organs, where they may encounter antigen for which they express specific receptors.

When naive lymphocytes recognize microbial antigens and also receive additional ("second") signals induced by microbes, the antigen-specific lymphocytes proliferate and differentiate into effector cells and memory cells (Fig. 1-13). Naive lymphocytes express receptors for antigens but do not perform the functions that are required to eliminate antigens. These cells reside in or circulate between peripheral lymphoid organs and survive for several days or months waiting to find and respond to antigen. Their differentiation into effector cells and memory cells is initiated by antigen recognition, thus ensuring that the immune response that develops is specific for the antigen. The effector cells in the B lymphocyte lineage are cells that secrete antibodies, called plasma cells. Effector CD4+ T cells produce proteins called cytokines that activate B cells and macrophages, thus mediating the helper function of this lineage, and effector CD8+ CTLs have the machinery to kill infected host cells. The development and functions of

these effector cells are discussed in later chapters. Most effector lymphocytes are short-lived and die as the antigen is eliminated, but some may migrate to special anatomic sites and live for long periods. This prolonged survival of effector cells is best documented for antibody-producing plasma cells, which develop in response to microbes in the peripheral lymphoid organs but may then migrate to the bone marrow and continue to produce small amounts of antibody long after the infection is eradicated. Memory cells,

Figure 1-13 Stages in the life history of lymphocytes. A. Naive lymphocytes recognize foreign antigens to initiate adaptive immune responses. Some of the progeny of these lymphocytes differentiate into effector cells, whose function is to eliminate antigens. The effector cells of the B lymphocyte lineage are antibody-secreting plasma cells. The effector cells of the CD4+ T lymphocyte lineage produce cytokines. (The effector cells of the CD8+ lineage are CTLs; these are not shown.) Other progeny of the antigen-stimulated lymphocytes differentiate into long-lived memory cells. B. The important characteristics of naive, effector, and memory cells in the B and T lymphocyte lineages are summarized. The processes of affinity maturation and class switching in B cells are described in Chapter 7.

Ⓐ

Cell type	Stage		
	Naive cells	Effector cells	Memory cells
B lymphocytes			
Helper T lymphocytes			

Ⓑ

Property	Stage		
	Naive cells	Effector cells	Memory cells
Antigen receptor	Yes	B cells: reduced T cells: yes	Yes
Life span	Months	Usually short (days)	Long (years)

Effector function	None	Yes
		  B cells: antibody secretion
		  Helper T cells:
		    cytokine secretion
		  CTLs: cytolysis
			None

Special characteristics			
B cells			
Affinity of Ig	Low	Variable	High (affinity maturation)
Isotype of Ig	Membrane-associated IgM, IgD	Membrane-associated and secreted IgM, IgG, IgA, IgE (class switching)	Various
T cells			
Migration	To lymph nodes	To peripheral tissues (sites of infection)	To lymph nodes and peripheral tissues

which are also generated from the progeny of antigen-stimulated lymphocytes, do survive for long periods of time in the absence of antigen. Memory cells are functionally silent: they do not perform effector functions unless stimulated by antigen. When memory cells encounter the same antigen that induced their development, the cells rapidly respond to give rise to secondary immune responses. Very little is known about the signals that generate memory cells, the factors that determine whether the progeny of antigen-stimulated lymphocytes will develop into effector or memory cells, or the mechanisms that keep memory cells alive in the absence of antigen or innate immunity.

Antigen-Presenting Cells

The common portals of entry for microbes, namely, the skin, gastrointestinal tract, and respiratory tract, contain specialized cells located in the epithelium that capture antigens and transport them to peripheral lymphoid tissues. This function of antigen capture is best understood for a cell type called **dendritic cells** because of their long dendrite-like processes. Dendritic cells capture protein antigens of microbes that enter through the epithelia and transport the antigens to regional lymph nodes. Here the antigen-bearing dendritic cells display portions of the antigens for recognition by T lymphocytes. If a microbe has invaded through the epithelium, it may be phagocytosed by macrophages that live in tissues and in various organs. Macrophages are also capable of displaying protein antigens to T cells. The process of antigen presentation to T cells is described in Chapter 3.

Cells that are specialized to display antigens to T lymphocytes have another important feature that gives them the ability to trigger T cell responses. These specialized cells respond to microbes by producing surface and secreted proteins that activate naive T lymphocytes, thus providing the "second signals" for T cell proliferation and differentiation (see Fig. 1-9). Specialized cells that display antigens to T cells and provide second signals are called "professional" APCs. The prototypic professional APCs are dendritic cells, but macrophages and a few other cell types may serve the same function. The

importance of second signals and APCs is discussed further in later chapters.

Much less is known about cells that may capture antigens for display to B lymphocytes, or even if such specialized cells exist. B lymphocytes may directly recognize antigens of microbes, or cells in lymphoid organs may capture antigens and deliver them to B cells. A type of dendritic cell called the follicular dendritic cell (FDC) resides in the germinal centers of lymphoid follicles in the peripheral lymphoid organs and displays antigens that stimulate the differentiation of B cells in the follicles. The role of FDCs is described in more detail in Chapter 7. FDCs do not present antigens to T cells and are quite different from the dendritic cells just described that function as professional APCs for T lymphocytes.

Effector Cells

The cells that eliminate microbes are called effector cells and consist of lymphocytes and other leukocytes. We have earlier referred to the effector cells of the B and T lymphocyte lineages. The elimination of microbes often requires the participation of other, nonlymphoid leukocytes, such as granulocytes and macrophages. These leukocytes may function as effector cells in both innate immunity and adaptive immunity. In innate immunity, macrophages and some granulocytes directly recognize microbes and eliminate them (see Chapter 2). In adaptive immunity, the products of B and T lymphocytes call in other leukocytes and activate the leukocytes to kill microbes.

Tissues of the Immune System

The tissues of the immune system consist of the generative (also called primary, or central) lymphoid organs, in which T and B lymphocytes mature and become competent to respond to antigens, and the peripheral (or secondary) lymphoid organs, in which adaptive immune responses to microbes are initiated (see Fig. 1-12). The generative lymphoid organs are described in Chapter 4, when we discuss the process of lymphocyte maturation. In the following section, we highlight some of the features of peripheral lymphoid organs that are important for the development of adaptive immunity.

Peripheral Lymphoid Organs

The peripheral lymphoid organs, which consist of the lymph nodes, the spleen, and the mucosal and cutaneous immune systems, are organized to concentrate antigen, APCs, and lymphocytes in a way that optimizes interactions among these cells and the development of adaptive immunity. The immune system has to locate microbes that enter at any site in the body and then respond to these microbes and eliminate them. In addition, as we have mentioned earlier, in the normal immune system very few T and B lymphocytes are specific for any one antigen, perhaps as few as 1 in 100,000 to 1 in 1 million cells. The anatomic organization of peripheral lymphoid organs enables lymphocytes in these organs to locate and respond to microbes. This organization is complemented by a remarkable ability of lymphocytes to circulate throughout the body in such a way that naive lymphocytes preferentially go to the specialized organs in which antigen is concentrated and effector cells go to sites of infection, from where microbes have to be eliminated. Furthermore, different types of lymphocytes often need to communicate to generate effective immune responses. For instance, helper T cells specific for an antigen interact with and help B lymphocytes specific for the same antigen, resulting in antibody production. An important function of lymphoid organs is to bring these rare cells together in a way that will enable them to interact productively.

Lymph nodes are nodular aggregates of lymphoid tissues located along lymphatic channels throughout the body (Fig. 1-14). Fluid from all epithelia and connective tissues and most parenchymal organs is drained by lymphatics, which transport this fluid, called lymph, from the tissues to the lymph nodes. Therefore, the lymph contains a mixture of substances that are absorbed from epithelia and tissues. As the lymph passes through lymph nodes, APCs in the nodes are able to sample the antigens of microbes that may enter through epithelia into tissues. In addition, dendritic cells pick up antigens of microbes from epithelia and transport these antigens to the lymph nodes. The net result of these processes of antigen capture and transport is that the antigens of microbes that enter through epithelia or colonize tissues become concentrated in draining lymph nodes.

The **spleen** (Fig. 1-15) is an abdominal organ that serves the same role in immune responses to blood-borne antigen as that of lymph nodes in responses to lymph-borne antigens. Blood entering the spleen flows through a network of channels (sinusoids). Blood-borne antigens are trapped and concentrated by dendritic cells and macrophages in the spleen. The spleen contains abundant phagocytes, which ingest and destroy microbes in the blood.

The cutaneous and mucosal lymphoid systems are located under the epithelia of the skin and the gastrointestinal and respiratory tracts, respectively. Pharyngeal tonsils and Peyer's patches of the intestine are two mucosal lymphoid tissues. Cutaneous and mucosal lymphoid tissues are sites of immune responses to antigens that breach epithelia, much as the lymph nodes and spleen are the sites of response to antigens that enter the lymph and blood.

Within the peripheral lymphoid organs, T lymphocytes and B lymphocytes are segregated into different anatomic compartments (Fig. 1-16). In lymph nodes, the B cells are concentrated in discrete structures, called follicles, located around the periphery, or cortex, of each node. If the B cells in a follicle have recently responded to an antigen, this follicle may contain a central region called a *germinal center*. The role of germinal centers in the production of antibodies is described in Chapter 7. The T lymphocytes are concentrated outside, but adjacent to, the follicles, in the paracortex. The follicles contain the FDCs that are involved in the activation of B cells, and the paracortex contains the dendritic cells that present antigens to T lymphocytes. In the spleen, T lymphocytes are concentrated in periarteriolar lymphoid sheaths surrounding small arterioles, and B cells reside in the follicles.

The anatomic organization of peripheral lymphoid organs is tightly regulated to allow immune responses to develop. B lymphocytes are located in the follicles because FDCs secrete a protein that belongs to a class of cytokines called chemokines ("chemoattractant cytokines"), for which naive B cells express a receptor. (Chemokines and other cytokines are discussed in

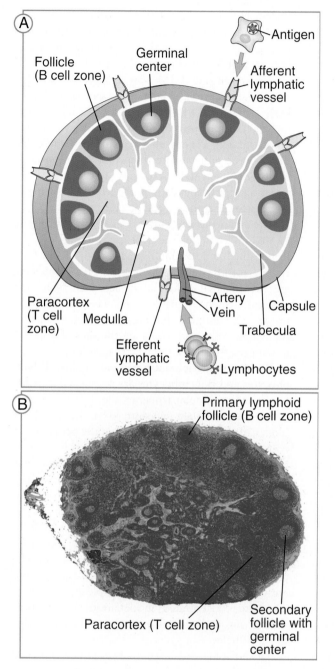

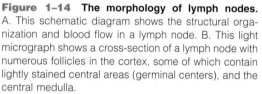

Figure 1-14 The morphology of lymph nodes. A. This schematic diagram shows the structural organization and blood flow in a lymph node. B. This light micrograph shows a cross-section of a lymph node with numerous follicles in the cortex, some of which contain lightly stained central areas (germinal centers), and the central medulla.

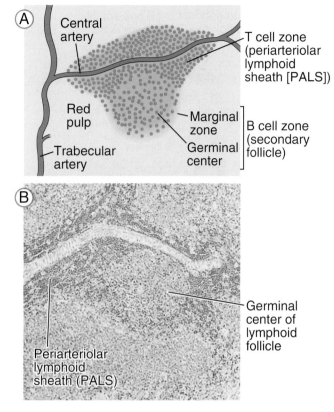

Figure 1–15 The morphology of the spleen.
A. This schematic diagram shows a splenic arteriole surrounded by the periarteriolar lymphoid sheath (PALS) and attached follicle containing a prominent germinal center. The PALS and lymphoid follicles together constitute the white pulp. B. This light micrograph of a section of a spleen shows an arteriole with the PALS and a secondary follicle. These are surrounded by the red pulp, which is rich in vascular sinusoids.

more detail in later chapters.) This chemokine is produced all the time, and it attracts B cells from the blood into the follicles of lymphoid organs. Similarly, T cells are segregated in the paracortex of lymph nodes and the periarteriolar lymphoid sheaths of the spleen, because T lymphocytes express receptors for a chemokine that is produced by cells that are present in these regions of the lymph nodes and spleen. As a result, T lymphocytes are recruited from the blood into the parafollicular cortex region of the lymph node and the periarteriolar lymphoid sheaths of the spleen. When the lymphocytes are activated by microbial antigens, they gradually reduce their expression of the chemokine receptors and are no longer constrained anatomically. As a result, the B cells and T cells migrate toward each other and meet at the edge of follicles, where helper T cells interact with and help B cells to differentiate into antibody-producing cells (see Chapter 7). The activated lymphocytes ultimately exit the node via efferent

lymphatic vessels and leave the spleen through veins. These activated lymphocytes end up in the circulation and can go to distant sites of infection.

Lymphocyte Recirculation

Lymphocytes constantly recirculate between tissues in such a way that naive lymphocytes traverse the peripheral lymphoid organs, where immune responses are initiated, and effector lymphocytes migrate to sites of infection, where infectious microbes are eliminated (Fig. 1-17). Thus, lymphocytes at distinct stages of their life histories migrate to the different sites where they are needed for their functions. This process of lymphocyte recirculation is best described for T lymphocytes. It is also most relevant for T cells, because effector T cells have to locate and eliminate microbes at any site of infection. By contrast, effector B lymphocytes remain in lymphoid organs and do not need to migrate to sites of

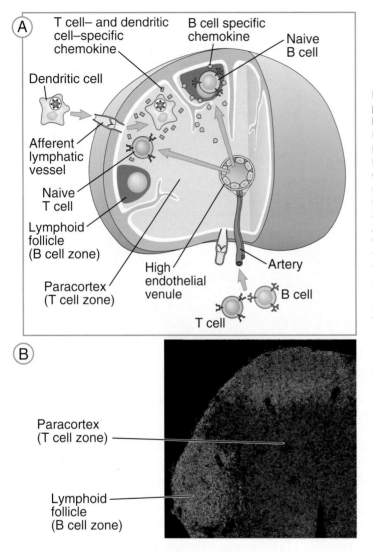

Figure 1-16 Segregation of T and B lymphocytes in different regions of peripheral lymphoid organs. A. The schematic diagram illustrates the path by which naive T and B lymphocytes migrate to different areas of a lymph node. The lymphocytes enter through a high endothelial venule (HEV), shown in cross-section, and are drawn to different areas of the node by chemokines that are produced in these areas and bind selectively to either cell type. Also shown is the migration of dendritic cells, which pick up antigens from epithelia, enter through afferent lymphatic vessels, and migrate to the T cell–rich areas of the node. B. In this section of a lymph node, the B lymphocytes, located in the follicles, are stained green, and the T cells, in the parafollicular cortex, are red. The method used to stain these cells is called immunofluorescence. In this technique, a section of the tissue is stained with antibodies specific for T or B cells that are coupled to fluorochromes that emit different colors when excited at the appropriate wavelengths. The anatomic segregation of T and B cells is also seen in the spleen (not shown). (Courtesy of Drs. Kathryn Pape and Jennifer Walter, University of Minnesota School of Medicine, Minneapolis.)

infection. Instead, B cells secrete antibodies, and the antibodies enter the blood and find microbes and microbial toxins in the circulation or distant tissues. Therefore, we will largely limit our discussion of lymphocyte recirculation to T lymphocytes.

Naive T lymphocytes that have matured in the thymus and entered the circulation migrate to lymph nodes where they can find antigens that enter through lymphatic vessels that drain epithelia and parenchymal organs. These naive T cells enter lymph nodes through specialized postcapillary venules, called **high endothelial venules** (HEVs), that are present in lymph nodes. Naive T cells express a surface receptor called L-selectin that binds to carbohydrate ligands that are expressed only on the endothelial cells of HEVs. (Selectins are a family of proteins involved in cell-cell adhesion that contain conserved structural features, including a lectin, or carbohydrate-binding, domain. More information about these proteins is in Chapter 6.) Because of the interaction of L-selectin with its ligand, naive T cells bind loosely to HEVs. In response to chemokines produced in the paracortical

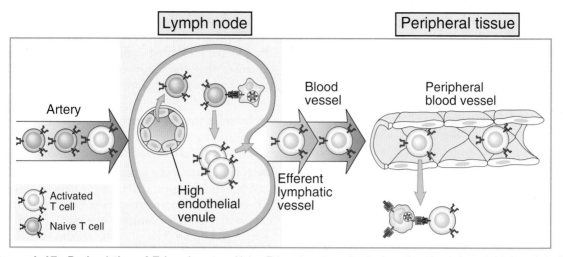

Figure 1–17   Recirculation of T lymphocytes. Naive T lymphocytes migrate from the blood through high endothelial venules (HEVs) into the T cell zones of lymph nodes, where the cells are activated by antigens. Activated T cells exit the nodes, enter the bloodstream, and migrate preferentially to peripheral tissues at sites of infection and inflammation. The adhesion molecules involved in the attachment of T cells to endothelial cells are described in Chapter 6.

regions of the lymph node, the naive T cells bind more firmly to and migrate through the HEVs into this region of the lymph nodes, where antigens are displayed by professional APCs.

If a naive T cell encounters the antigen that it specifically recognizes, that T cell is activated. Such an encounter between an antigen and a specific lymphocyte is likely to be a random event, but most T cells in the body circulate through some lymph nodes at least once a day. As a result, some of the cells in the total population of T lymphocytes have an excellent chance of encountering antigens that these cells recognize. As we mentioned earlier and will describe in more detail in Chapter 3, the likelihood of the correct T cell finding its antigen is increased in peripheral lymphoid organs, particularly lymph nodes, because microbial antigens are concentrated in the same regions of these organs through which naive T cells circulate. In response to the microbial antigen, the naive T cells are activated to proliferate and differentiate. During this process, the expression of adhesion molecules and chemokine receptors on the T cells changes such that differentiated effector T cells tend to leave the lymph nodes and enter the circulation. These effector cells preferentially migrate into the tissues that are colonized by infec-

tious ·microbes, where the T lymphocytes perform their function of eradicating the infection. This process is described in more detail in Chapter 6, where cell-mediated immune reactions are discussed.

Memory T cell populations appear to consist of some cells that recirculate through lymph nodes, where they can mount secondary responses to captured antigens, and other cells that migrate to sites of infection, where they can respond rapidly to eliminate the infection.

We do not know much about lymphocyte circulation through the spleen or other lymphoid tissues or about the circulation pathway of naive and activated B lymphocytes. B lymphocytes appear also to enter lymph nodes through HEVs, but after they respond to antigen, their differentiated progeny either remain in the lymph nodes or migrate mainly to the bone marrow. The spleen does not contain HEVs, but the general pattern of lymphocyte migration through this organ is probably similar to migration through lymph nodes.

SUMMARY

▶ The physiologic function of the immune system is to protect individuals against infections.

▶ Innate immunity is the early line of defense, mediated by cells and molecules that are always present and ready to eliminate infectious microbes. Adaptive immunity is the form of immunity that is stimulated by microbes, has a fine specificity for foreign substances, and responds more effectively against each successive exposure to a microbe.

▶ Lymphocytes are the cells of adaptive immunity, and the only cells with clonally distributed receptors for antigens.

▶ Adaptive immunity consists of humoral immunity, in which antibodies neutralize and eradicate extracellular microbes and toxins, and cell-mediated immunity, in which T lymphocytes eradicate intracellular microbes.

▶ Adaptive immune responses consist of sequential phases: antigen recognition by lymphocytes, activation of the lymphocytes to proliferate and to differentiate into effector and memory cells, elimination of the microbes, decline of the immune response, and long-lived memory.

▶ There are different populations of lymphocytes that serve distinct functions and may be distinguished by the expression of particular membrane molecules.

▶ B lymphocytes are the only cells that produce antibodies. B lymphocytes express membrane antibodies that recognize antigens, and effector B cells secrete the antibodies that neutralize and eliminate the antigen.

▶ T lymphocytes recognize peptide fragments of protein antigens displayed on other cells. Helper T lymphocytes activate phagocytes to destroy ingested microbes and activate B lymphocytes to produce antibodies. Cytolytic (cytotoxic) T lympho-

cytes kill infected cells harboring microbes in the cytoplasm.

▶ Antigen-presenting cells capture antigens of microbes that enter through epithelia, concentrate these antigens in lymphoid organs, and display the antigens for recognition by T cells.

▶ Lymphocytes and antigen-presenting cells are organized in peripheral lymphoid organs, where immune responses are initiated and develop.

▶ Naive lymphocytes circulate through the peripheral lymphoid organs searching for foreign antigens. Effector T lymphocytes migrate to peripheral sites of infection, where they function to eliminate infectious microbes. Effector B lymphocytes remain in lymphoid organs and the bone marrow, from where they secrete antibodies that enter the circulation and find and eliminate microbes.

Review Questions

1 What are the two types of adaptive immunity, and what types of microbes do these adaptive immune responses combat?

2 What are the principal classes of lymphocytes, how do they differ in function, and how may they be identified and distinguished?

3 What are the important differences among naive, effector, and memory T and B lymphocytes?

4 Where are T and B lymphocytes located in lymph nodes, and how is their anatomic separation maintained?

5 How do naive and effector T lymphocytes differ in their patterns of migration?

Innate Immunity

The Early Defense Against Infections

2

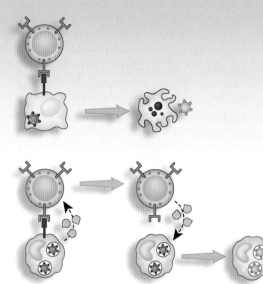

All multicellular organisms, including plants, invertebrates, and vertebrates, possess intrinsic mechanisms for defending themselves against microbial infections. Because these defense mechanisms are always present, ready to recognize and eliminate microbes, they are said to constitute **innate immunity** (also called natural, or native, immunity). The components of innate immunity make up the innate immune system. The shared characteristic of the mechanisms of innate immunity is that they recognize and respond to microbes but do not react against nonmicrobial substances. Innate immunity may also be triggered by host cells that are damaged by microbes. Innate immunity contrasts to adaptive immunity, which must be stimulated by and adapts to encounter with microbes before it can be effective. Furthermore, adaptive immune responses may be directed against microbial as well as nonmicrobial antigens.

For many years it was believed that innate immunity is nonspecific and weak and is not effective in combating most infections. We now know that, in fact, innate immunity specifically targets microbes and is a powerful early defense mechanism capable of controlling and even eradicating infections before adaptive immunity becomes active. Innate immunity not only provides the early defense against infections but also instructs the adaptive immune system to respond to different microbes in ways that are effective at combating these microbes. Conversely, the adaptive immune response often uses mechanisms of innate immunity to eradicate infections. Thus, there is a constant bidirectional cross-talk between innate immunity and adaptive immunity. For these reasons,

21

there is great interest in defining the mechanisms of innate immunity and learning how to harness these mechanisms for optimizing defense against infections.

Most of this book is devoted to a description of the adaptive immune system and how lymphocytes, the cells of adaptive immunity, recognize and respond to infectious microbes. Before starting a discussion of adaptive immunity, the early defense reactions of innate immunity are discussed in this chapter. The discussion focuses on three main questions:

- How does the innate immune system recognize microbes?
- How do the different components of innate immunity function to combat different kinds of microbes?
- How do innate immune reactions stimulate adaptive immune response?

Recognition of Microbes by the Innate Immune System

The specificity of innate immunity is different in several respects from the specificity of lymphocytes, the recognition systems of adaptive immunity (Fig. 2-1).

The components of innate immunity recognize structures that are shared by various classes of microbes and are not present on host cells. Each component of innate immunity may recognize many bacteria, or viruses, or fungi. For instance, phagocytes express receptors for bacterial lipopolysaccharide (LPS, also called endotoxin), which is present in many bacterial species but is not produced by mammalian cells. Other receptors of phagocytes recognize terminal mannose residues on glycoproteins; many bacterial glycoproteins have terminal mannose, unlike mammalian glycoproteins, which end with sialic acid or N-acetylgalactosamine. Phagocytes recognize and respond to double-stranded RNA, which is found in many viruses but not in mammalian cells, and to unmethylated CpG nucleotides, which are common in bacterial DNA but are not found in mammalian DNA. The microbial molecules that are the targets of innate immunity are sometimes called molecular patterns, to indicate that they are shared by microbes of the same type. The receptors of innate immunity that recognize these shared structures are

called pattern recognition receptors. Some components of innate immunity are capable of binding to host cells but are prevented from being activated by these cells. For instance, if the plasma proteins of the complement system are deposited on host cells, the activation of these complement proteins is blocked by regulatory molecules that are present on the host cells but are not present on microbes. These and other examples of innate immune recognition are discussed later in this chapter. In contrast to innate immunity, the adaptive immune system is specific for structures, called antigens, that may be microbial or nonmicrobial, and are not necessarily shared by classes of microbes but may differ among microbes of the same type.

Another characteristic of innate immunity that makes it a highly effective defense mechanism is that the components of innate immunity have evolved to recognize structures of microbes that are often essential for the survival and infectivity of these microbes. Therefore, a microbe cannot evade innate immunity simply by mutating or not expressing the targets of innate immune recognition: microbes that do not express functional forms of these structures lose their ability to infect and colonize the host. In contrast, microbes frequently evade adaptive immunity by mutating the antigens that are recognized by lymphocytes, because these antigens are usually not required for the life of the microbes.

The receptors of the innate immune system are encoded in the germline and are not produced by somatic recombination of genes. These germline-encoded pattern recognition receptors have evolved as a protective adaptation to potentially harmful microbes. In contrast, the antigen receptors of lymphocytes, namely, antibodies and T cell receptors, are produced by recombination of receptor genes during the maturation of these cells (see Chapter 4). Gene recombination can generate many more structurally different receptors than can be produced from inherited germline genes, but these different receptors cannot have a predetermined specificity for microbes. Therefore, the specificity of adaptive immunity is much more diverse than that of innate immunity, and the adaptive immune system is capable of recognizing many more chemically distinct structures. It is estimated that the total population of lymphocytes can

	Innate immunity	Adaptive immunity
Specificity	For structures shared by classes of microbes ("molecular patterns") 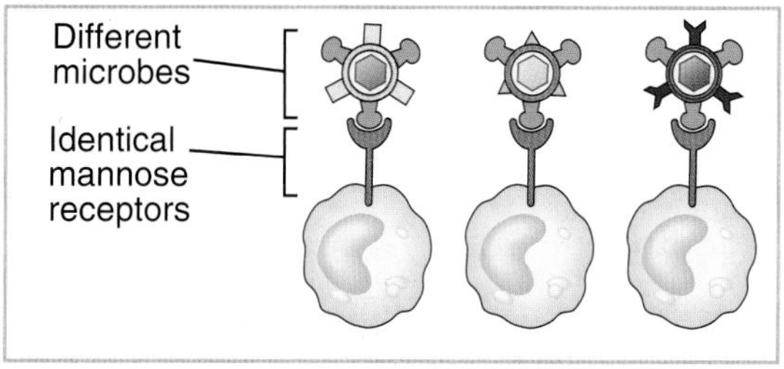	For structural detail of microbial molecules (antigens); may recognize nonmicrobial antigens 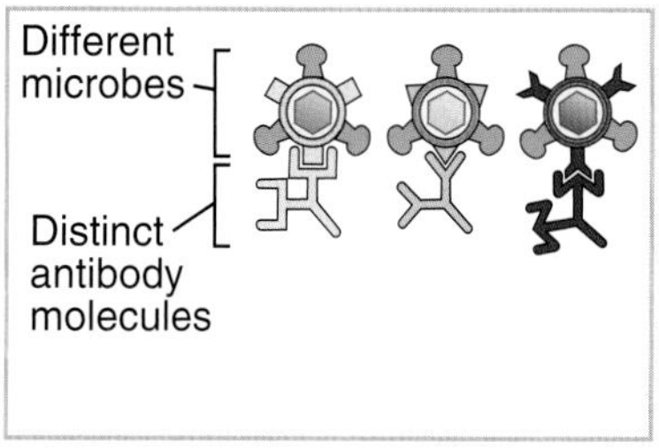
Receptors	Encoded in germline; limited diversity 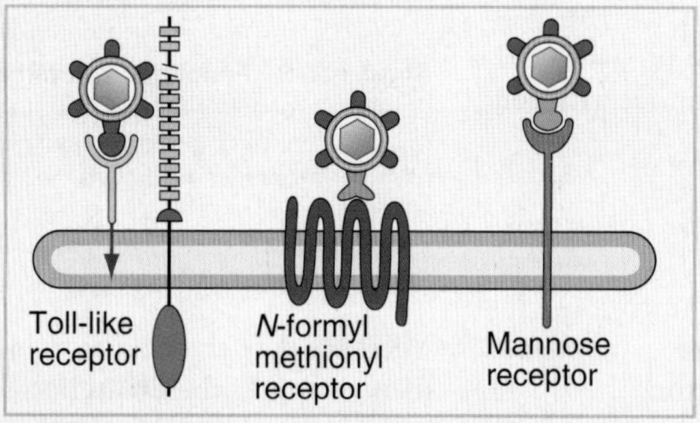	Encoded by genes produced by somatic recombination of gene segments; greater diversity 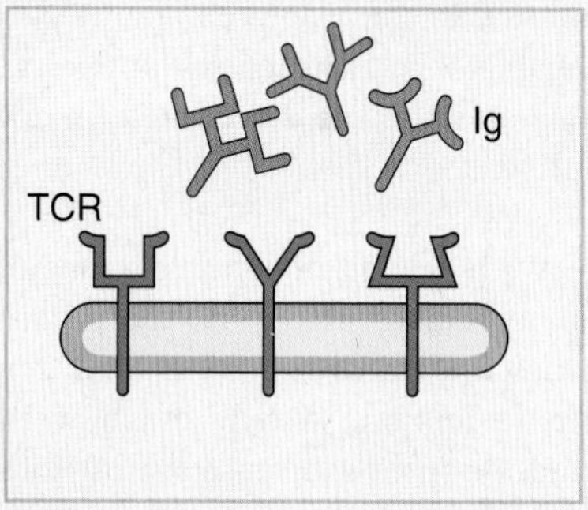
Distribution of receptors	Nonclonal: identical receptors on all cells of the same lineage	Clonal: clones of lymphocytes with distinct specificities express different receptors
Discrimination of self and nonself	Yes; host cells are not recognized or they may express molecules that prevent innate immune reactions	Yes; based on selection against self-reactive lymphocytes; may be imperfect (giving rise to autoimmunity)

Figure 2–1 The specificity of innate immunity and adaptive immunity. The important features of the specificity and receptors of innate and adaptive immunity are summarized, with selected examples, some of which are illustrated in the boxed panels.

recognize over a billion different antigens; in contrast, all the receptors of innate immunity probably recognize less than a thousand microbial patterns. Furthermore, the receptors of the adaptive immune system are clonally distributed, meaning that each clone of lymphocytes (B cells and T cells) has a different receptor specific for a particular antigen. In contrast, in the innate immune system the receptors are nonclonally distributed; that is, identical receptors are expressed on all the cells of a particular type, such as macrophages. Therefore, many cells of innate immunity may recognize the same microbe.

The innate immune system responds in the same way to repeat encounters with a microbe, whereas

the adaptive immune system responds more efficiently to each successive encounter with a microbe. In other words, the adaptive immune system remembers, and adapts to, encounters with a microbe. This is the phenomenon of immunologic memory. It ensures that host defense reactions are highly effective against repeated or persistent infections. Memory is a defining characteristic of adaptive immunity and is not seen in innate immunity.

The innate immune system does not react against the host. This inability of the innate immune system to react against an individual's own, or self, cells and molecules is partly because of the inherent specificity of innate immunity for microbial structures and partly because mammalian cells express regulatory molecules that prevent innate immune reactions. The adaptive immune system also discriminates between self and nonself; in the adaptive immune system, lymphocytes capable of recognizing self antigens are produced but they are killed or inactivated on encounter with self antigens.

With this introduction to some of the characteristics of innate immunity, the discussion proceeds to a description of the individual components of the innate immune system and how these components function in host defense against infections.

Components of Innate Immunity

The innate immune system consists of epithelia, which provide barriers to infection, cells in the circulation and tissues, and several plasma proteins. These components play different but complementary roles in blocking the entry of microbes and in eliminating microbes that enter the tissues of the host.

Epithelial Barriers

The common portals of entry of microbes, namely, the skin, gastrointestinal tract, and respiratory tract, are protected by continuous epithelia that provide physical and chemical barriers against infection (Fig. 2-2). The three major interfaces between the body and the external environment are the skin, the gastrointestinal tract, and the respiratory tract.

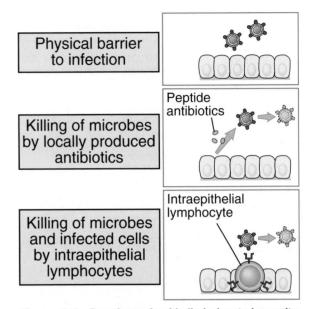

Figure 2–2 Functions of epithelia in innate immunity. Epithelia present at the portals of entry of microbes provide physical barriers, produce antimicrobial substances, and harbor lymphocytes that are believed to kill microbes and infected cells.

Microbes may enter hosts from the external environment through these interfaces by physical contact, ingestion, and breathing. All three portals of entry are lined by continuous epithelia that physically interfere with the entry of microbes. Epithelial cells also produce peptide antibiotics that kill bacteria. In addition, epithelia contain a type of lymphocyte, called intraepithelial lymphocytes, which belong to the T cell lineage but express antigen receptors of limited diversity. Some of these T cells express receptors composed of two chains, called γ and δ chains, that are similar, but not identical, to the highly diverse $\alpha\beta$ T cell receptors expressed on the majority of T lymphocytes (see Chapters 4 and 5). Intraepithelial lymphocytes, including $\gamma\delta$ T cells, often recognize microbial lipids and other structures that are shared by microbes of the same type. Intraepithelial lymphocytes presumably serve as sentinels against infectious agents that attempt to breach the epithelia, but the specificity and functions of these cells remain poorly understood. A population of B lymphocytes, called B-1 cells, resembles intraepithelial T cells in the limited diversity of their antigen receptors. B-1 cells are found not in epithelia but mostly in the peritoneal cavity, where they may respond to microbes and microbial toxins that pass through the walls of the intestine. Most of the circulating IgM antibodies found in the blood of normal individuals, called natural antibodies, are the products of B-1 cells, and many of these antibodies are specific for carbohydrates that are present in the cell walls of many bacteria.

Phagocytes: Neutrophils and Monocytes/Macrophages

The two types of circulating phagocytes, neutrophils and monocytes, are blood cells that are recruited to sites of infection, where they recognize and ingest microbes for intracellular killing. Neutrophils (also called polymorphonuclear leukocytes or PMNs) are the most abundant leukocytes in the blood, numbering 4000 to 10,000 per mm^3 (Fig. 2-3). In response to infections, the production of neutrophils from the bone marrow increases rapidly, and their number may rise to 20,000 per mm^3 of blood. The production of neutrophils is stimulated by cytokines, known as colony-stimulating factors, that are produced by many cell types in response to infections and act on bone marrow stem cells to stimulate proliferation and maturation of neutrophil precursors. Neutrophils are the first cell type to respond to most infections, particularly bacterial and fungal infections. They ingest microbes in the circulation, and they rapidly enter extravascular tissues at sites of infection,

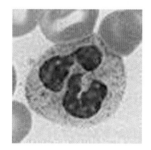

Figure 2–3 Morphology of neutrophils. The light micrograph of a blood neutrophil shows the multilobed nucleus, because of which these cells are also called polymorphonuclear leukocytes, and the faint cytoplasmic granules (mostly lysosomes).

where they also ingest microbes and die after a few hours.

Monocytes are less abundant than neutrophils, numbering 500 to 1000 per mm^3 of blood (Fig. 2-4). They, too, ingest microbes in the blood and in tissues. Unlike neutrophils, monocytes that enter extravascular tissues survive in these sites for long periods; in the tissues, these monocytes differentiate into cells called **macrophages** (see Fig. 2-4). Blood monocytes and tissue macrophages are two stages of the same cell lineage, which is often called the mononuclear phagocyte system. Resident macrophages are found in connective tissues and in every organ in the body, where they serve the same function as mononuclear phagocytes newly recruited from the circulation.

Neutrophils and monocytes migrate to extravascular sites of infection by binding to endothelial adhesion molecules and in response to chemoattractants that are produced on encounter with microbes (Fig. 2-5). If an infectious microbe breaches an epithelium and enters the subepithelial tissue, resident macrophages recognize the microbe and respond by producing soluble proteins called cytokines (described in more detail later). Two of these cytokines, called tumor necrosis factor (TNF) and interleukin-1 (IL-1), act on the endothelium of small vessels at the site of infection. These cytokines stimulate the endothelial cells to rapidly express two adhesion molecules called E-selectin and P-selectin (the name "selectin" referring to the carbohydrate-binding, or lectin, property of these molecules). Circulating neutrophils and monocytes express surface carbohydrates that bind weakly to the selectins. The neutrophils become tethered to the endothelium, flowing blood disrupts this binding, the bonds re-form downstream, and so on, resulting in the rolling of the leukocytes on the endothelial surface. Leukocytes express another set of adhesion molecules that are called integrins because they "integrate" extrinsic signals into cytoskeletal alterations. Integrins are present in a low-affinity state on unactivated leukocytes. As these cells are rolling on the endothelium, tissue macrophages that encountered the microbe, and the endothelial cells responding to the macrophage-derived TNF and IL-1, produce cytokines called chemokines (chemoattractant cytokines). Chemokines bind to the luminal surface

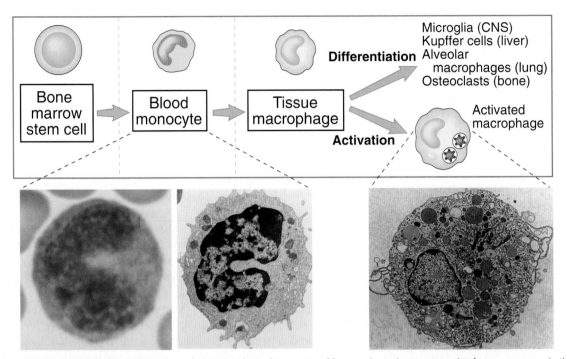

Figure 2–4   Stages in the maturation of mononuclear phagocytes. Mononuclear phagocytes arise from precursors in the bone marrow. The circulating blood stage is the monocyte; a light micrograph and an electron micrograph of a blood mono-cyte are shown, illustrating the phagocytic vacuoles and lysosomes. In the tissues, these cells become macrophages; they may be activated by microbes, and they may differentiate into specialized forms that are resident in different tissues. The electron micrograph of a portion of an activated macrophage shows numerous phagocytic vacuoles and cytoplasmic organelles. (From Fawcett DW. Bloom and Fawcett Textbook of Histology, 12th ed. WB Saunders, Philadelphia, 1994.)

endothelial cells and are thus displayed at a high concentration to the leukocytes that are rolling on the endothelium. These chemokines stimulate a rapid increase in the affinity of the leukocyte integrins for their ligands on the endothelium. Concurrently, TNF and IL-1 act on the endothelium to stimulate expression of ligands for integrins. The firm binding of integrins to their ligands arrests the rolling leukocytes on the endothelium. The cytoskeleton of the leukocytes is reorganized, and the cells spread out on the endothelial surface. Chemokines also stimulate the motility of leukocytes. As a result, the leukocytes begin to migrate through the vessel wall and along the chemokine concentration gradient to the site of infection. The sequence of selectin-mediated rolling, integrin-mediated firm adhesion, and chemokine-mediated motility leads to the migration of blood leukocytes to an extravascular site of infection within minutes after the infection. (As we shall see in Chapter 6, the same sequence of events is responsible for the migration of activated T lymphocytes into infected tissues.) The accumulation of leukocytes at sites of infection, with attendant vascular dilatation and increased vascular permeability, is called inflammation. Inherited deficiencies in integrins and selectin ligands lead to defective leukocyte recruitment to sites of infection and increased susceptibility to infections. These disorders are called leukocyte adhesion deficiencies.

Neutrophils and macrophages recognize microbes in the blood and extravascular tissues by surface receptors that are specific for microbial products (Fig. 2-6). There are several different types of receptors, specific for different structures or patterns that

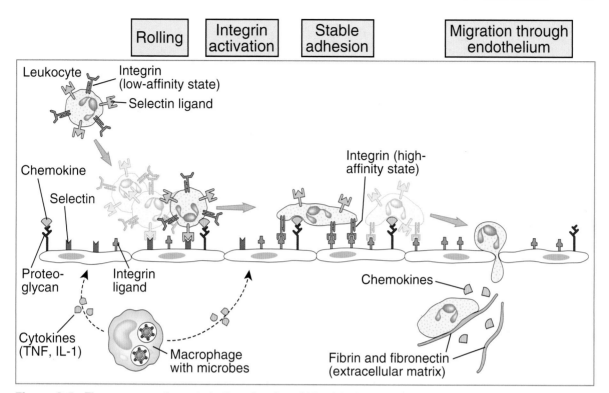

Figure 2–5   **The sequence of events in the migration of blood leukocytes to sites of infection.** At sites of infection, macrophages that have encountered microbes produce cytokines (e.g., TNF and IL-1) that activate the endothelial cells of nearby venules to produce selectins, ligands for integrins, and chemokines. Selectins mediate weak tethering and rolling of blood neutrophils on the endothelium; integrins mediate firm adhesion of neutrophils; and chemokines activate the neutrophils and stimulate their migration through the endothelium to the site of infection. Blood monocytes and activated T lymphocytes use the same mechanisms to migrate to sites of infection.

are frequently found on microbial molecules. **Toll-like receptors** (TLRs) are homologous to a *Drosophila* protein called Toll, which is essential for protecting the flies against infections. TLRs are specific for different components of microbes. For instance, TLR-2 is essential for macrophage responses to several bacterial lipoglycans, TLR-4 for bacterial lipopolysaccharide (LPS, or endotoxin), TLR-5 for a component of bacterial flagella called flagellin, and TLR-9 for unmethylated CpG nucleotides also found in bacteria. Signals generated by engagement of TLRs activate a transcription factor called NF-κB (nuclear factor κB), which stimulates production of cytokines, enzymes, and other proteins involved in the antimicrobial functions of activated phagocytes (discussed later). Neutrophils and macrophages express receptors

that recognize other microbial structures and that promote phagocytosis and killing of the microbes. These receptors include one that recognizes N-formylmethionine-containing peptides (produced by microbes but not host cells), mannose receptors (mentioned earlier), integrins (mainly one called Mac-1), and scavenger receptors (specific for several pathogen and host molecules). Macrophages also express receptors for cytokines, such as interferon-γ (IFN-γ), which are produced during innate and adaptive immune responses. IFN-γ is a powerful activator of the microbicidal functions of phagocytes. In addition, phagocytes express receptors for products of complement activation and for antibodies, and these receptors avidly bind microbes that are coated with complement proteins or antibodies (the latter only in

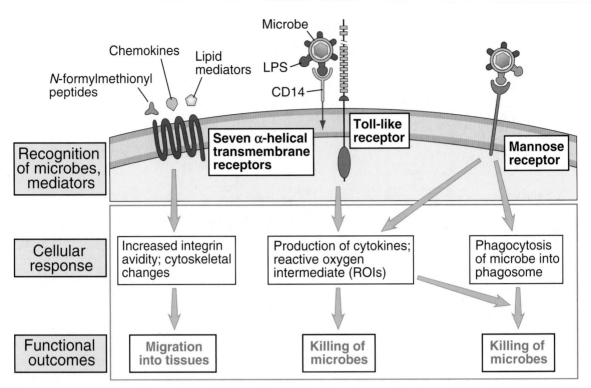

Figure 2–6   Receptors and responses of phagocytes. Neutrophils and macrophages use diverse membrane receptors to recognize microbes, microbial products, and substances produced by the host in infections. These receptors activate cellular responses that function to stimulate inflammation and eradicate microbes. Note that only selected examples of receptors of different classes are shown. LPS, lipopolysaccharide.

adaptive immunity). The process of coating microbes for efficient recognition by phagocytes is called opsonization.

The recognition of microbes by neutrophils and macrophages leads to phagocytosis of the microbes and activation of the phagocytes to kill the ingested microbes (Fig. 2-7). Phagocytosis is a process in which the phagocyte extends its plasma membrane around the recognized microbe, the membrane closes up and pinches off, and the particle is internalized in a membrane-bound vesicle, called a phagosome. The phagosomes fuse with lysosomes to form phagolysosomes. At the same time as the microbe is being bound by the phagocyte's receptors and ingested, the receptors deliver signals that activate several enzymes in the phagolysosomes. One of these enzymes, called phagocyte oxidase, converts molecular oxygen into superoxide anion and free radicals. These substances are

called reactive oxygen intermediates (ROIs), and they are toxic to the ingested microbes. A second enzyme, called inducible nitric oxide synthase, catalyzes the conversion of arginine to nitric oxide (NO), also a microbicidal substance. The third set of enzymes are lysosomal proteases, which break down microbial proteins. All these microbicidal substances are produced mainly within lysosomes and phagolysosomes, where they act on the ingested microbes but do not damage the phagocytes. In strong reactions, the same enzymes may be liberated into the extracellular space and may injure host tissues. This is the reason why inflammation, normally a protective host response to infections, may cause tissue injury as well. Inherited deficiency of the phagocyte oxidase enzyme is the cause of an immunodeficiency disease called chronic granulomatous disease. In this disorder, phagocytes are unable to eradicate intracellular

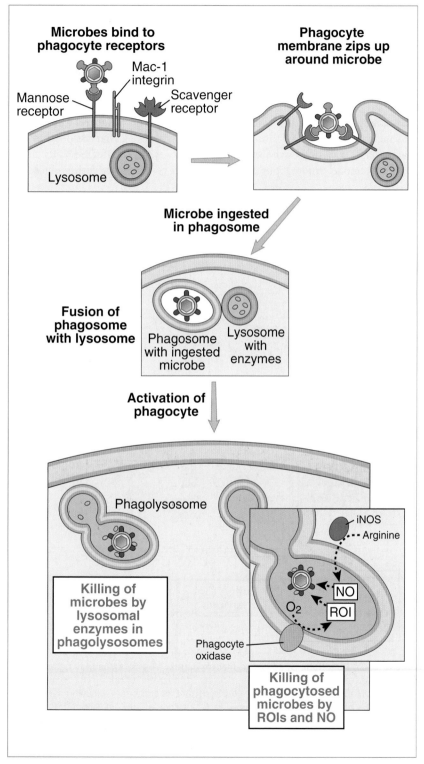

Figure 2–7 **Phagocytosis and intracellular killing of microbes.** Macrophages and neutrophils express many surface receptors that may bind microbes for subsequent phagocytosis; selected examples of such receptors are shown. Microbes are ingested into phagosomes, which fuse with lysosomes, and the microbes are killed by enzymes and several toxic substances produced in the phagolysosomes. The same substances may be released from the phagocytes and may kill extracellular microbes (not shown). iNOS, inducible nitric oxide synthase; NO, nitric oxide; ROI, reactive oxygen intermediate.

microbes, and the host tries to contain the infection by calling in more macrophages and lymphocytes, resulting in collections of cells around the microbes that are called granulomas.

In addition to killing phagocytosed microbes, macrophages perform several functions that play important roles in defense against infections (Fig. 2-8). Macrophages produce cytokines that are important mediators of host defense (see later discussion). Macrophages secrete growth factors and enzymes that serve to remodel injured tissue and replace it with connective tissue. Macrophages also stimulate T lymphocytes and respond to products of T cells: these reactions are important in cell-mediated immunity and are described in Chapter 6.

Natural Killer Cells

Natural killer (NK) cells are a class of lymphocytes that respond to intracellular microbes by killing infected cells and by producing the macrophage-activating cytokine, IFN-γ (Fig. 2-9). Natural killer

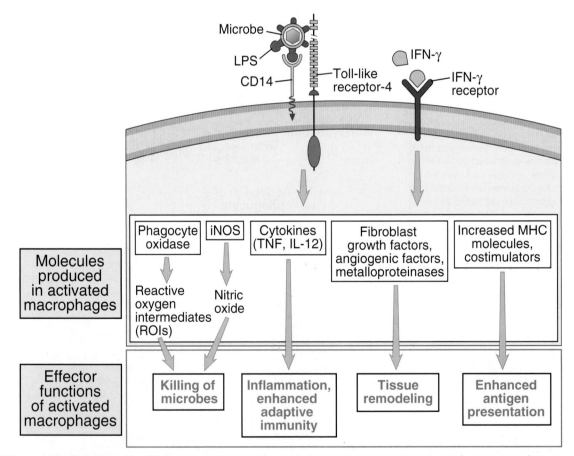

Figure 2–8 Functions of activated macrophages. Macrophages may be activated by signals from many surface receptors. The two examples shown are the receptor for bacterial endotoxin (LPS), which transduces signals via an attached Toll-like receptor, and the receptor for the most important macrophage-activating cytokine, IFN-γ. Signals from activating receptors stimulate the production of several proteins, which mediate the important functions of macrophages. Different macrophage surface receptors may stimulate distinct or overlapping responses. The biochemical signaling pathways used by these receptors are complex; their common feature is that they stimulate the production of transcription factors, which result in the production of various proteins.

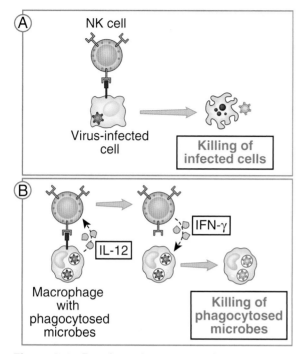

Figure 2–9   Functions of natural killer (NK) cells. A. NK cells kill host cells infected by intracellular microbes, thus eliminating reservoirs of infection. B. NK cells respond to IL-12 produced by macrophages and secrete IFN-γ, which activates the macrophages to kill phagocytosed microbes.

occur because NK cells also express inhibitory receptors that recognize normal host cells and inhibit the activation of the NK cells. These inhibitory receptors are specific for various alleles of self class I major histocompatibility complex (MHC) molecules, which are proteins expressed on all nucleated cells in every individual. (In Chapter 3 the important function of MHC molecules in displaying peptide antigens to T lymphocytes is described.) Two major families of NK cell inhibitory receptors are the killer cell immunoglobulin-like receptors (KIRs), so called because they share structural homology to immunoglobulin molecules (described in Chapter 4), and receptors consisting of a protein called CD94 and a lectin subunit called NKG2. Both families of inhibitory receptors contain in their cytoplasmic domains structural motifs called immunoreceptor tyrosine-based inhibitory motifs (ITIMs), which become phosphorylated on tyrosine residues when the receptors bind class I MHC molecules. The phosphorylated ITIMs bind and promote the activation of cytoplasmic protein tyrosine phosphatases. These phosphatases remove phosphate groups from the tyrosine residues of various signaling molecules and thus block the activation of NK cells through activating receptors. Therefore, when the inhibitory receptors of NK cells encounter self MHC molecules, the NK cells are shut off (Fig. 2-10). Many viruses have mechanisms to block expression of class I molecules in infected cells, which allows them to evade killing by virus-specific CD8+ cytolytic T lymphocytes (CTLs) (see Chapter 6). When this happens, the NK cell inhibitory receptors are not engaged, and they become activated to eliminate cells infected by such viruses. The ability of NK cells to protect against infections is enhanced by cytokines secreted by macrophages that have encountered microbes. One of these NK-activating cytokines produced by macrophages is called interleukin-12 (IL-12). Natural killer cells also express receptors for the Fc portions of some IgG antibodies and use these receptors to bind to cells coated with antibodies. The role of this reaction in antibody-mediated humoral immunity is described in Chapter 8.

When NK cells are activated, they respond in two ways (see Fig. 2-9). First, activation triggers the discharge of proteins contained in the NK cells' cyto-

cells comprise about 10% of the lymphocytes in the blood and peripheral lymphoid organs. These cells contain abundant cytoplasmic granules and express characteristic surface markers, but they do not express immunoglobulins or T cell receptors, the antigen receptors of B and T lymphocytes, respectively. NK cells recognize host cells that have been altered by microbial infection. Although the mechanisms of NK recognition are incompletely understood, it is known that NK cells express various receptors for molecules on host cells, and some of these receptors activate the NK cells and some inhibit the NK cells. Among the activating receptors are those that recognize cell surface molecules that are commonly expressed on host cells infected with viruses and on phagocytes harboring viruses and intracellular bacteria. Other activating NK cell receptors recognize normal host cell surface molecules, which could theoretically activate NK cells to kill normal cells. This does not usually

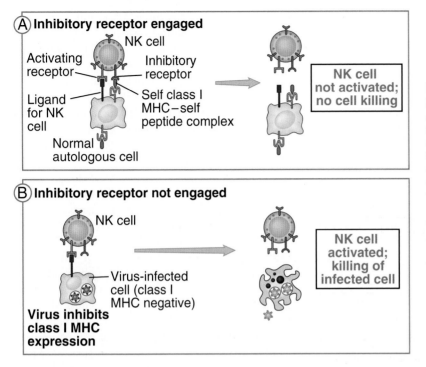

(A) **Inhibitory receptor engaged**

NK cell

Activating receptor

Inhibitory receptor

Ligand for NK cell

Self class I MHC–self peptide complex

Normal autologous cell

NK cell not activated; no cell killing

(B) **Inhibitory receptor not engaged**

NK cell

Virus-infected cell (class I MHC negative)

Virus inhibits class I MHC expression

NK cell activated; killing of infected cell

Figure 2–10 The function of inhibitory receptors of NK cells. A. The inhibitory receptors of NK cells recognize self class I MHC molecules, thus ensuring that NK cells do not attack normal host cells (which always express class I MHC molecules containing bound self peptides). B. NK cells are activated by infected cells in which class I MHC expression is reduced, because the inhibitory receptors are not engaged in the absence of class I MHC molecules. The result is that the infected cells are killed.

plasmic granules toward the infected cells. These NK cell granule proteins include molecules that create holes in the plasma membrane of the infected cells and other molecules that enter the infected cells and activate enzymes that induce apoptotic death. The cytolytic mechanisms of NK cells are the same as the mechanisms used by CTLs to kill infected cells (see Chapter 6). The net result of these reactions is that NK cells kill infected host cells. By killing infected host cells, NK cells, like CTLs, function to eliminate cellular reservoirs of infection and thus eradicate infections by obligate intracellular microbes, such as viruses. Second, activated NK cells synthesize and secrete the cytokine, IFN-γ. IFN-γ activates macrophages to become more effective at killing phagocytosed microbes. Thus, NK cells and macrophages function cooperatively to eliminate intracellular microbes: macrophages ingest microbes and produce IL-12, IL-12 activates NK cells to secrete IFN-γ, and IFN-γ in turn activates the macrophages to kill the ingested microbes. As is discussed in Chapter 6, essentially the same sequence of reactions involving macrophages and T lymphocytes is central to the cell-mediated arm of adaptive immunity.

Thus, hosts and microbes are engaged in a constant evolutionary struggle: the host uses CTLs to recognize MHC-displayed viral antigens, viruses shut off MHC expression, and NK cells have evolved to respond to the absence of MHC molecules. Whether the host or the microbe wins this kind of evolutionary struggle, of course, determines the outcome of the infections.

The Complement System

The complement system is a collection of circulating and membrane-associated proteins that are important in defense against microbes. Many complement proteins are proteolytic enzymes, and complement activation involves the sequential activation of these enzymes, sometimes called an enzymatic cascade. The complement cascade may be activated by one of three pathways (Fig. 2-11). The **alternative pathway** is triggered when some complement proteins are activated on microbial surfaces and cannot be controlled because complement regulatory proteins are not present on microbes (but are present on host cells). This pathway is a component of innate immunity. The **classical pathway** is triggered after antibodies

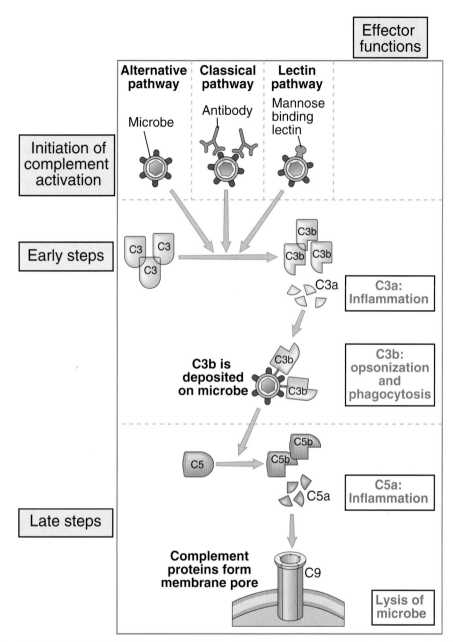

Figure 2–11 Pathways of complement activation. The activation of the complement system may be initiated by three distinct pathways, all of which lead to the production of C3b (the early steps). C3b initiates the late steps of complement activation, culminating in the production of numerous peptides and polymerized C9 (which forms the "membrane attack complex," so called because it creates holes in plasma membranes). The principal functions of proteins produced at different steps are shown. The activation, functions, and regulation of the complement system are discussed in much more detail in Chapter 8.

bind to microbes or other antigens and is thus a component of the humoral arm of adaptive immunity. The **lectin pathway** is activated when a plasma protein, mannose-binding lectin, binds to terminal mannose residues on the surface glycoproteins of microbes. This lectin activates proteins of the classical pathway, but because it is initiated in the absence of antibody it is a component of innate immunity. Activated complement proteins function as proteolytic enzymes to cleave other complement proteins. The central component of complement is a plasma protein called C3, which is cleaved by enzymes generated in the early steps. The major proteolytic fragment of C3, called C3b, becomes covalently attached to microbes and is able to activate downstream complement proteins on the microbial surface. The three pathways of complement activation differ in how they are initiated, but they share the late steps and perform the same effector functions.

The complement system serves three functions in host defense. First, C3b coats microbes and promotes the binding of these microbes to phagocytes, by virtue of receptors for C3b that are expressed on the phagocytes. Second, some breakdown products of complement proteins are chemoattractants for neutrophils and monocytes and promote inflammation at the site of complement activation. Third, complement activation culminates in the formation of a polymeric protein complex that inserts into the microbial cell membrane, forming pores that lead to the influx of water and ions and death of the microbe. A more detailed discussion of the activation and functions of complement is in Chapter 8, where the effector mechanisms of humoral immunity are considered.

Cytokines of Innate Immunity

In response to microbes, macrophages and other cells secrete proteins called cytokines that mediate many of the cellular reactions of innate immunity (Fig. 2-12). Cytokines are soluble proteins that mediate immune and inflammatory reactions and are responsible for communications between leukocytes and between leukocytes and other cells. Most of the molecularly defined cytokines are called interleukins, by convention, implying that these molecules are pro-

duced by leukocytes and act on leukocytes. (In reality, this is too limited a definition, because many cytokines are produced by or act on cells other than leukocytes, and many cytokines that fulfill these criteria are given other names for historical reasons.) In innate immunity, the principal sources of cytokines are macrophages activated by recognition of microbes. For instance, binding of LPS to its receptor on macrophages is a powerful stimulus for cytokine secretion by the macrophages. Bacteria elicit much the same response via other macrophage receptors, many of which are members of the Toll-like receptor family. Cytokines are also produced in cell-mediated immunity. In this type of adaptive immunity, the major sources of cytokines are helper T lymphocytes (see Chapter 5).

All cytokines are produced in small amounts in response to an external stimulus, such as a microbe. Cytokines bind to high-affinity receptors on target cells. Most cytokines act on the cells that produce them (called autocrine actions) or on adjacent cells (paracrine actions). In innate immune reactions against infections, enough macrophages may be activated that large amounts of cytokines are produced, and they may be active distant from their site of secretion.

The cytokines of innate immunity serve various functions in host defense. As discussed earlier in this chapter, TNF, IL-1, and chemokines are the principal

Figure 2-12   Cytokines of innate immunity. A. Macrophages responding to microbes produce cytokines that stimulate inflammation (leukocyte recruitment) and activate NK cells to produce the macrophage-activating cytokine IFN-γ. B. Some important characteristics of the major cytokines of innate immunity are listed. Note that IFN-γ is a cytokine of both innate and adaptive immunity and is referred to again in Chapter 5. The name "tumor necrosis factor" (TNF) arose from an experiment showing that a cytokine induced by LPS killed tumors in mice. We now know that this effect is the result of TNF-induced thrombosis of tumor blood vessels, which is an exaggerated form of a reaction seen in inflammation. The name "interferon" arose from the ability of these cytokines to interfere with viral infection. IFN-γ is a weak antiviral cytokine compared with the type I IFNs.

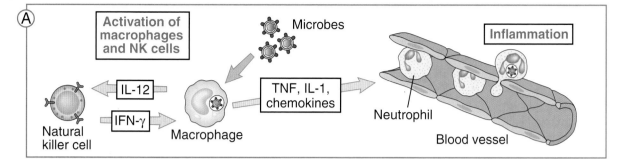

Cytokine	Principal cell source(s)	Principal cellular targets and biologic effects
Tumor necrosis factor (TNF)	Macrophages, T cells	Endothelial cells: activation (inflammation, coagulation) Neutrophils: activation Hypothalamus: fever Liver: synthesis of acute phase proteins Muscle, fat: catabolism (cachexia) Many cell types: apoptosis
Interleukin (IL-1)	Macrophages, endothelial cells, some epithelial cells	Endothelial cells: activation (inflammation, coagulation) Hypothalamus: fever Liver: synthesis of acute phase proteins
Chemokines	Macrophages, endothelial cells, T lymphocytes, fibroblasts, platelets	Leukocytes: chemotaxis, activation
Interleukin-12 (IL-12)	Macrophages, dendritic cells	NK cells and T cells: IFN-γ synthesis, increased cytolytic activity T cells: T_H1 differentiation
Interferon-γ (IFN-γ)	NK cells, T lymphocytes	Activation of macrophages Stimulation of some antibody responses
Type I IFNs (IFN-α, IFN-β)	IFN-α: Macrophages IFN-β: Fibroblasts	All cells: antiviral state, increased class I MHC expression NK cells: activation
Interleukin-10 (IL-10)	Macrophages, T cells (mainly T_H2)	Macrophages: inhibition of IL-12 production, reduced expression of costimulators and class II MHC molecules
Interleukin-6 (IL-6)	Macrophages, endothelial cells, T cells	Liver: synthesis of acute phase proteins B cells: proliferation of antibody-producing cells
Interleukin-15 (IL-15)	Macrophages, others	NK cells: proliferation T cells: proliferation
Interleukin-18 (IL-18)	Macrophages	NK cells and T cells: IFN-γ synthesis

cytokines involved in recruiting blood neutrophils and monocytes to sites of infection. At high concentrations, TNF promotes thrombosis of blood and reduces blood pressure by a combination of reduced myocardial contractility and vascular dilatation. Severe, disseminated gram-negative bacterial infections sometimes lead to a potentially lethal clinical syndrome called **septic shock,** which is characterized by low blood pressure (shock), disseminated intravascular coagulation, and metabolic disturbances. All the clinical and pathologic manifestations of septic shock are caused by very high levels of TNF, which is produced by macrophages responding to the bacterial LPS. Macrophages also produce IL-12 in response to LPS and many phagocytosed microbes. The role of IL-12 in activating NK cells, ultimately leading to macrophage activation, has been mentioned previously. Natural killer cells produce IFN-γ, whose function as a macrophage-activating cytokine has also been described earlier. Because IFN-γ is produced by T cells as well, it is considered a cytokine of both innate immunity and adaptive immunity. In viral infections, macrophages and other infected cells produce cytokines called type I interferons, which inhibit viral replication and prevent spread of the infection to uninfected cells. A type I IFN called IFN-α is used clinically to treat chronic viral hepatitis.

Other Plasma Proteins of Innate Immunity

Several circulating proteins in addition to complement proteins are involved in defense against infections. Plasma mannose-binding lectin (MBL) is a protein that recognizes microbial carbohydrates and can coat microbes for phagocytosis or activate the complement cascade by the lectin pathway. MBL belongs to the collectin family of proteins, which share homology to collagen and contain a carbohydrate-binding (lectin) domain. Surfactant proteins in the lung also belong to the collectin family and protect the airways from infection. C-reactive protein (CRP) binds to phosphorylcholine on microbes and coats the microbes for phagocytosis by macrophages, which express a receptor for CRP. The circulating levels of many of these plasma proteins increase

rapidly after infection. This protective response is called the **acute phase response** to infection.

Innate immune responses to different types of microbes may vary and are designed to best eliminate these microbes. Extracellular bacteria and fungi are combated by phagocytes and the complement system and by acute phase proteins. Defense against intracellular bacteria and viruses is mediated by phagocytes and NK cells, with cytokines providing the communications between the phagocytes and NK cells.

Evasion of Innate Immunity by Microbes

Pathogenic microbes have evolved to resist the mechanisms of innate immunity and are thus able to enter and colonize their hosts (Fig. 2-13). Some intracellular bacteria resist destruction inside phagocytes. *Listeria monocytogenes* produces a protein that enables it to escape from phagocytic vesicles and enter the cytoplasm of infected cells, where it is no longer susceptible to reactive oxygen intermediates and nitric oxide (which are produced mainly in phagolysosomes). The cell walls of mycobacteria contain a lipid that inhibits fusion of vesicles containing ingested bacteria with lysosomes. Other microbes have cell walls that are resistant to the actions of complement proteins. As discussed in Chapters 6 and 8, the same mechanisms enable microbes to resist the effector mechanisms of cell-mediated and humoral immunity, the two arms of adaptive immunity.

Role of Innate Immunity in Stimulating Adaptive Immune Responses

So far we have focused on how the innate immune system recognizes microbes and functions to combat infections. We mentioned at the beginning of this chapter that, in addition to its defense functions, the innate immune response to microbes serves an important warning function by alerting the adaptive immune system that an effective immune response is needed. In this final section of the chapter, some of the mechanisms by which innate immune responses stimulate adaptive immune responses are summarized.

Mechanism of immune evasion	Organism (example)	Mechanism
Resistance to phagocytosis	*Pneumococcus*	Capsular polysaccharide inhibits phagocytosis
Resistance to reactive oxygen intermediates in phagocytes	Staphylococci	Production of catalase, which breaks down reactive oxygen intermediates
Resistance to complement activation (alternative pathway)	*Neisseria meningitides*	Sialic acid expression inhibits C3 and C5 convertases
	Streptococcus	M protein blocks C3 binding to organism and C3b binding to complement receptors
Resistance to antimicrobial peptide antibiotics	*Pseudomonas*	Synthesis of modified LPS that resists action of peptide antibiotics

Figure 2–13 Evasion of innate immunity by microbes. Selected examples by which microbes may evade or resist innate immunity are shown.

Innate immune responses generate molecules that function as "second signals," together with antigens, to activate T and B lymphocytes. In Chapter 1 we introduced the concept that full activation of antigen-specific lymphocytes requires two signals: antigen itself is "signal 1," and microbes, innate immune responses to microbes, and host cells damaged by microbes may all provide "signal 2" (see Fig. 1-9, Chapter 1). This requirement for microbe-dependent second signals ensures that lymphocytes respond to infectious agents and not to harmless, non-infectious substances. In experimental situations or for vaccination, adaptive immune responses may be induced by antigens without microbes. In all these cases, the antigens have to be administered with substances, called **adjuvants,** that elicit the same innate immune reactions as microbes do. In fact, many potent adjuvants are the products of microbes. The nature and mechanisms of action of second signals are described in detail in the discussion of the activation of T and B lymphocytes (see Chapters 5 and 7). At this time, it is useful to describe two illustrative examples of second signals that are generated during innate immune reactions (Fig. 2-14).

Microbes, or IFN-γ produced by NK cells in response to microbes, stimulate dendritic cells and macrophages to produce two types of second signals that can activate T lymphocytes. First, the dendritic cells and macrophages express surface molecules called **costimulators,** which bind to receptors on naive T cells and function together with antigen recognition to activate the T cells. Second, the dendritic cells and macrophages secrete the cytokine IL-12, which stimulates the differentiation of naive T cells into the effector cells of cell-mediated adaptive immunity.

Blood-borne microbes activate the complement system by the alternative pathway. One of the proteins produced during complement activation, called C3d, becomes covalently attached to the microbe. When B lymphocytes recognize microbial antigens by their antigen receptors, at the same time the B cells recognize the C3d bound to the microbe by a receptor for C3d. The combination of antigen recognition and C3d recognition initiates the process of B cell differentiation into antibody-secreting cells. Thus, a complement product serves as the second signal for humoral immune responses.

These examples illustrate an important feature of second signals, namely, that these signals not only stimulate adaptive immunity but also guide the nature of the adaptive immune response. Intracellular and

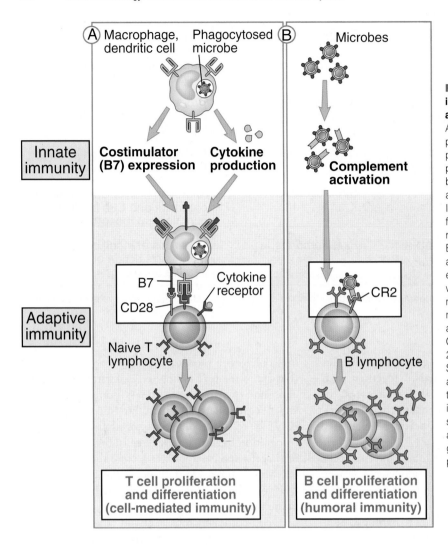

Figure 2–14 **The role of innate immunity in stimulating adaptive immune responses.** A. Macrophages respond to phagocytosed microbes by expressing costimulators (e.g., B7 proteins, which are recognized by the CD28 receptor of T cells) and by secreting cytokines (e.g., IL-12). Costimulators and IL-12 function, together with antigen recognition, to activate the T cells. B. The complement system is activated by microbes and generates proteins, such as C3d, which become attached to the microbes. B lymphocytes recognize microbial antigens by their antigen receptors and recognize C3d by a receptor called the type 2 complement receptor (CR2). Signals from the antigen receptor and CR2 function cooperatively to activate the B cells. Note that, in both examples, the second signals act on lymphocytes that also specifically recognize antigens of microbes, this recognition providing "signal 1."

phagocytosed microbes need to be eliminated by cell-mediated immunity, the adaptive response mediated by T lymphocytes. Microbes that are ingested by or live in macrophages induce the second signals, namely, costimulators and IL-12, that stimulate T cell responses. In contrast, blood-borne microbes need to be combated by antibodies, which are produced by B lymphocytes during humoral immune responses. Blood-borne microbes activate the plasma complement system, which in turn stimulates B cell activation and antibody production. Thus, different types of microbes induce different innate immune responses, which then stimulate the types of adaptive immunity that are best able to combat different infectious pathogens.

SUMMARY

▶ All multicellular organisms contain intrinsic mechanisms of defense against infections, which constitute innate immunity.

▶ The mechanisms of innate immunity respond to microbes and not to nonmicrobial substances, are specific for structures present on various classes of microbes, are mediated by receptors encoded in the germline, and are not enhanced by repeat exposures to microbes.

▶ The principal components of innate immunity are epithelia, phagocytes and natural killer (NK) cells, cytokines, and plasma proteins, including the proteins of the complement system.

▶ Epithelia provide physical barriers against microbes, produce antibiotics, and contain lymphocytes that may prevent infections.

▶ The principal phagocytes, neutrophils and monocytes/macrophages, are blood cells that are recruited to sites of infection, where they recognize microbes by several receptors. Neutrophils and macrophages ingest microbes for intracellular destruction, secrete cytokines, and respond in other ways that contribute to elimination of microbes and repair of infected tissues.

▶ Natural killer cells kill host cells infected by intracellular microbes and produce the cytokine IFN-γ, which activates macrophages to kill phagocytosed microbes.

▶ The complement system is a family of proteins that are activated sequentially on encounter with some microbes and by antibodies (in the humoral arm of adaptive immunity). Complement proteins coat (opsonize) microbes for phagocytosis, stimulate inflammation, and lyse microbes.

▶ Cytokines of innate immunity function to stimulate inflammation (TNF, IL-1, chemokines), activate NK cells (IL-12), activate macrophages (IFN-γ), and prevent viral infections (type I IFN).

▶ In addition to providing the early defense against infections, innate immune responses provide "second signals" for the activation of B and T lymphocytes. The requirement for these second signals ensures that adaptive immunity is elicited by microbes (the natural inducers of innate immune reactions) and not by non-microbial substances.

Review Questions

1 How does the specificity of innate immunity differ from that of adaptive immunity?

2 Give three examples of the ability of innate immune mechanisms to recognize microbes but not mammalian cells.

3 What are the mechanisms by which the epithelium of the skin prevents the entry of microbes?

4 How do phagocytes ingest and kill microbes?

5 What is the role of MHC molecules in the recognition of infected cells by NK cells, and what is the physiologic significance of this recognition?

6 What are the roles of the following cytokines in defense against infections: (a) TNF, (b) IL-12, and (c) type I interferon?

7 How do innate immune responses enhance adaptive immunity?

Antigen Capture and Presentation to Lymphocytes

What Lymphocytes See

3

Adaptive immune responses are initiated when the antigen receptors of lymphocytes recognize antigens. B and T lymphocytes differ in the types of antigens they recognize. The antigen receptors of B lymphocytes, namely, membrane-bound antibodies, can recognize a wide variety of macromolecules (proteins, polysaccharides, lipids, and nucleic acids) as well as small chemicals in soluble or cell surface–associated form. Therefore, B cell–mediated humoral immune responses may be generated against many types of microbial cell wall and soluble antigens. Most T lymphocytes, on the other hand, can only see peptide fragments of protein antigens, and only when these peptides are presented by specialized peptide display molecules on host cells. Therefore, T cell–mediated immune responses may be generated only against the protein antigens of microbes that are associated with host cells. This chapter focuses on the nature of the antigens that are recognized by lymphocytes. Chapter 4 describes the receptors that lymphocytes use to detect these antigens.

The induction of immune responses by antigens is a remarkable process that has to overcome many seemingly insurmountable barriers. The first of these barriers is the low frequency of naive lymphocytes in the body specific for any one antigen, which may be less than about 1 in every 10^5. This small fraction of the body's lymphocytes has to locate and react rapidly to the antigen, wherever it is introduced. Second, different kinds of microbes need to be combated by different types of adaptive immune responses. In fact, the immune system has to react in different ways even to the same microbe at different stages of its life. For instance, if a microbe, such as a virus, has entered the circulation and is free in the blood, the immune system needs to produce antibodies that bind the microbe, prevent it from infecting host cells, and help to eliminate it. But after the microbe has infected host cells, antibodies are no longer effective, and it may be necessary to activate cytolytic T lymphocytes (CTLs) to kill the infected cells and eliminate the reservoir of infection. Thus, we are faced with two important questions.

- How do the rare lymphocytes specific for any microbial antigen find that microbe, especially considering that microbes may enter anywhere in the body?

- How does the immune system produce the effector cells and molecules best able to eradicate a particular type of infection, such as antibodies against extracellular microbes and CTLs to kill infected cells harboring microbes in their cytoplasm?

The answer to both questions is that the immune system has developed a highly specialized system for capturing and displaying antigens to lymphocytes. A large amount of research by immunologists, cell biologists, and biochemists has led to a sophisticated understanding of how protein antigens are captured, broken down, and displayed for recognition by T lymphocytes. This is the major topic of discussion in this chapter. We know much less about how antigens are captured for recognition by B lymphocytes, and at the end of the chapter our limited understanding of how protein and nonprotein antigens are seen by B cells is summarized.

Antigens Recognized by T Lymphocytes

The majority of T lymphocytes recognize peptide antigens that are bound to and displayed by the **major histocompatibility complex (MHC) molecules of antigen-presenting cells (APCs).** The MHC is a genetic locus whose principal products function as the peptide display molecules of the immune system. In every individual, different clones of T cells can see peptides only when these peptides are displayed by that individual's MHC molecules. This property of T cells is called **MHC restriction.** Thus, each T cell has a dual specificity: the T cell receptor (TCR) recognizes some residues of peptide antigen and also recognizes residues of the MHC molecule that is displaying that peptide (Fig. 3-1). The properties of MHC molecules and the significance of MHC restriction are described later in this chapter. How T cells learn to recognize peptides presented only by self MHC molecules is described in Chapter 4. It should be noted that there are relatively small subpopulations of T cells that may recognize lipid and other nonpeptide antigens displayed by nonpolymorphic class I MHC–like molecules, but the functions of these T cells are poorly understood.

The specialized cells that capture microbial antigens and display them for recognition by T lymphocytes are called **antigen-presenting cells.** Naive T lymphocytes need to see antigens presented by "professional" APCs to initiate immune responses against protein antigens. (As mentioned in Chapter 1, the

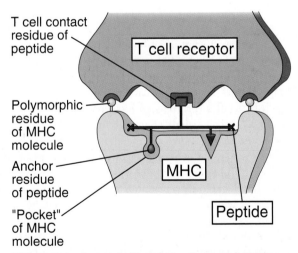

Figure 3–1   A model of how a T cell receptor (TCR) recognizes a complex of a peptide antigen displayed by a major histocompatibility (MHC) molecule. MHC molecules are expressed on antigen-presenting cells and function to display peptides derived from protein antigens. Peptides bind to the MHC molecules by anchor residues, which attach the peptides to pockets in the MHC molecules. The TCR of every T cell recognizes some residues of the peptide and some (polymorphic) residues of the MHC molecule.

term *professional* refers to the ability of these cells to both display antigens for T cells and provide the additional signals needed to activate naive T cells.) Differentiated effector T cells again need to see antigens presented by various APCs, to activate the effector functions of the T cells in humoral and cell-mediated immune responses. The way in which APCs present antigens to trigger immune responses is described first, and then the role of MHC molecules in these processes is discussed.

Capture of Protein Antigens by Antigen-Presenting Cells

Protein antigens of microbes that enter the body are captured by professional APCs and concentrated in the peripheral lymphoid organs where immune responses are initiated (Fig. 3-2). Microbes enter the body mainly through the skin (by contact), the gastrointestinal tract (by ingestion), and the respiratory tract (by inhalation). (Some insect-borne microbes may be injected into the blood stream as a result of insect bites.) All the interfaces between the body and the external environment are lined by continuous epithelia, whose principal function is to provide a physical barrier to infection. The epithelia contain a population of professional APCs that belong to the lineage of dendritic cells; the same cells are present in the T cell–rich areas of peripheral lymphoid organs and, in smaller numbers, in most other organs (Fig. 3-3). In the skin, the epidermal dendritic cells are called Langerhans cells. These epithelial dendritic cells are

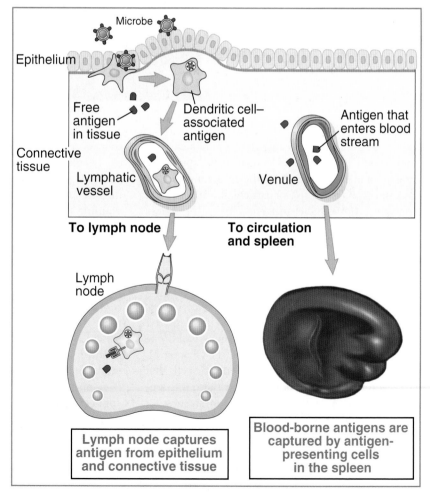

Figure 3–2 The capture and display of microbial antigens. Microbes enter through an epithelium and are captured by antigen-presenting cells resident in the epithelium, or they enter lymphatic vessels or blood vessels. The microbes and their antigens are transported to peripheral lymphoid organs, the lymph nodes, and the spleen, where protein antigens are displayed for recognition by T lymphocytes.

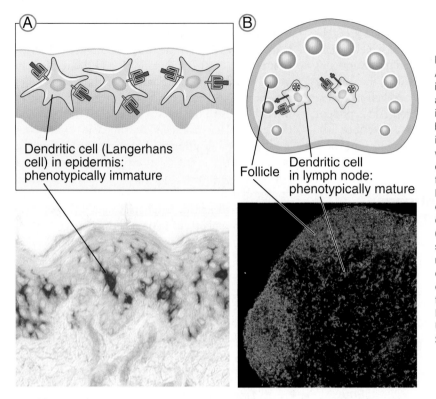

Dendritic cell (Langerhans cell) in epidermis: phenotypically immature

Follicle   Dendritic cell in lymph node: phenotypically mature

Figure 3–3 Dendritic cells. A. Immature dendritic cells reside in epithelia, such as the skin, and form a network of cells with interdigitating processes, seen as blue cells on the section of skin immunohistochemically stained with an antibody that recognizes dendritic cells. (The micrograph of the skin is courtesy of Dr. Y-J. Liu, DNAX, Palo Alto, Calif.) B. Mature dendritic cells reside in the T cell–rich areas of lymph nodes (and spleen, not shown) and are seen in the section of a lymph node stained with fluorochrome-conjugated antibodies against dendritic cells (*red*) and B cells in follicles (*green*). (Courtesy of Drs. Kathryn Pape and Jennifer Walter, University of Minnesota Medical School, Minneapolis.)

said to be "immature," because they are inefficient at stimulating T lymphocytes. Dendritic cells capture the antigens of microbes that enter the epithelium, by the processes of phagocytosis (for particulate antigens) and pinocytosis (for soluble antigens) (Fig. 3-4). These cells may express receptors that enable them to bind microbes. One such receptor recognizes terminal mannose residues on glycoproteins, a typical feature of microbial but not mammalian glycoproteins. When macrophages and epithelial cells in tissues encounter microbes, these cells respond by producing cytokines, such as tumor necrosis factor (TNF) and interleukin-1 (IL-1). The production of these cytokines is part of the innate immune response to microbes (see Chapter 2). TNF and IL-1 act on the epithelial dendritic cells that have captured microbial antigens and cause the dendritic cells to round up and lose their adhesiveness for the epithelium. Now the dendritic cells are ready to leave the epithelium with their cargo of antigen.

Dendritic cells also express surface receptors for a group of chemoattracting cytokines (chemokines) that are normally produced in the T cell–rich areas of lymph nodes. These chemokines direct the dendritic cells that have exited the epithelium to migrate via lymphatic vessels to the lymph nodes draining that epithelium (see Fig. 3-4). During the process of migration, the dendritic cells mature from cells designed to capture antigens into APCs capable of stimulating T lymphocytes. This maturation is reflected in increased synthesis and stable expression of MHC molecules, which display antigen to T cells, and of other molecules, called costimulators, that are required for full T cell responses (discussed later in the chapter). The maturation of dendritic cells is presumably a response to the products of the microbes that these cells encountered. If a microbe breaches the epithelium and enters connective tissues or parenchymal organs, it may be captured by immature dendritic cells that live in these tissues and again transported to lymph nodes. Soluble antigens in the lymph are picked up by dendritic cells that reside in the lymph nodes, and blood-borne

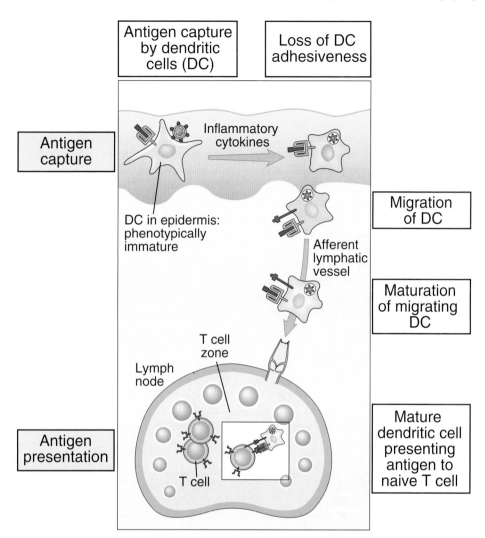

Figure 3–4   The capture and presentation of protein antigens by dendritic cells. Immature dendritic cells in the epithelium (skin, in the example shown, where the dendritic cells are called Langerhans cells) capture microbial antigens and leave the epithelium. The dendritic cells migrate to draining lymph nodes, being attracted there by chemokines produced in the nodes. During their migration, and probably in response to the microbe, the dendritic cells mature; and in the lymph nodes, the dendritic cells present antigens to naive T lymphocytes. Dendritic cells at different stages of their maturation may express different membrane proteins. Immature dendritic cells express surface receptors that capture microbial antigens, whereas mature dendritic cells express high levels of MHC molecules and costimulators, which function to stimulate T cells.

antigens are handled in essentially the same way by dendritic cells in the spleen.

The net result of this sequence of events is that the protein antigens of microbes that enter the body are transported to and concentrated in the regions of lymph nodes where the antigens are most likely to encounter T lymphocytes. Recall that naive T lymphocytes continuously recirculate through lymph nodes, and it is estimated that every naive T cell in the body may cycle through some lymph nodes at least once a day. Therefore, professional APCs bearing captured antigen and naive T cells poised to recognize antigens come together in lymph nodes. This process is very efficient; it is estimated that if microbial antigens are introduced at any site in the body, a T cell response to these antigens begins in the lymph nodes draining that site within 12 to 18 hours.

Different types of APCs serve distinct functions in T cell–dependent immune responses. Dendritic cells are the principal inducers of such responses, because dendritic cells are the most potent APCs for activating naive T lymphocytes. Dendritic cells not only initiate T cell responses but may also influence the nature of the response. For instance, there are subsets of dendritic cells that can direct the differentiation of naive CD4+ T cells into distinct populations that function in defense against different types of microbes (see Chapter 5). Another important type of APC is the macrophage, which is abundant in all tissues. In cell-mediated immune reactions, macrophages phagocytose microbes and display the antigens of these microbes to effector T cells, which activate the macrophages to kill the microbes (see Chapter 6). B lymphocytes ingest protein antigens and display them to helper T cells; this process is important for the development of humoral immune responses (see Chapter 7). As is discussed later in this chapter, all nucleated cells can present antigens derived from microbes in the cytoplasm to CTLs.

Professional APCs may also be involved in initiating the responses of CD8+ T lymphocytes to the antigens of intracellular microbes. The sequence of antigen capture and transport to lymphoid organs is best understood for the presentation of antigens of extracellular microbes to CD4+ T lymphocytes. But some microbes, such as viruses, rapidly infect host cells and can only be eradicated by CTLs destroying the infected cells. The immune system, and especially CD8+ T lymphocytes, must be able to recognize and respond to the antigens of these intracellular microbes. However, viruses may infect any type of host cells, not only professional APCs, and these infected cells may not produce all the signals that are needed to initiate T cell activation. How then are naive CD8+ T lymphocytes able to respond to the intracellular antigens of infected cells? A likely mechanism is that professional APCs ingest infected cells and display the antigens present in the infected cells for recognition by CD8+ T lymphocytes (Fig. 3-5). This process is called **cross-presentation** (or cross-priming), to indicate that one cell type, the professional APCs, can present the antigens of other cells, the infected cells, and prime (or activate) naive T

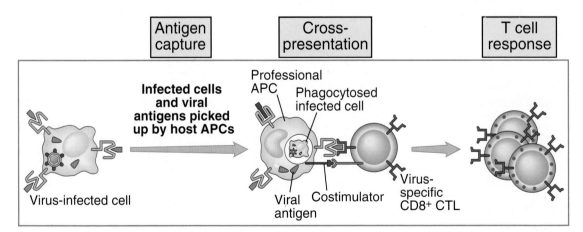

Figure 3–5   Cross-presentation of microbial antigens from infected cells by professional APCs. Cells infected with intracellular microbes, such as viruses, are ingested (captured) by professional APCs, and the antigens of the infectious microbes are broken down and presented in association with the MHC molecules of the APCs. T cells recognize the microbial antigens and costimulators expressed on the APCs, and the T cells are activated. In this example, we show CD8+ T cells (CTL) recognizing class I MHC–associated antigens; the same cross-presenting APC may display class II MHC–associated antigens from the microbe for recognition by CD4+ helper T cells.

lymphocytes specific for these antigens. The professional APCs that ingest infected cells may also present the microbial antigens to CD4+ helper T lymphocytes. Thus, both classes of T lymphocytes, CD4+ and CD8+ cells, specific for the same microbe are activated close to one another. As we shall see in Chapter 6, this process may be important for the antigen-stimulated differentiation of naive CD8+ T cells to effector CTLs, which often requires help from CD4+ cells. Once the CD8+ T cells have differentiated into CTLs, they kill infected host cells without any need for professional APCs or signals other than recognition of antigen (see Chapter 6).

Now that we know how protein antigens are captured, transported to, and concentrated in peripheral lymphoid organs, the next question is how are these antigens displayed to T lymphocytes? To answer this question, we first need to understand what MHC molecules are and how they function in immune responses.

The Structure and Function of MHC Molecules

The MHC molecules are membrane proteins on APCs that display peptide antigens for recognition by T lymphocytes. The MHC was discovered as the genetic locus that is the principal determinant of acceptance or rejection of tissue grafts exchanged between individuals. In other words, individuals that are identical at their MHC locus (inbred animals and identical twins) will accept grafts from one another, and individuals that differ at their MHC loci will reject such grafts. Graft rejection is, of course, not a natural biologic phenomenon, and therefore MHC genes, and the molecules they encode, could not have evolved only to mediate graft rejection. We now know that the physiologic function of MHC molecules is to display peptides derived from protein antigens to antigen-specific T lymphocytes. This function of MHC molecules is the explanation for the phenomenon of MHC restriction of T cells, which was mentioned earlier.

The MHC locus is a collection of genes found in all mammals (Fig. 3-6). Human MHC proteins are called **human leukocyte antigens (HLA),** because these proteins were discovered as antigens of leukocytes that could be identified with specific antibodies. The genes encoding these molecules make up the HLA locus. In all species, the MHC locus contains two sets of highly polymorphic genes, called the class I and class II MHC genes. These genes encode the class I and class II MHC molecules that display

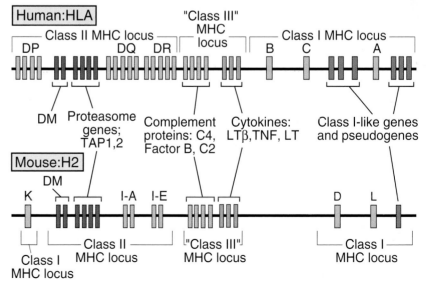

Figure 3–6 The genes of the MHC locus. Schematic maps of the human MHC (called the HLA complex) and the mouse MHC (called the H2 complex) are shown, illustrating the major genes that code for molecules involved in immune responses. Sizes of genes and distances between them are not drawn to scale.

peptides to T cells. In addition to the polymorphic genes, the MHC locus contains many nonpolymorphic genes. Some of these nonpolymorphic genes code for proteins involved in antigen presentation, and others code for proteins whose function is not known.

Class I and class II MHC molecules are membrane proteins that each contains a peptide-binding cleft at its amino-terminal end. Although the subunit composition of class I and class II molecules is different, their overall structure is very similar (Fig. 3-7). Each class I molecule consists of an α chain noncovalently attached to a protein called β_2-microglobulin that is encoded by a gene outside the MHC. The amino-terminal $\alpha 1$ and $\alpha 2$ domains of the class I MHC molecule form a peptide-binding cleft, or groove, that is large enough to accommodate peptides of 8 to 11 amino acids. The floor of the peptide-binding cleft is the region that binds peptides for display to T lymphocytes, and the sides and tops of the cleft are the regions that are contacted by the T cell receptor (which, of course, contacts part of the displayed peptide as well) (see Fig. 3-1). The polymorphic residues of class I molecules, that is, the amino acids that differ among different individuals' MHC molecules, are located in the $\alpha 1$ and $\alpha 2$ domains of the α chain. Some of these polymorphic residues contribute to variations in the floor of the peptide-binding cleft and thus in the ability of different MHC molecules to bind peptides. Other polymorphic residues contribute to variations in the tops of the clefts and thus influence recognition by T cells. The $\alpha 3$ domain is invariant and contains the binding site for the T cell coreceptor CD8. As we shall see in Chapter 5, T cell activation requires recognition of MHC-associated peptide antigen by the TCR and simultaneous recognition of the MHC molecule by the coreceptor. Therefore, CD8$^+$ T cells can only respond to peptides displayed by class I MHC molecules, the MHC molecules to which the CD8 coreceptor binds.

Each class II MHC molecule consists of two chains, called α and β. The amino-terminal regions of both chains, called the $\alpha 1$ and $\beta 1$ domains, contain polymorphic residues and form a cleft that is large enough to accommodate peptides of 10 to 30 residues. The nonpolymorphic $\beta 2$ domain contains the binding site for the T cell coreceptor CD4. Because CD4 binds to class II MHC molecules, CD4$^+$ T cells can only respond to peptides presented by class II MHC molecules.

There are several features of MHC genes and molecules that are important for the normal function of these molecules (Fig. 3-8).

MHC genes are codominantly expressed, meaning that the alleles inherited from both parents are expressed equally. Because there are three polymorphic class I genes, called HLA-A, HLA-B, and HLA-C in humans, and each person inherits one set of these genes from each parent, any cell can express six different class I molecules. There are also three sets of polymorphic class II genes, called HLA-DR, HLA-DQ, and HLA-DP, but in this case both the α chain and the β chain are polymorphic, and the α chain from one allele may associate with the β chain from the other allele. This kind of mixing may give rise to some "hybrid" class II molecules, so that up to 10 to 20 different class II molecules may be expressed.

MHC genes are highly polymorphic, meaning that there are many different alleles present among the different individuals in the population. The polymorphism is so great that no two individuals in the usual outbred population have exactly the same set of MHC genes and molecules. Because the polymorphic residues determine which peptides are presented by which MHC molecules, the existence of multiple alleles ensures that there are always some members of the population that will be able to present any particular microbial protein antigen. It has been suggested that the evolution of MHC polymorphism ensures that a population will not succumb to a new microbe or to an old microbe that mutates its proteins, because at least some individuals will be able to mount effective immune responses to the peptide antigens of newly introduced or mutated microbes. MHC molecules are encoded by inherited DNA sequences, and variations (accounting for the polymorphism) are not induced by gene recombination (as they are in antigen receptors; see Chapter 4).

Class I molecules are expressed on all nucleated cells, but class II molecules are expressed mainly on professional APCs, such as dendritic cells, and on macrophages and B lymphocytes. The physiologic significance of this strikingly different expression pattern is described later in the chapter.

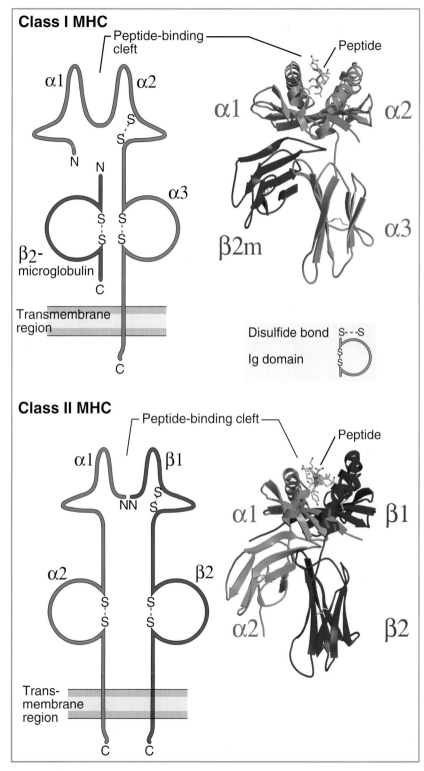

Figure 3–7 The structure of class I MHC and class II MHC molecules. The schematic diagrams and models of the crystal structures of class I MHC and class II MHC molecules illustrate the domains of the molecules and the fundamental similarities between them. Both types of MHC molecules contain peptide-binding clefts and invariant portions that bind CD8 (the α3 domain of class I) or CD4 (the β2 domain of class II). β2m, β2-microglobulin. (Crystal structures courtesy of Dr. P. Bjorkman, California Institute of Technology, Pasadena.)

Feature	Significance	
Co-dominant expression: Both parental alleles of each MHC gene are expressed	Increases number of different MHC molecules that can present peptides to T cells	
Polymorphic genes: Many different alleles are present in the population	Ensures that different individuals are able to present and respond to different microbial peptides	
MHC-expressing cell types: Class II: Professional APCs, macrophages, B cells	CD4+ helper T lymphocytes interact with dendritic cells, macrophages, B lymphocytes	
Class I: All nucleated cells	CD8+ CTLs can kill any virus-infected cell	

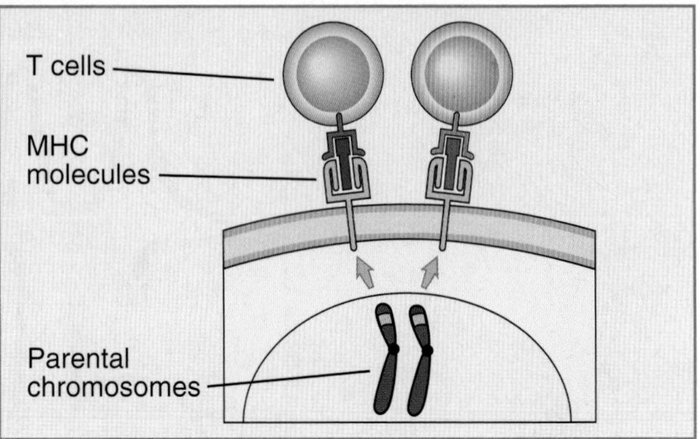

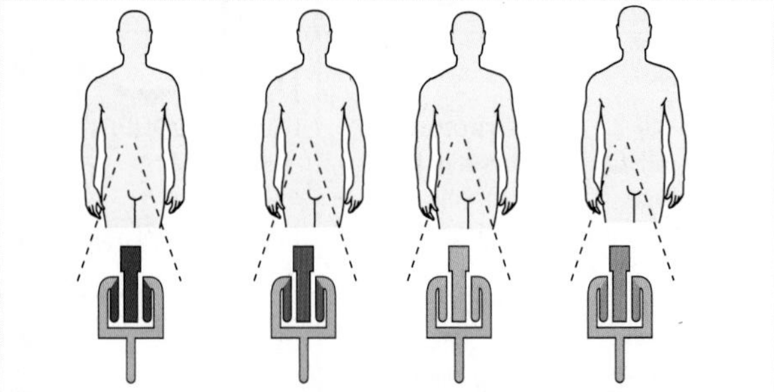

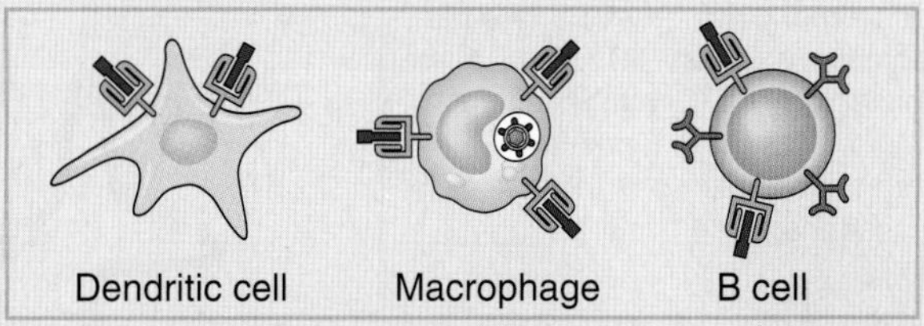

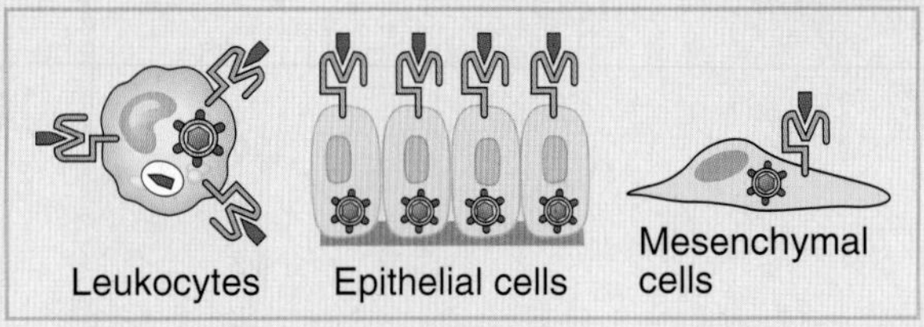

Figure 3–8   Properties of MHC molecules and genes. Some of the important features of MHC molecules are listed, with their significance for immune responses.

The peptide-binding clefts of MHC molecules bind peptides derived from protein antigens and display these peptides for recognition by T cells (Fig. 3-9). There are pockets in the floors of the peptide-binding clefts of most MHC molecules. The side chains of amino acids in the peptide antigens fit into these MHC pockets and anchor the peptides in the cleft of the MHC molecule. Peptides that are anchored in the cleft by these side chains (also called anchor residues) contain some residues that bow upward and are recognized by the antigen receptors of T cells.

Several features of the interaction of peptide antigens with MHC molecules are important for understanding the peptide display function of MHC molecules (Fig. 3-10).

Each MHC molecule can present only one peptide at a time, because there is only one cleft, but each MHC molecule is capable of presenting many different peptides. As long as the pockets of the MHC molecule can accommodate the anchor residues of the peptide, that peptide can be displayed by the MHC molecule. Therefore, only one or two residues in a peptide have to fit into an MHC molecule's cleft. Thus, MHC molecules are said to have a "broad" specificity for peptide binding: each molecule can bind many but not all possible peptides. This, of course, is an essential feature, because each individual has only a few different MHC molecules that must be able to present a vast number and variety of antigens. Except for rare exceptions, MHC molecules bind only peptides and not other types of antigens. This is why MHC-restricted CD4$^+$ T cells and CD8$^+$ T cells can only recognize and respond to protein antigens, the natural source of peptides. The binding of peptides to MHC molecules is a low-affinity interaction with a very slow off-rate, up to hours or days in solution. The low affinity required for binding ensures that there are few structural constraints on this binding, so that many different peptides can bind to the same MHC molecule. The slow off-rate ensures that once an MHC molecule has acquired a peptide, it will display the peptide for a long time, maximizing the chance that a T cell will find the peptide and initiate a response.

MHC molecules acquire their peptide cargo during their biosynthesis and assembly inside cells.

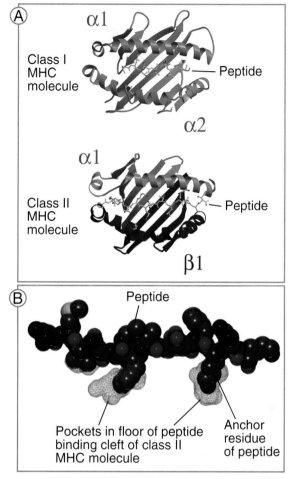

Figure 3–9 Binding of peptides to MHC molecules. A. These top views of the crystal structures of MHC molecules show how peptides (in *yellow*) lie on the floors of the peptide-binding clefts and are available for recognition by T cells. (Courtesy of Dr. P. Bjorkman, California Institute of Technology, Pasadena.) B. The side view of a cut-out of a peptide bound to a class II MHC molecule shows how anchor residues of the peptide hold it in the pockets in the cleft of the MHC molecule. (From Scott CA, PA Peterson, L Teyton, and IA Wilson. Crystal structures of two I-A^d-peptide complexes reveal that high affinity can be achieved without large anchor residues. Immunity 8:319-329, 1998. © Cell Press; with permission.) These structures are the basis for the schematic view of peptide recognition by T cells shown in Figure 3-1.

Feature	Significance	
Each MHC molecule displays one peptide at a time	Each T cell responds to a single peptide bound to an MHC molecule	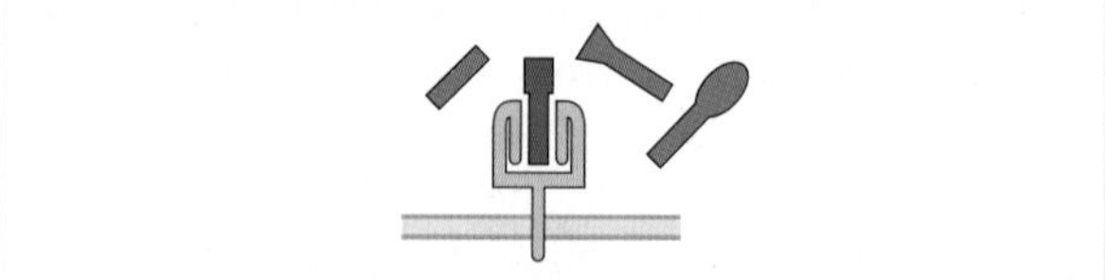
Peptides are acquired during intracellular assembly	Class I and class II MHC molecules display peptides from different cellular compartments	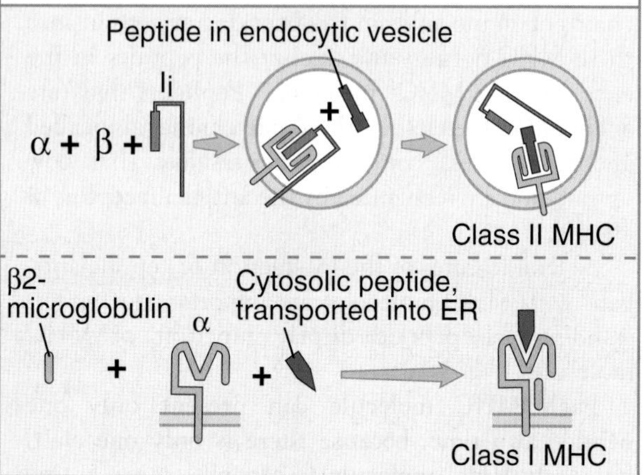
Low affinity, broad specificity	Many different peptides can bind to the same MHC molecule	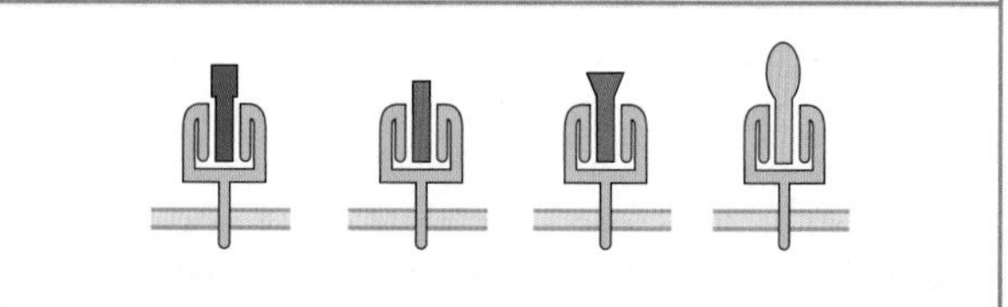
Very slow off-rate	MHC molecule displays bound peptide for long enough to be located by T cell	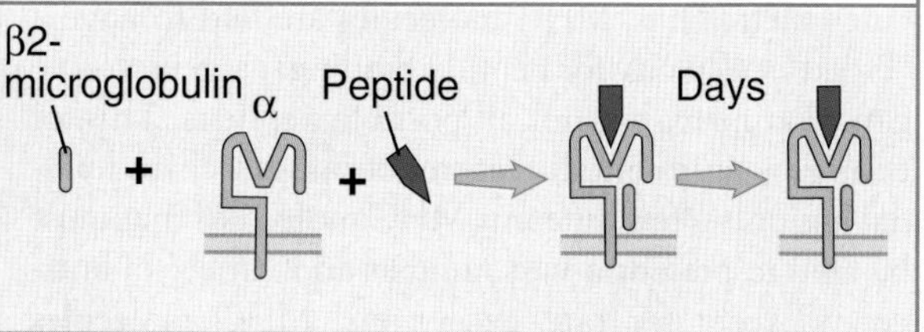
Stable expression requires peptide	Only MHC molecules that are displaying peptides are expressed for recognition by T cells.	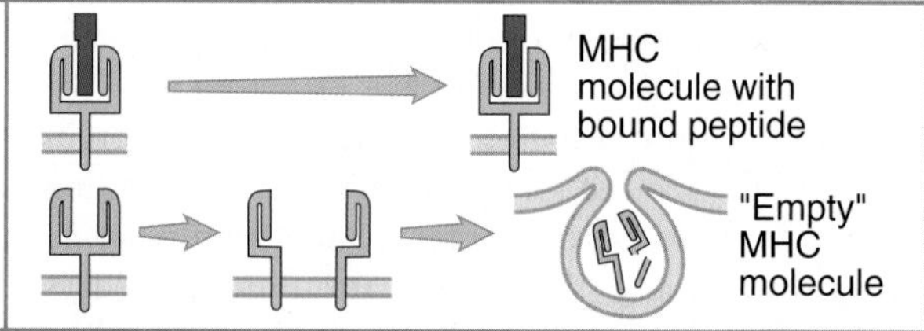
MHC molecules bind only peptides	MHC-restricted T cells respond only to protein antigens, and not to other chemicals	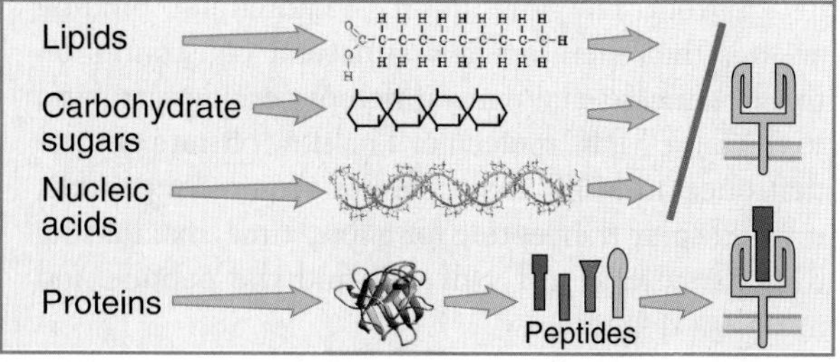

Figure 3–10 Features of peptide binding to MHC molecules. Some of the important features of peptide binding to MHC molecules are listed, with their significance for immune responses.

Therefore, MHC molecules display peptides derived from microbes that are inside host cells, and this is why MHC-restricted T cells recognize cell-associated microbes and are the mediators of immunity to intracellular microbes. Also, class I MHC molecules acquire peptides from cytosolic proteins and class II molecules from proteins in intracellular vesicles. The mechanisms and significance of these processes are discussed later in the chapter. Only peptide-loaded MHC molecules are stably expressed on cell surfaces. The reason for this is that MHC molecules must assemble both their chains and bound peptides to achieve a stable structure and "empty" molecules are degraded inside cells. This requirement for peptide binding ensures that only "useful" MHC molecules, that is, those that are displaying peptides, are expressed on cell surfaces for recognition by T cells.

In each individual, the MHC molecules can display peptides derived from foreign, that is, microbial, proteins as well as peptides from that individual's own proteins. This inability of MHC molecules to discriminate between foreign antigens and self antigens raises two questions. First, at any time the quantity of self proteins is certain to be much greater than that of any microbial antigens. Why then are the available MHC molecules not constantly occupied by self peptides and unable to present foreign antigens? The likely answer is that new MHC molecules are constantly being synthesized, ready to accept peptides, and they are adept at capturing any peptides that are present in cells. Also, a single T cell may only need to see a peptide displayed by as few as 0.1% to 1% of the approximately 10^5 MHC molecules on an APC, so that even rare MHC molecules displaying a peptide are enough to initiate an immune response. The second problem is, if MHC molecules are constantly displaying self peptides, why do we not develop immune responses to self antigens, so-called autoimmune responses? The answer to this question is that T cells specific for self antigens are either killed or inactivated; this process is discussed in Chapter 9. Although it seems puzzling that MHC molecules present self peptides, this is actually the key to the normal surveillance function of T cells. Thus, T cells are constantly patrolling the body looking at MHC-associated peptides, not reacting to peptides derived from self proteins but able to respond to rare microbial peptides.

MHC molecules are capable of displaying peptides but not intact microbial protein antigens. It follows that there must be mechanisms for converting naturally occurring proteins into peptides able to bind to MHC molecules. This conversion is called **antigen processing,** and it is described in the next section.

Processing of Protein Antigens

Extracellular proteins that are internalized by professional APCs into vesicles are processed and displayed by class II MHC molecules, whereas proteins in the cytosol of nucleated cells are processed and displayed by class I MHC molecules (Fig. 3-11). These two pathways of antigen processing involve different cellular organelles and proteins (Fig. 3-12). They are designed to sample all the proteins present in the extracellular and intracellular environments. The segregation of antigen processing pathways also ensures that different classes of T lymphocytes recognize antigens from different compartments, as is discussed later.

Processing of Internalized Antigens for Display by Class II MHC Molecules

APCs may internalize extracellular microbes or microbial proteins by several mechanisms (Fig. 3-13). Microbes may bind to surface receptors specific for microbial products or to receptors that recognize antibodies or products of complement activation that are attached to the microbes. B lymphocytes internalize proteins that specifically bind to the cells' antigen receptors (see Chapter 7). Some APCs may phagocytose microbes or pinocytose proteins without any specific recognition event. After internalization into APCs by any of these pathways, the microbial proteins enter intracellular vesicles called endosomes or phagosomes, which may fuse with lysosomes. In these vesicles the proteins are broken down by proteolytic enzymes, generating many peptides of varying lengths and sequences.

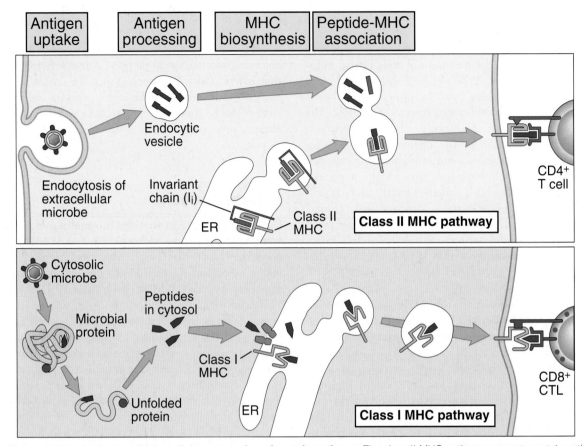

Figure 3–11   Pathways of intracellular processing of protein antigens. The class II MHC pathway converts protein antigens that are endocytosed into vesicles of APCs into peptides that bind to class II MHC molecules for recognition by CD4+ T cells. The class I MHC pathway converts proteins in the cytoplasm into peptides that bind to class I MHC molecules for recognition by CD8+ T cells. ER, endoplasmic reticulum.

APCs constantly synthesize class II MHC molecules in the endoplasmic reticulum (ER). Each newly synthesized class II molecule carries with it an attached protein called the invariant chain, which contains a sequence (called the class II invariant chain peptide, or CLIP) that binds tightly to the peptide-binding cleft of the class II molecule. Thus, the cleft of the newly synthesized class II molecule is occupied. This "inaccessible" class II molecule begins its transport to the cell surface in an exocytic vesicle, which then fuses with the endosomal vesicle containing broken-down peptides derived from ingested extracellular proteins. The same endosomal vesicle

contains a class II–like protein called DM, whose function is to remove CLIP from the class II MHC molecule. After removal of CLIP, the cleft of the class II molecule becomes available to accept peptides. If the class II MHC molecule is able to bind one of the peptides generated from the ingested proteins, the complex becomes stable and is delivered to the cell surface. If the MHC molecule does not find a peptide it can bind, the empty molecule is unstable and is degraded by proteases in the endosomes. Any one protein antigen may give rise to many peptides, only a few of which (perhaps only one or two) may bind to the MHC molecules present in the individual.

Feature	Class II MHC Pathway	Class I MHC pathway
Composition of stable peptide-MHC complex	Polymorphic α and β chains, peptide 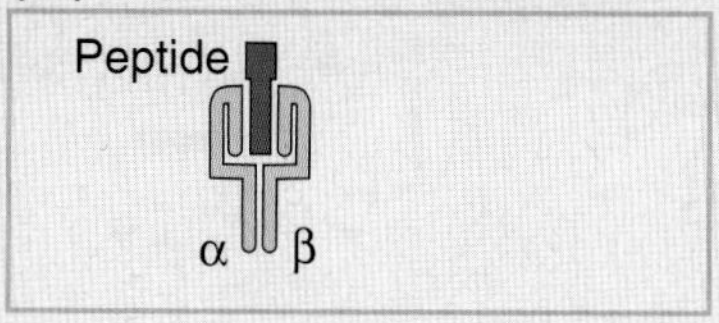	Polymorphic α chain, β2-microglobulin, peptide 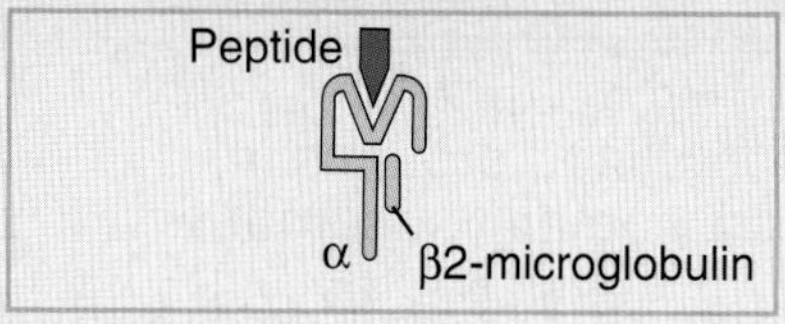
Types of APCs	Dendritic cells, mononuclear phagocytes, B lymphocytes; endothelial cells, thymic epithelium	All nucleated cells
Responsive T cells	CD4+ T cells (mostly helper T cells) 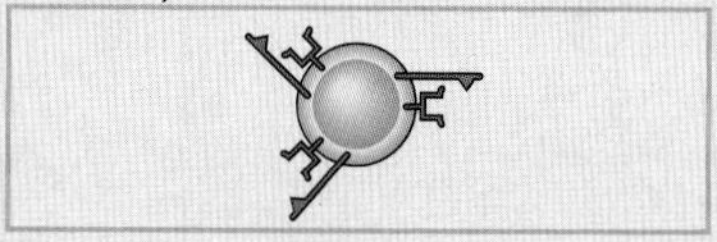	CD8+ T cells 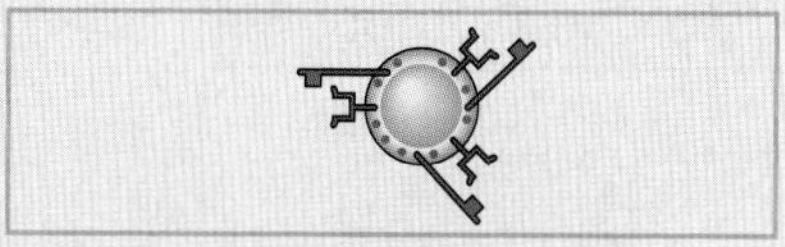
Source of protein antigens	Endosomal/lysosomal proteins (mostly internalized from extracellular environment)	Cytosolic proteins (mostly synthesized in the cell; may enter cytosol from phagosomes)
Enzymes responsible for peptide generation	Endosomal and lysosomal proteases (e.g., cathepsins)	Cytosolic proteasome
Site of peptide loading of MHC	Specialized vesicular compartment	Endoplasmic reticulum
Molecules involved in transport of peptides and loading of MHC molecules	Invariant chain, DM	TAP

Figure 3–12 **Features of the pathways of antigen processing.**

Therefore, only these peptides from the intact antigen stimulate immune responses in that individual; such peptides are said to be the **immunodominant epitopes** of the antigen.

Processing of Cytosolic Antigens for Display by Class I MHC Molecules

Antigenic proteins may be produced in the cytoplasm from viruses that are living inside infected cells, from some phagocytosed microbes that may break through vesicles and escape into the cytoplasm, and from mutated or altered host genes, as in tumors. All these proteins, as well as the cell's own cytoplasmic proteins that have outlived their usefulness, are targeted for destruction by proteolysis. These proteins are unfolded, covalently tagged with a small peptide called ubiquitin, and "threaded" through a proteolytic organelle called the proteasome, where the unfolded proteins are degraded by enzymes (Fig. 3-14). Some classes of proteasomes efficiently cleave cytosolic

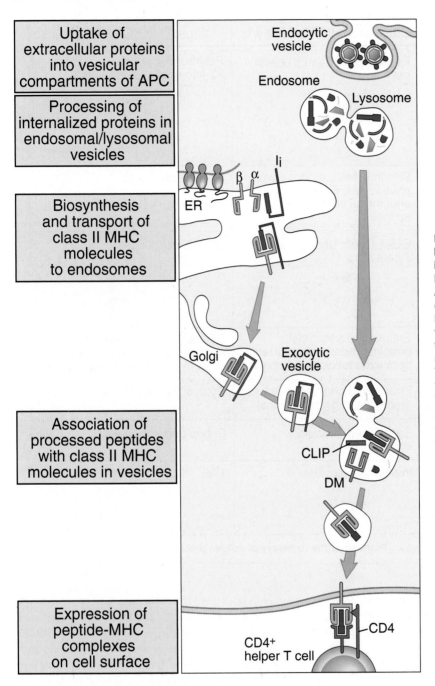

Uptake of extracellular proteins into vesicular compartments of APC

Processing of internalized proteins in endosomal/lysosomal vesicles

Biosynthesis and transport of class II MHC molecules to endosomes

Association of processed peptides with class II MHC molecules in vesicles

Expression of peptide-MHC complexes on cell surface

Endocytic vesicle

Endosome

Lysosome

Ii

β α

ER

Golgi

Exocytic vesicle

CLIP

DM

CD4

CD4+ helper T cell

Figure 3–13 The class II MHC pathway of processing of internalized vesicular antigens. Protein antigens are ingested by APCs into vesicles, where they are degraded into peptides. Class II MHC molecules enter the same vesicles and lose the CLIP peptide that occupies the cleft of newly synthesized class II molecules. These class II molecules are able to bind peptides derived from the endocytosed protein. The peptide–class II MHC complexes are transported to the cell surface and are recognized by CD4+ T cells.

Figure 3–14 The class I MHC pathway of processing of cytosolic antigens. Proteins enter the cytoplasm of cells either from phagocytosed microbes or from endogenous synthesis by microbes, such as viruses, that reside in the cytoplasm of infected cells. Cytoplasmic proteins are unfolded, ubiquitinated, and degraded in proteasomes. The peptides that are produced are transported by the TAP transporter into the endoplasmic reticulum (ER), where the peptides bind to newly synthesized class I MHC molecules. The peptide–class I MHC complexes are transported to the cell surface and are recognized by CD8+ T cells.

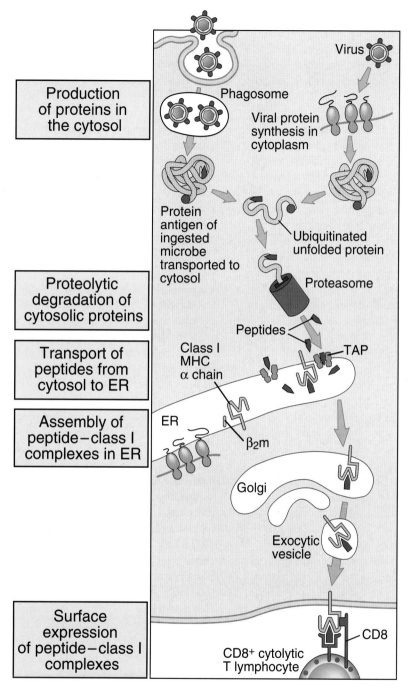

Production of proteins in the cytosol

Proteolytic degradation of cytosolic proteins

Transport of peptides from cytosol to ER

Assembly of peptide–class I complexes in ER

Surface expression of peptide–class I complexes

Virus

Phagosome

Viral protein synthesis in cytoplasm

Protein antigen of ingested microbe transported to cytosol

Ubiquitinated unfolded protein

Proteasome

Peptides

Class I MHC α chain

TAP

ER

β2m

Golgi

Exocytic vesicle

CD8

CD8+ cytolytic T lymphocyte

proteins into peptides with the size and sequence properties typical of class I MHC–binding peptides. But the cell faces another challenge: the peptides are in the cytoplasm while the MHC molecules are being synthesized in the ER, and the two have to come together. This problem is overcome by a specialized transport molecule, called the transporter associated with antigen processing (TAP), which picks up peptides from the cytoplasm and actively pumps the peptides across the ER membrane into the interior of the ER. (This, of course, is the reverse of the normal direction of protein traffic, which is from the site of synthesis in the ER out into the cytoplasm or to the plasma membrane.) Newly synthesized class I MHC molecules are loosely attached to the interior face of the TAP molecule. Thus, as peptides enter the ER, they can be captured by the class I molecules. (Recall that in the ER, the class II molecules are not able to bind peptides because of the invariant chain.) If a class I molecule finds a peptide with the right fit, the complex is stabilized and transported to the cell surface. During this transport, the class I–peptide complex may intersect endosomes, but now the class I molecule is not available to bind peptides, and, being stable, it is able to resist proteolysis by endosomal proteases. If a class I molecule does not find a peptide in the ER, the molecule becomes unstable and is degraded by proteases.

The constant struggle between microbes and their hosts is well illustrated by the numerous strategies that viruses have developed to block the class I MHC pathway of antigen presentation. These strategies include removing newly synthesized MHC molecules from the ER, inhibiting the transcription of MHC genes, and blocking peptide transport by the TAP transporter. By inhibiting the class I MHC pathway, viruses reduce presentation of their own antigens to CD8$^+$ T cells and are thus able to evade the adaptive immune system. These viral evasion strategies are partly counterbalanced by the ability of natural killer cells of the innate immune system to recognize and kill virally infected cells that have lost class I MHC expression (see Chapter 2). Further discussion of these mechanisms of immune evasion by viruses is found in Chapter 6.

The Physiologic Significance of MHC-Associated Antigen Presentation

It is expected that such a precisely regulated system for protein antigen processing and presentation plays an important role in stimulating immune responses. In fact, many fundamental features of T cell–mediated immunity are closely linked to the peptide display function of MHC molecules.

The advantage of the restriction of T cell recognition to MHC-associated peptides is that T cells will see and respond only to cell-associated antigens. This is partly because MHC molecules are cell membrane proteins and partly because peptide loading and subsequent expression of MHC molecules are dependent on intracellular biosynthetic and assembly steps. In other words, MHC molecules can be loaded with peptides only inside cells, where the antigens of phagocytosed and intracellular pathogens are present. Therefore, T lymphocytes can only recognize the antigens of phagocytosed and intracellular microbes, which are the types of microbes that have to be combated by T cell–mediated immunity.

By segregating the class I and class II pathways of antigen processing, the immune system is able to respond to extracellular and intracellular microbes in ways best able to combat these microbes (Fig 3-15). Extracellular microbes are captured by APCs, including B lymphocytes and macrophages, and are presented by class II molecules, which, of course, are expressed mainly on these APCs (and on dendritic cells). Because of the specificity of CD4 for class II, class II–associated peptides are recognized by CD4$^+$ T lymphocytes, which function as helper cells. These helper T cells help B lymphocytes to produce antibodies, and they help phagocytes to ingest and destroy microbes, thus activating the two effector mechanisms best able to eliminate extracellular and ingested microbes. Neither of these mechanisms is effective against viruses that live in the cytoplasm of host cells. Cytosolic antigens are processed and displayed by class I MHC molecules, which are expressed on all nucleated cells—again, as expected, because all nucleated cells can be infected with some viruses. Class I–associated peptides are recognized by CD8$^+$ T

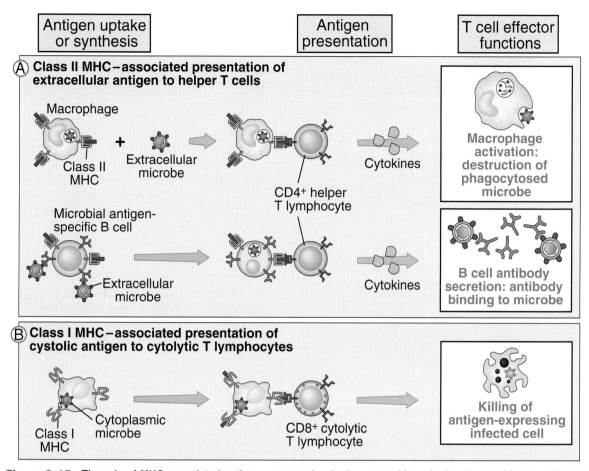

Figure 3–15   The role of MHC-associated antigen presentation in the recognition of microbes by CD4+ and CD8+ T cells. A. Protein antigens of microbes that are endocytosed from the extracellular environment by macrophages and B lymphocytes enter the class II MHC pathway of antigen processing. As a result, these proteins are recognized by CD4+ helper T lymphocytes, whose functions are to activate macrophages to destroy phagocytosed microbes and activate B cells to produce antibodies against extracellular microbes and toxins. B. Protein antigens of microbes that live in the cytoplasm of infected cells enter the class I MHC pathway of antigen processing. As a result, these proteins are recognized by CD8+ CTLs, whose function is to kill infected cells.

lymphocytes, which differentiate into CTLs. The CTLs kill the infected cells and eradicate the infection, this being the most effective mechanism for eliminating cytoplasmic microbes. Thus, the nature of the protective immune response to different microbes is optimized by linking several features of antigen presentation and T cell recognition: the pathways of processing of vesicular and cytosolic antigens, the cellular expression of class II and class I MHC molecules, the specificity of CD4 and CD8 coreceptors for class II and class I molecules, and the functions of CD4+ cells as helper cells and of CD8+ cells as CTLs.

This chapter began with two questions: how do rare antigen-specific lymphocytes find antigens, and how are the appropriate immune responses generated against extracellular and intracellular microbes? Understanding the biology of APCs and the role of MHC molecules in displaying the peptides of protein antigens has provided satisfying answers to both questions, specifically for T cell–mediated immune responses.

Functions of Antigen-Presenting Cells in Addition to Antigen Display

APCs not only display peptides for recognition by T cells but, in response to microbes, also express "second signals" for T cell activation. The "two-signal" concept of lymphocyte activation was introduced in Chapter 1 and will be returned to when the responses of T and B cells are discussed (see Chapters 5 and 7). Recall that antigen is the necessary signal 1, and signal 2 is provided by microbes or APCs reacting to microbes. The requirement for "signal 2" ensures that adaptive immune responses are generated against microbes and not against harmless noninfectious substances, even though there may be lymphocytes capable of recognizing such substances. Different types of microbial products and innate immune responses may activate APCs to express second signals for lymphocyte activation. For instance, many bacteria produce a substance called lipopolysaccharide (LPS, also called endotoxin). When the bacteria are captured by APCs for presentation of their protein antigens, LPS acts on the same APCs and stimulates two changes. In response to LPS, the APCs express surface proteins, called **costimulators,** that are recognized by receptors on T cells, and the APCs secrete cytokines that are recognized by cytokine receptors on T cells. The costimulators and cytokines act in concert with antigen recognition by the TCR to stimulate the proliferation and differentiation of the T cells. In this case, antigen is signal 1 and costimulators and cytokines provide signal 2 for the development of T cell–mediated immunity.

Antigens Recognized by B Lymphocytes

B lymphocytes use membrane-bound antibodies to recognize a wide variety of antigens, including proteins, polysaccharides, lipids, and small chemicals. These antigens may be expressed on microbial surfaces (e.g., capsular or envelope antigens) or they may be in soluble form (e.g., secreted toxins). B cells differentiate in response to antigen and other signals into cells that secrete antibodies (see Chapter 7). The secreted antibodies enter the circulation and mucosal fluids and bind to the antigens, leading to their neutralization and elimination. The antigen receptors of B cells and the antibodies that are secreted usually recognize antigens in the native conformation, without any requirement for antigen processing or display by a specialized system. There is also no apparent requirement for a specialized population of APCs to present antigens to naive B cells. Therefore, antigen recognition by B cells appears to be much less regulated than that by T lymphocytes. Because B cell activation occurs in the peripheral lymphoid organs, such as the spleen and lymph nodes, there may well be mechanisms for capturing microbes and even nonmicrobial foreign antigens of diverse chemical composition in these organs. Clearly, if there are such mechanisms, they must keep the antigens in their native conformation and make these antigens available to B lymphocytes. But little is known about how B lymphocytes specific for a particular antigen (which are as rare as T cells specific for a peptide) find that antigen in the lymphoid organs.

The B cell–rich lymphoid follicles of the lymph nodes and spleen contain a population of cells called follicular dendritic cells (FDCs), whose function is to display antigens to activated B cells. FDCs use their Fc receptors to bind antigens that are coated with antibodies, and their receptors for the C3d complement protein, to bind antigens with attached complement. These antigens are seen by specific B lymphocytes during humoral immune responses, and they function mainly to select B cells that bind the antigens with high affinity. This process is discussed in Chapter 7.

SUMMARY

▶ The induction of immune responses to the protein antigens of microbes is dependent on a specialized system for capturing and displaying these antigens for recognition by the rare naive T cells specific for any antigen. Microbes and microbial antigens that enter the body through epithelia are captured by professional antigen-presenting cells (APCs), mainly dendritic cells, located in the epithelia and transported to regional lymph nodes, or are captured by APCs resident in lymph nodes and spleen. The protein antigens of the microbes are displayed by the APCs to naive T lymphocytes that recirculate through the lymphoid organs.

▶ The function of displaying peptides derived from protein antigens is performed by molecules encoded in the major histocompatibility complex (MHC).

▶ Proteins that are ingested by APCs from the extracellular environment are proteolytically degraded within the vesicles of the APCs, and the peptides that are generated bind to the clefts of newly synthesized class II MHC molecules. Class II MHC molecules are recognized by CD4, because of which CD4+ helper T cells are specific for class II MHC–associated peptides that are derived mainly from extracellular proteins.

▶ Proteins that are produced by microbes living in the cytoplasm of infected cells, or enter the cytoplasm from phagocytosed microbes, are degraded by cytosolic proteases and bind to the clefts of newly synthesized class I MHC molecules. Class I MHC molecules are recognized by CD8, because of which CD8+ cytolytic T lymphocytes are specific for class I MHC–associated peptides derived from cytosolic proteins.

▶ The role of MHC molecules in antigen display ensures that T cells only see cell-associated protein antigens, and the correct type of T cell (helper or cytolytic cell) responds to the type of microbe that T cell is best able to combat.

▶ Microbes activate APCs to express membrane proteins (called costimulators) and to secrete cytokines that provide signals that function in concert with antigens to stimulate specific T cells. The requirement for these second signals ensures that T cells respond to microbial antigens and not to harmless, nonmicrobial substances.

▶ B lymphocytes recognize proteins as well as nonprotein antigens, even in their native conformations. It is not known if a specialized system of antigen display is essential for the induction of B cell responses. Follicular dendritic cells (FDCs) display antigens to germinal center B cells and select the high-affinity B cells during humoral immune responses.

⇄ Review Questions

1 When antigens enter through the skin, in what organs are they concentrated? What cell type(s) play important roles in this process of antigen capture?

2 What are MHC molecules? What are human MHC molecules called? How were they discovered, and what is their function?

3 What are the differences between the antigens that are displayed by class I and class II MHC molecules?

4 Describe the sequence of events by which class I and class II MHC molecules acquire antigens for display.

5 Which functional subsets of T cells recognize antigens presented by class I and class II MHC molecules? What molecules on T cells contribute to their specificity for either class I or class II MHC–associated peptide antigens?

Antigen Recognition in the Adaptive Immune System

Structure of Lymphocyte Antigen Receptors and the Development of Immune Repertoires

4

Antigen Receptors of Lymphocytes
- Antibodies
- T Cell Receptors for Antigens

Development of Immune Repertoires
- Maturation of Lymphocytes
- Production of Diverse Antigen Receptors
- Maturation and Selection of B Lymphocytes
- Maturation and Selection of T Lymphocytes

Summary

Adaptive immune responses are specific for the antigens that initiate these responses, because the activation of lymphocytes is triggered by recognition of antigens. **Specific antigen recognition is the task of two structurally similar types of cell surface proteins of lymphocytes: membrane-bound antibodies on B cells and T cell receptors (TCRs) on T lymphocytes.**

Cellular receptors in the immune system, as in other biologic systems, serve two functions: they detect external stimuli (antigens, for the adaptive immune system), and they trigger responses of the cells on which the receptors are expressed. To recognize a large number and variety of antigens, the antigen receptors of lymphocytes must be able to bind to and distinguish between many, often closely related, chemical structures. Antigen receptors are clonally distributed, meaning that each clone of lymphocytes having a particular specificity has a unique receptor, different from the receptors of all other clones. (Recall that a clone consists of a parent cell and its progeny.) The total number, or repertoire, of lymphocyte specificities is very large, because the immune system consists of many clones with distinct specificities. Although each clone of B lymphocytes or T lymphocytes recognizes a different antigen, all B or T cells respond in essentially the same way to recognition of antigens.

To link antigen recognition to lymphocyte activation, the antigen receptors transmit biochemical signals that are fundamentally the same in all lymphocytes and are unrelated to specificity. These features of lymphocyte recognition and antigen receptors raise two important questions:

- How do the antigen receptors of lymphocytes recognize extremely diverse antigens and transmit quite conserved activating signals to the cells?
- How is the vast diversity of receptor structures generated in lymphocytes? The diversity of antigen recognition implies the existence of many structurally different antigen receptor proteins, more than can be reasonably encoded in the inherited genome (germline). Therefore, there must be special mechanisms for generating this diversity.

In this chapter, we describe the structures of the antigen receptors of B and T lymphocytes and how these receptors recognize antigens. Also to be discussed is how the diversity of antigen receptors is generated during the process of lymphocyte maturation, thus giving rise to the repertoire of mature lymphocytes. The process of antigen-induced lymphocyte activation is described in later chapters.

Antigen Receptors of Lymphocytes

The antigen receptors of B and T lymphocytes have several features that are important for the functions of these receptors in adaptive immunity (Fig. 4-1).

The antigen receptors of B and T lymphocytes recognize chemically different structures. B lymphocytes are able to recognize the shapes, or conformations, of native macromolecules, including proteins, lipids, carbohydrates, and nucleic acids, as well as simple small chemical groups and parts of macromolecules. In striking contrast, most T cells see only peptides, and only when these peptides are displayed on antigen-presenting cells (APCs) bound to membrane proteins encoded in the major histocompatibility complex (MHC) genetic locus. The properties and functions of MHC molecules were described in Chapter 3.

Antigen receptor molecules consist of regions, or domains, that are involved in antigen recognition and, therefore, vary between clones of lymphocytes

and other regions that are required for structural integrity and for effector functions and are relatively conserved among all clones. The antigen-recognizing portions of the receptors are called the **variable (V) regions,** and the conserved portions are the **constant (C) regions.** Even within the V regions, much of the sequence variability is concentrated within short stretches, which are called hypervariable regions, or complementarity determining regions (CDRs), because they form the parts of the receptor that bind antigens (i.e., they are complementary to the shapes of antigens). By concentrating sequence variation in small regions of the receptor, it is possible to maximize the variability while retaining the basic structures of the receptors. Furthermore, as will be seen later in this chapter, there are special genetic mechanisms for introducing variations in the antigen-recognizing regions of these receptors while using a limited set of genes to code for most of the receptor polypeptides.

Antigen receptors are noncovalently attached to other invariant molecules whose function is to deliver to the inside of the cell the activation signals that are triggered by antigen recognition (see Fig. 4-1). Thus, the two functions of lymphocyte receptors for antigen—specific antigen recognition and signal transduction—are mediated by different polypeptides. This again allows variability to be segregated in one set of molecules (the receptors themselves) while leaving the conserved function of signal transduction in other, invariant, proteins. The collection of antigen receptors and signaling molecules in B lymphocytes is called the **B cell receptor (BCR)**

Figure 4–1 Properties of antibodies and T cell antigen receptors (TCRs). Antibodies (also called immunoglobulins, or Ig) may be expressed as membrane receptors or secreted proteins; TCRs only function as membrane receptors. When Ig or TCR molecules recognize antigens, signals are delivered to the lymphocytes by proteins associated with the antigen receptors. The antigen receptors and attached signaling proteins form the B cell receptor (BCR) and TCR complexes. Note that single antigen receptors are shown recognizing antigens, but signaling requires the cross-linking of two or more receptors by binding to adjacent antigen molecules. The important characteristics of these antigen-recognizing molecules are summarized.

Feature or function	Antibody (Immunoglobulin)	T cell receptor (TCR)
Forms of antigens recognized	Macromolecules (proteins, polysaccharides, lipids, nucleic acids), small chemicals Conformational and linear epitopes	Peptides displayed by MHC molecules on APCs Linear epitopes
Diversity	Each clone has a unique specificity; potential for >10^9 distinct specificities	Each clone has a unique specificity; potential for >10^{11} distinct specificities
Antigen recognition is mediated by:	Variable (V) regions of heavy and light chains of membrane Ig	Variable (V) regions of α and β chains
Signaling functions are mediated by:	Proteins (Igα and Igβ) associated with membrane Ig	Proteins (CD3 and ζ) associated with TCR
Effector functions are mediated by:	Constant (C) regions of secreted Ig	TCR does not perform effector functions

complex, and in T lymphocytes it is called the **T cell receptor (TCR) complex.** When adjacent antigen receptors of lymphocytes bind to two or more antigen molecules, the receptors are pulled together into an aggregate. This process is called cross-linking, and it brings the associated signaling proteins of the receptor complexes into close proximity. When this happens, enzymes attached to the cytoplasmic portions of the signaling proteins catalyze the phosphorylation of other proteins. Phosphorylation triggers complex signaling cascades that culminate in the production of numerous molecules that mediate the responses of the lymphocytes. We will return to the processes of T and B lymphocyte activation in Chapters 5 and 7, respectively.

Antibodies may be membrane-bound antigen receptors of B cells or secreted proteins, but TCRs exist only as membrane receptors of T cells. Secreted antibodies are present in the blood and mucosal secretions, where they function to neutralize and eliminate microbes and toxins (i.e., they are the effector molecules of humoral immunity). Antibodies are also called **immunoglobulins (Ig),** referring to immunity-conferring proteins with the characteristic electrophoretic mobility of plasma globulins. Secreted antibodies recognize microbial antigens and toxins by their variable domains just like the membrane-bound antigen receptors of B lymphocytes. The constant regions of some secreted antibodies have the ability to bind to other molecules that participate in the elimination of antigens; these molecules include receptors on phagocytes and proteins of the complement system. Thus, antibodies serve two functions in humoral immunity: B cell membrane-bound antibodies recognize antigens to initiate humoral immune responses, and secreted antibodies eliminate antigens in the effector phase of such responses. In cell-mediated immunity, the effector function of microbe elimination is performed by T lymphocytes themselves. The antigen receptors of T cells are involved only in antigen recognition and T cell activation, and these proteins do not mediate effector functions and are not secreted.

With this introduction, we proceed to a description of the antigen receptors of lymphocytes, first antibodies and then TCRs.

Antibodies

An antibody molecule is composed of four polypeptide chains, including two identical heavy (H) chains and two identical light (L) chains, with each chain containing one variable region and one constant region (Fig. 4-2). The four chains are assembled to form a Y-shaped molecule. Each light chain is attached to one heavy chain, and the two heavy chains are attached to each other, all by disulfide bonds. A light chain is made up of one V and one C domain, and a heavy chain has one V and three or four C domains. Each domain folds into a characteristic three-dimensional shape, which is called the immunoglobulin (Ig) domain. Ig domains are present in many other proteins in the immune system as well as outside the immune system, and most of these proteins are involved in sensing signals from the environment and from other cells. All these proteins are said to be members of the Ig superfamily, and they may have evolved from a common ancestral gene.

Each variable region of the heavy chain (called V_H) or of the light chain (called V_L) contains three hypervariable regions, or CDRs. Of these three, the greatest variability is in CDR3, which is located at the junction of the V and C regions. As expected, CDR3 is also the portion of the Ig molecule that contributes most to antigen binding. Regions of antibody molecules are often named based on the properties of proteolytic fragments of immunoglobulins. The fragment of an antibody that contains a whole light chain (with its single V and C domains) attached to the V and first C domains of a heavy chain contains the portion of the antibody required for antigen recognition and is therefore called Fab (fragment antigen binding). The remaining heavy chain C domains make up the Fc region, with Fc referring to fragment crystalline (so named because this fragment tends to crystallize in solution). In each Ig molecule, there are two identical Fab regions that bind antigen and one Fc region that is responsible for most of the biologic activity and effector functions of the antibodies. (As will be seen later, some antibodies consist of two or five Ig molecules attached to one another.) Between the Fab and Fc regions of most antibody molecules is a flexible portion called the hinge region. The hinge allows the two antigen-binding Fab regions of each antibody

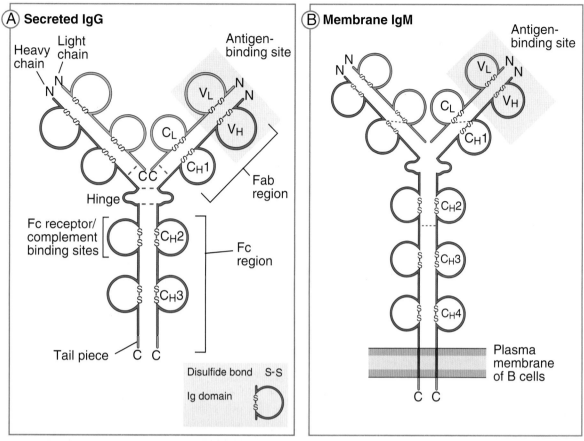

Crystal structure of secreted IgG

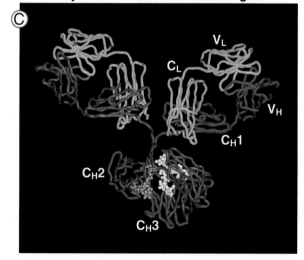

Figure 4–2 The structure of antibodies. Schematic diagrams of a secreted IgG (A) and a membrane form of IgM (B) are shown, illustrating the domains of the heavy and light chains and the regions of the proteins that participate in antigen recognition and effector functions. N and C refer to the amino-terminal and carboxy-terminal ends of the polypeptide chains, respectively. The crystal structure of a secreted IgG molecule (C) illustrates the domains and their spatial orientation. In the crystal structure, the heavy chains are colored *blue* and *red*, and the light chains are colored *green*; carbohydrates are shown in *gray*. (Courtesy of Dr. Alex McPherson, University of California, Irvine.)

molecule to move, enabling them to simultaneously bind antigen epitopes that are separated from one another by varying distances. The C-terminal end of the heavy chain may be anchored in the plasma membrane, as seen in B cell receptors, or it may terminate in a tail piece that lacks the membrane anchor so that the antibody is produced as a secreted protein. Light chains are not attached to cell membranes.

There are two types of light chains, called κ and λ, that differ in their C regions but do not differ in function. There are five types of heavy chains, called μ, δ, γ, ε, and α, that also differ in their C regions. Each type of light chain may complex with any type of heavy chain in an antibody molecule. Antibodies that contain different heavy chains are said to belong to different **isotypes,** or **classes,** and are named according to their heavy chains (i.e., IgM, IgD, IgG, IgE, and IgA), regardless of the light chain class. Different isotypes differ in their physical and biologic properties and in their effector functions (Fig. 4-3). The antigen receptors of naive B lymphocytes, which are mature B cells that have not encountered antigen, are membrane-bound IgM and IgD. After stimulation by antigen and helper T lymphocytes, the antigen-specific clone of B lymphocytes may expand and differentiate into progeny that secrete antibodies. Some of the progeny of IgM- and IgD-expressing B cells may secrete IgM, and other progeny of the same B cells may produce antibodies of other heavy chain classes. This change in Ig isotype production is called **heavy chain class (or isotype) switching,** and its mechanism and importance are discussed further in Chapter 7. Although heavy chain C regions may switch during humoral immune responses, each clone of B cells maintains its specificity, because the V regions do not change. The light chain class (i.e., κ or λ) also remains fixed throughout the life of each B cell clone.

Antibodies are capable of binding a wide variety of antigens, including macromolecules and small chemicals. The reason for this is that the antigen-binding region of antibody molecules forms a flat surface capable of accommodating many different shapes (Fig. 4-4). Antibodies bind to antigens by reversible, noncovalent interactions, including hydrogen bonds and charge interactions. The parts of antigens that are recognized by antibodies are called **epitopes,** or **determinants.** Different antigenic determinants may be recognized based on sequence (linear determinants) or shape (conformational determinants). Some of these epitopes are hidden within antigen molecules and are exposed as a result of a physicochemical change (neodeterminants).

The strength with which one antigen-binding surface of an antibody binds to one epitope of an antigen is called the **affinity** of the interaction. Affinity is often expressed as the dissociation constant (K_d), which is the molar concentration of an antigen required to occupy half the available antibody molecules in a solution; the lower the K_d, the higher the affinity. Most antibodies produced in a primary immune response have a K_d in the range of 10^{-6} to 10^{-9} M, but with repeated stimulation (e.g., in a secondary immune response) the affinity increases to a K_d of 10^{-8} to 10^{-11} M. This increase in antigen-binding strength is called **affinity maturation;** its mechanisms and importance are discussed in Chapter 7. Each IgG, IgD, and IgE antibody molecule has two antigen-binding sites. Secreted IgA is a dimer and therefore has four antigen-binding sites, and secreted IgM is a pentamer, with 10 antigen-binding sites. Therefore, each antibody molecule can bind 2 to 10 epitopes of an antigen, as long as identical epitopes are present sufficiently close together, e.g., on a cell surface, in an aggregated antigen or in some lipids, polysaccharides, and nucleic acids that contain multiple repeated epitopes. The total strength of binding is much greater than the affinity of a single antigen-antibody bond and is called the **avidity** of the interaction. Antibodies produced against one antigen may bind other, structurally similar, antigens. Such binding to similar epitopes is called a **cross-reaction.**

In mature B lymphocytes, membrane-associated Ig molecules recognize antigens, but this recognition is not enough to activate the B cells. The Ig molecules are noncovalently attached to two other proteins, called Igα and Igβ, that make up the B cell receptor complex. When the Ig receptor recognizes antigen, the associated proteins transmit the signals to the interior of the B cell that initiate the process of B cell activation. These and other signals in humoral immune responses are discussed further in Chapter 7.

The realization that one clone of B cells makes an antibody of one specificity has been exploited to

Isotype of antibody	Subtypes	H chain	Serum concentr. (mg/mL)	Serum half-life (days)	Secreted form	Functions
IgA	IgA1,2	α(1 or 2)	3.5	6	Monomer, dimer, trimer **IgA (dimer)** 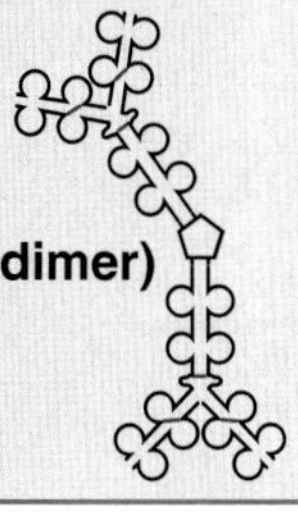	Mucosal immunity, neonatal passive immunity
IgD	None	δ	Trace	3	None	Naive B cell antigen receptor
IgE	None	ε	0.05	2	Monomer **IgE** 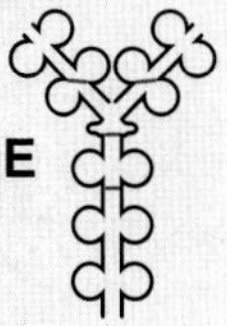	Mast cell activation (immediate hypersensitivity)
IgG	IgG1-4	γ (1,2,3 or 4)	13.5	23	Monomer **IgG1** 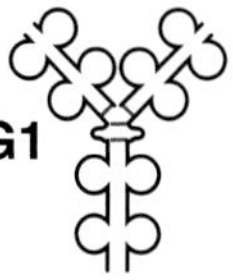	Opsonization, complement activation, antibody-dependent cell-mediated cytotoxicity, neonatal immunity, feedback inhibition of B cells
IgM	None	μ	1.5	5	Pentamer **IgM** 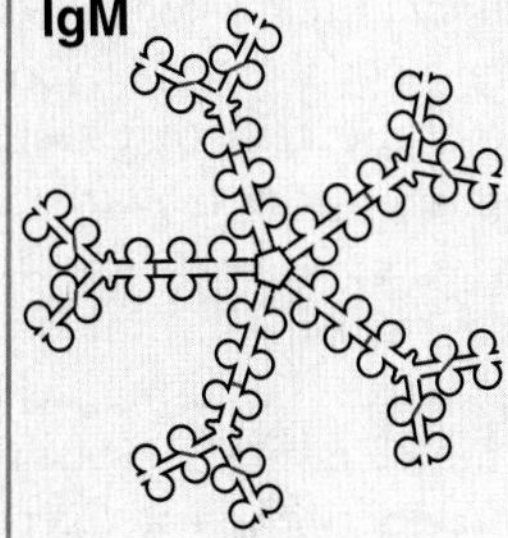	Naive B cell antigen receptor, complement activation

Figure 4–3 Features of the major isotypes (classes) of antibodies. The table summarizes some important features of the major antibody isotypes of humans. Isotypes are classified on the basis of their heavy chains; each isotype may contain either κ or λ light chain. The schematic diagrams illustrate the distinct shapes of the secreted forms of these antibodies. Note that IgA consists of two subclasses, called IgA1 and IgA2, and IgG consists of four subclasses, called IgG1, IgG2, IgG3, and IgG4. (IgG subclasses are given different names in other species, for historical reasons; in mice, they are called IgG1, IgG2a, IgG2b, and IgG3.) The serum concentrations are average values in normal individuals.

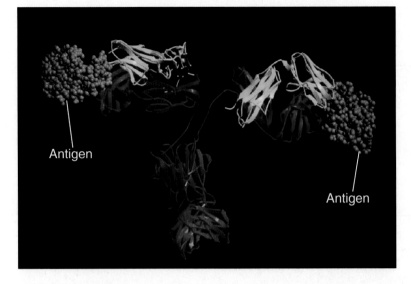

Antigen

Antigen

Figure 4–4 Binding of an antigen by an antibody. This model of a protein antigen bound to an antibody molecule shows how the antigen-binding site can accommodate soluble macromolecules in their native (folded) conformation. The heavy chains of the antibody are *red,* the light chains are *yellow,* and the antigen is colored *blue.* (Courtesy of Dr. Dan Vaughn, Cold Spring Harbor Laboratory, Cold Spring Harbor, NY.)

produce **monoclonal antibodies,** one of the most important technical advances in immunology, with far-reaching implications for clinical medicine and research. To produce monoclonal antibodies, B cells from an animal immunized with an antigen are fused with myeloma cells (tumors of plasma cells). The myeloma cell line is mutated to lack an enzyme, because of which it does not grow in the presence of a certain toxic drug, but fused cells do grow as the normal B cells provide the enzyme. Thus, by fusing the two cell populations and selecting them by culture with the drug, it is possible to grow out fused cells derived from the B cells and the myeloma, which are called **hybridomas.** From a population of hybridomas, one can select and clone the cells that secrete the antibody of desired specificity; such antibodies are monoclonal antibodies. It is possible to make mono-clonal antibodies against virtually any antigen. Most of these antibodies are made by fusing cells from immunized mice with mouse myelomas. Such mouse monoclonal antibodies cannot be injected repeatedly into humans, because humans see the mouse Ig as foreign and make an immune response to the injected antibodies. This problem has been overcome by retaining the antigen-binding V regions of the mouse monoclonal antibody and replacing the rest of the Ig with human Ig; such "humanized" antibodies are suit-able for administration to humans. More recently,

monoclonal antibodies have been synthesized by using recombinant DNA technology to clone the DNA complementary to messenger RNA encoding human antibodies and by selecting antibodies of desired specificity. Another recent approach is to express human antibody genes in mice whose own Ig genes have been deleted and then immunize these mice with an antigen. Monoclonal antibodies are now in widespread use as therapeutic and diagnostic reagents in many diseases.

T Cell Receptors for Antigens

The TCR for peptide antigen displayed by MHC molecules is a heterodimer composed of an α chain and a β chain, each chain containing one variable (V) region and one constant (C) region (Fig. 4-5). The V and C regions are homologous to immunoglob-ulin V and C regions. In the V region of each TCR chain there are three hypervariable, or complemen-tarity-determining, regions. As in antibodies, CDR3 is the most variable among different TCRs. Unlike anti-bodies, both TCR chains are anchored in the plasma membrane, and TCRs are not produced in a secreted form. Also, TCRs do not undergo class switching or affinity maturation during the life of a T cell clone.

Both the α chain and the β chain of the TCR participate in specific recognition of MHC molecules

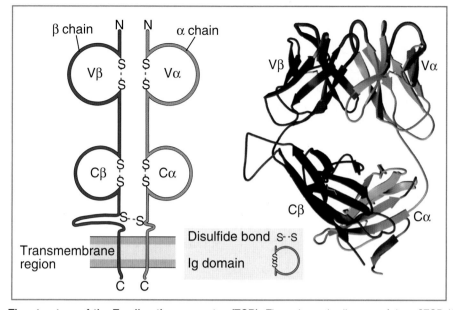

Figure 4–5   The structure of the T cell antigen receptor (TCR). The schematic diagram of the αβTCR (*left*) shows the domains of a typical TCR specific for a peptide-MHC complex. The antigen-binding portion of the TCR is formed by the Vα and Vβ domains. N and C refer to the amino-terminal and carboxy-terminal ends of the polypeptides. The ribbon diagram (*right*) shows the structure of the extracellular portion of a TCR as revealed by x-ray crystallography. (From Bjorkman PJ. MHC restriction in three dimensions: a view of T cell receptor/ligand interactions. Cell 89:167-170, 1997. © Cell Press; with permission.)

and bound peptides (Fig. 4-6). One of the remarkable features of T cell antigen recognition that has emerged from x-ray crystallographic analyses of TCRs bound to MHC-peptide complexes is that each TCR recognizes as few as one to three residues of the MHC-associated peptide. We also know that only a few peptides of even complex microbes, called the immunodominant epitopes, are actually recognized by the immune system. This means that T cells can tell the difference between complex microbes based on very few amino acid differences between the immunodominant epitopes of the microbes. It is surprising that the exquisite specificity of T cells is maintained on the basis of such small differences in antigenic peptides.

Five to 10 percent of T cells in the body express receptors composed of γ and δ chains, which are structurally similar to the αβ TCR but have very different specificities. The γδ TCR may recognize a variety of protein and nonprotein antigens, usually not displayed by classical MHC molecules. T cells expressing γδ TCRs are abundant in epithelia. This observation suggests that γδ T cells recognize microbes that are commonly encountered at epithelial surfaces, but neither the specificity nor the function of these T cells is well established. Another subpopulation of T cells, making up less than 5% of all T cells, express markers of natural killer (NK) cells and are called NK-T cells. NK-T cells express αβ TCRs, but they recognize glycolipid and other nonpeptide antigens displayed by nonpolymorphic MHC-like molecules. The functions of NK-T cells are also not well understood.

The TCR recognizes antigen, but it, like membrane Ig on B cells, is incapable of transmitting signals to the T cell. Associated with the TCR is a complex of proteins, called the CD3 molecules and the ζ chain, that make up the TCR complex (see Fig. 4-1). The CD3 and ζ chains transmit some of the signals that are initiated when the TCR recognizes antigen. In addition, T cell activation requires engagement of

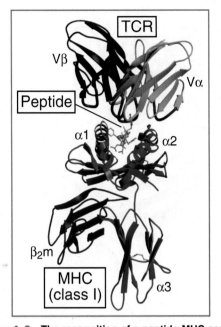

Figure 4–6   The recognition of a peptide-MHC complex by a T cell antigen receptor. This ribbon diagram is drawn from the crystal structure of the extracellular portion of a peptide-MHC complex bound to a TCR that is specific for the peptide displayed by the MHC molecule. The peptide can be seen attached to the cleft at the top of the MHC molecule, and one residue of the peptide contacts the V region of a TCR. The structure of MHC molecules and their function as peptide display proteins is described in Chapter 3. (From Bjorkman PJ. MHC restriction in three dimensions: a view of T cell receptor/ligand interactions. Cell 89:167-170, 1997. © Cell Press; with permission.)

the coreceptor molecules, CD4 or CD8, which recognize nonpolymorphic portions of MHC molecules. The functions of these TCR-associated proteins and coreceptors are discussed in Chapter 5.

The antigen receptors of B and T lymphocytes have many similarities, but they are also different in important ways (Fig. 4-7). Antibodies bind the greatest variety of antigens with the highest affinities, which is why antibodies can bind to and neutralize many different microbes and toxins that may be present at low concentrations in the circulation. The affinity of TCRs is low, which is why the binding of T cells to APCs has to be strengthened by so-called accessory molecules (see Chapter 5).

Development of Immune Repertoires

Now that we know what the antigen receptors of B and T lymphocytes are composed of and how these receptors recognize antigens, the next question that arises concerns how the enormous diversity of these receptors is produced. As the clonal selection theory predicted, there are many clones of lymphocytes with distinct specificities, perhaps as many as 10^9, and these clones arise before encounter with antigen. If every possible receptor were encoded by one gene, a large fraction of the genome would be devoted to coding for antigen receptors only. This is obviously unreasonable. In fact, the immune system has developed mechanisms for generating extremely diverse repertoires of B and T lymphocytes, and the generation of diverse receptors is intimately linked to the process of lymphocyte maturation. The remainder of this chapter discusses the way in which mature B and T lymphocytes with their highly variable receptors are generated.

Maturation of Lymphocytes

The maturation of lymphocytes from bone marrow stem cells consists of three types of processes: proliferation of immature cells, expression of antigen receptor genes, and selection of lymphocytes that express useful antigen receptors (Fig. 4-8). These events are common to B and T lymphocytes, even though B lymphocytes mature in the bone marrow and T lymphocytes mature in a specialized organ called the thymus. Each of the three processes that occur during lymphocyte maturation plays a special role in the generation of the lymphocyte repertoire.

Immature lymphocytes undergo tremendous proliferation at several stages during their maturation. The proliferation of developing lymphocytes maximizes the number of cells that are available to express useful antigen receptors and to mature into functionally competent lymphocytes. Proliferation of the earliest lymphocyte precursors is stimulated mainly by the growth factor, interleukin-7 (IL-7), which is produced by stromal cells in the bone marrow and the thymus. IL-7 stimulates proliferation of B and T lymphocyte progenitors before they express antigen

Feature	Antigen-binding molecule	
	Immunoglobulin (Ig)	T cell receptor (TCR)
	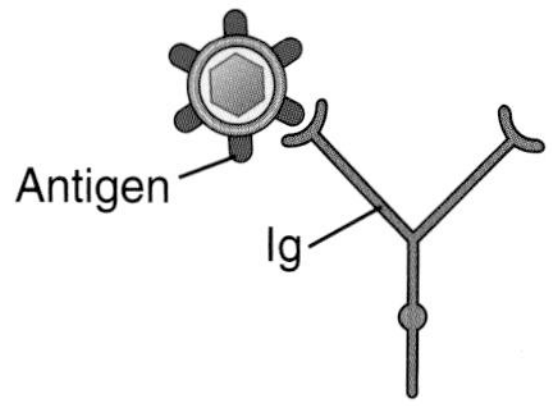	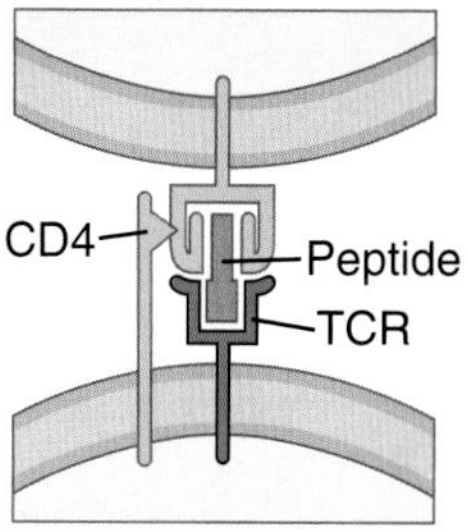
Antigen binding	Made up of three CDRs in V_H and three CDRs in V_L	Made up of three CDRs in $V\alpha$ and three CDRs in $V\beta$
Structure of antigens bound	Linear and conformational determinants of macro-molecules and small chemicals	Only 1-3 amino acid residues of a peptide and polymorphic residues of an MHC molecule
Affinity of antigen binding	K_d 10^{-7}-10^{-11} M; average affinity of Igs increases during immune response	K_d 10^{-5}-10^{-7} M
On-rate and off-rate	Rapid on-rate, variable off-rate	Slow on-rate, slow off-rate
Accessory molecules involved in binding	None	CD4 or CD8 simultaneously binds MHC molecule

Figure 4–7   Features of antigen recognition by antibodies and T cell antigen receptors (TCRs). A summary is presented of the important features of antigen recognition by Ig and TCR molecules, the antigen receptors of B and T lymphocytes, respectively.

receptors, thus generating a large pool of cells in which diverse antigen receptors may be produced. After antigen receptor proteins are expressed, these receptors take over the function of delivering the signals for proliferation, ensuring that only the clones with intact receptors are selected to expand.

Antigen receptors are produced from several gene segments that are separate from one another in the germline and recombine during lymphocyte maturation. Diversity is generated during this recombination process mainly by varying the nucleotide sequences at the site of recombination. The expression of diverse antigen receptors is the central event in lymphocyte maturation and is described in the next section.

Maturing lymphocytes are selected at several steps during their maturation to preserve the useful specificities. Selection is based on the expression of intact antigen receptor components and what they recognize. Prelymphocytes that fail to express antigen receptors die by apoptosis (see Fig. 4-8). Immature T cells are selected to recognize self MHC molecules;

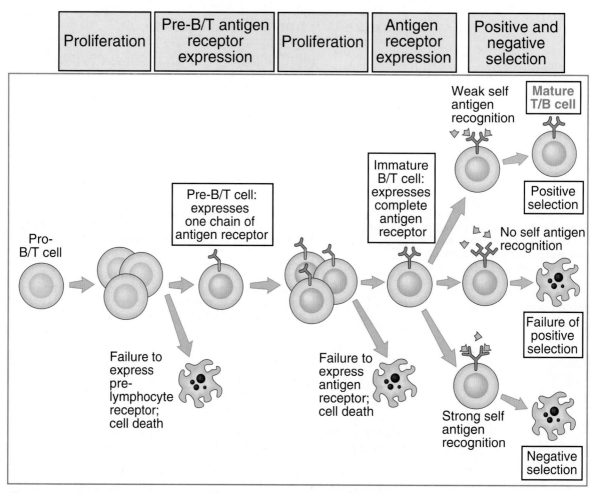

Figure 4–8   Steps in the maturation of lymphocytes. During their maturation, B and T lymphocytes go through cycles of proliferation and expression of receptor chains by gene recombination. Cells that fail to express useful receptors die by apoptosis, because they do not receive necessary survival signals. At the end of the process, the cells undergo positive and negative selection. The lymphocytes shown may be B or T cells.

this process is called **positive selection.** After they mature, these T cells need to recognize the same MHC molecules to be activated. The basis for positive selection is that antigen receptors on developing lymphocytes recognize MHC molecules in the thymus and deliver signals for the survival and proliferation of the cells, ensuring that cells with the correct (self MHC-restricted) antigen receptors complete the maturation process. Immature B and T lymphocytes are also selected against high-affinity recognition of self antigens present in the bone marrow and thymus,

respectively. This process, called **negative selection,** eliminates potentially dangerous lymphocytes that may be capable of reacting against self antigens that are present throughout the body, including in the generative lymphoid organs.

The processes of lymphocyte maturation and selection are best understood separately for B and T cells. We start, however, with the central event that is common to both lineages, namely, the recombination and expression of antigen receptor genes.

Production of Diverse Antigen Receptors

The expression of B and T lymphocyte antigen receptors is initiated by somatic recombination of gene segments that code for the variable regions of the receptors, and diversity is generated during this process. Hematopoietic stem cells in the bone marrow, and early lymphoid progenitors, contain Ig and TCR genes in their inherited, or germline, configuration. In this configuration, Ig heavy chain and light chain loci and the TCR α chain and β chain loci each contain multiple variable region (V) genes, numbering up to a few hundred, and one or a few constant region (C) genes (Fig. 4-9). Between the V and C genes are several small stretches of nucleotides, which are called joining (J) and diversity (D) gene segments. (All antigen receptor gene loci contain V, J, and C genes, but only the Ig heavy chain and TCR β loci also contain D gene segments.) The commitment of a lymphocyte progenitor to become a B lymphocyte is associated with recombination of one Ig V_H gene segment with one D and one J segment, the segments being selected randomly (Fig. 4-10). Thus, the committed but immature B cell now has a recombined V-D-J gene in the heavy chain locus. This gene is transcribed; and in the primary RNA, the V-D-J complex is spliced onto the first C region RNA, which happens to encode the μ chain, to form the complete μ mRNA. This μ mRNA is translated to produce the μ heavy chain, which is the first Ig protein synthesized during B cell maturation. A similar sequence of DNA recombination and RNA splicing leads to production of a light chain in B cells and of the TCR α and β chains in T lymphocytes.

The somatic recombination of V and J, or V, D, and J, gene segments is mediated by a collection of enzymes called the **V(D)J recombinase.** The lymphoid-specific component of the V(D)J recombinase, which is composed of the recombinase-activating gene (RAG)-1 and RAG-2 proteins, recognizes DNA sequences that flank all antigen receptor V, D, and J gene segments. As a result of this recognition, the recombinase brings the V, D, and J segments close together. Exonucleases then cut the DNA at the ends of the segments, and the DNA breaks are repaired by

ligases, producing a full-length recombined V-J or V-D-J gene (see Fig. 4-10). The lymphoid-specific component of the V(D)J recombinase is expressed only in immature B and T lymphocytes. Although the same enzymes can mediate recombination of all Ig and TCR genes, intact Ig H and L chain genes are expressed only in B cells, and TCR α and β genes are expressed only in T cells. The mechanisms responsible for this lineage specificity of receptor expression are not known.

Diversity of antigen receptors is produced by the use of different combinations of V, D, and J gene segments in different clones of lymphocytes (called combinatorial diversity) and even more by changes in nucleotide sequences introduced at the junctions of V, (D), and J gene segments (called junctional diversity) (Fig. 4-11). Combinatorial diversity is limited by the number of available V, D, and J gene segments, but junctional diversity is almost unlimited. This junctional diversity is produced by two types of sequence changes, both of which generate more sequences than are present in the germline genes. First, exonucleases may remove nucleotides from V, D, and J gene segments at the time of recombination, and if the resulting recombined sequences do not contain stop or nonsense codons, many different and new sequences may be produced. Second, an enzyme called terminal deoxyribonucleotidyl transferase (TdT) takes nucleotides that are not parts of germline genes and adds these nucleotides randomly to the sites of V(D)J recombination forming the so-called N regions. In addition, during an intermediate stage of the process of V(D)J recombination, overhanging DNA sequences may be generated that are then filled in by "P-nucleotides," introducing even more variability at the sites of recombination. As a result of junctional diversity, every antibody and TCR differs from every other antibody and TCR in the nucleotide sequence at the site of V(D)J recombination. This junction encodes the amino acids of CDR3, which was mentioned as the most variable of the CDRs and the one most important for antigen recognition. Thus, junctional diversity maximizes the variability in the antigen-binding regions of antibodies and TCRs. In the process of creating junctional diversity, many genes may be produced that cannot code for proteins and are, therefore, useless. This is a price the immune

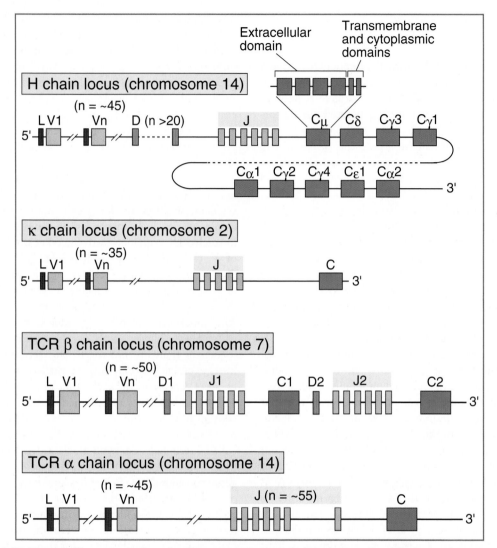

Figure 4–9   The germline organization of antigen receptor gene loci. In the germline, inherited antigen receptor gene loci contain coding segments (exons, shown as *blocks of varying sizes*) that are separated by segments that are not expressed (introns, shown as *lines*). Each Ig heavy chain constant (C) region and TCR C region consists of multiple exons that encode the domains of the C regions; the organization of the Cμ exon in the Ig heavy chain locus is shown as an example. The diagrams illustrate the antigen receptor gene loci in humans; the basic organization is the same in all species, although the precise order and number of gene segments may vary. The sizes of the segments and the distances between them are not drawn to scale. L, leader sequence (a small stretch of nucleotides that guides proteins through the endoplasmic reticulum and is cleaved from the mature proteins); C, constant segments; D, diversity; J, joining; V, variable.

system pays for generating tremendous diversity. The risk of producing nonfunctional genes is also the reason why the process of lymphocyte maturation contains several checkpoints at which cells with useful receptors are selected to survive.

Maturation and Selection of B Lymphocytes

The maturation of B lymphocytes occurs mainly in the bone marrow (Fig. 4-12). Progenitors committed

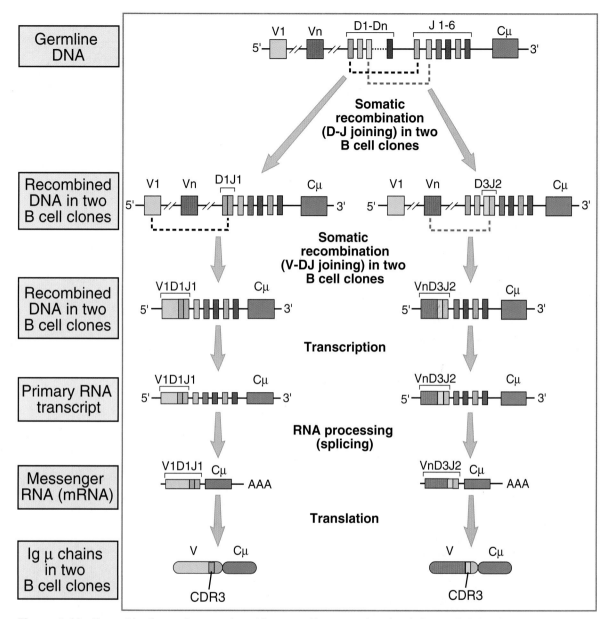

Figure 4–10 Recombination and expression of Ig genes. The expression of an Ig heavy chain involves two gene recombination events (D-J joining, followed by joining of a V region to the DJ complex, with deletion and loss of intervening gene segments). The recombined gene is transcribed, and the VDJ segment is spliced onto the first heavy chain RNA (which is μ), to give rise to the μ mRNA. The mRNA is translated to produce the μ heavy chain protein. The recombination of other antigen receptor genes, that is, the Ig light chain and the TCR α and β chains, follows essentially the same sequence, except that in loci lacking D segments (Ig light chains and TCR α) a V gene recombines directly with a J gene segment.

	Immunoglobulin		T cell receptor	
	Heavy chain	κ	α	β
Number of V gene segments	45	35	45	50
Number of diversity (D) gene segments	23	0	0	2
Number of joining (J) gene segments	6	5	~50	12

Mechanism

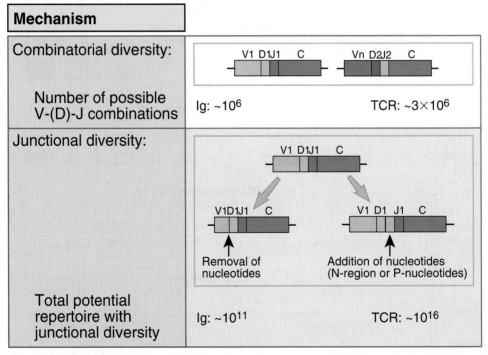

Combinatorial diversity:	
Number of possible V-(D)-J combinations	Ig: ~10^6 TCR: ~3×10^6
Junctional diversity:	
Total potential repertoire with junctional diversity	Ig: ~10^{11} TCR: ~10^{16}

Figure 4–11   Mechanisms of diversity in antigen receptors. Diversity in immunoglobulins (Ig) and T cell receptors (TCRs) is produced by random combinations of V, D, and J gene segments, which is limited by the numbers of these segments, and by removal and addition of nucleotides at the V-J or V-D-J junctions, which is almost unlimited. Both mechanisms maximize diversity in the CDR3 regions of the antigen receptor proteins. The estimated contributions of these mechanisms to the potential size of the mature B and T cell repertoires are shown. Also, diversity is increased by the ability of different Ig heavy and light chains, or different TCR α and β chains, to associate in different cells, forming different receptors (not shown). Although the upper limit on the number of Ig and TCR proteins that may be expressed is very large, it is estimated that each individual contains on the order of only 10^7 clones of B cells and T cells with distinct specificities and receptors; in other words, only a fraction of the potential repertoire may actually be expressed. (Adapted from Davis MM, and PJ Bjorkman. T-cell antigen receptor genes and T-cell recognition. Nature 334:395-402, 1988. © 1988, Macmillan Magazines Ltd; with permission.)

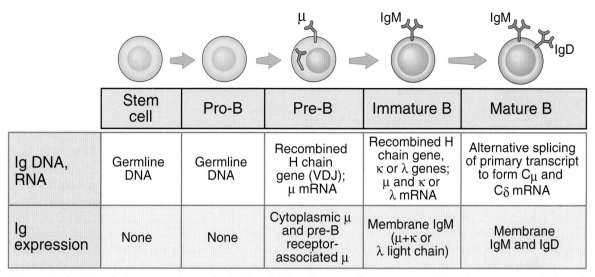

	Stem cell	Pro-B	Pre-B	Immature B	Mature B
Ig DNA, RNA	Germline DNA	Germline DNA	Recombined H chain gene (VDJ); μ mRNA	Recombined H chain gene, κ or λ genes; μ and κ or λ mRNA	Alternative splicing of primary transcript to form C_μ and C_δ mRNA
Ig expression	None	None	Cytoplasmic μ and pre-B receptor-associated μ	Membrane IgM (μ+κ or λ light chain)	Membrane IgM and IgD

Figure 4–12   Steps in the maturation and selection of B lymphocytes. The maturation of B lymphocytes proceeds through sequential steps, each of which is characterized by particular changes in Ig gene expression and in the patterns of Ig protein expression. At the pro-B cell and pre-B cell stages, failure to express functional antigen receptors (Ig heavy chain and Ig light chain, respectively) results in death of the cells by a default pathway of apoptosis.

to the B cell lineage proliferate under the influence of IL-7, giving rise to a large number of precursors of B cells, called *pro-B cells*. In the next stage of maturation, called *pre-B cells*, Ig genes in the heavy chain locus of one chromosome recombine and give rise to the μ heavy chain protein. Most of this protein remains in the cytoplasm, and cytoplasmic μ is the hallmark of pre-B cells. Some of the μ protein is expressed on the cell surface in association with two other, invariant, proteins that resemble light chains, to form the pre-B cell receptor (pre-BCR) complex. It is not clear what, if anything, the pre-BCR recognizes, and simply the assembly of the components of this complex may deliver signals that promote the survival and proliferation of the cells on which the pre-B cell receptor is expressed. This is the first checkpoint in B cell development, and it selects and expands all the pre-B cells that express a functional μ heavy chain. If the μ chain protein is not produced, perhaps because of faulty recombination of the μ gene, the cell cannot be selected, and it dies by programmed cell death (apoptosis).

The μ protein and the pre-BCR complex signal two other processes. One process shuts off recombi-

nation of Ig heavy chain genes on the second chromosome, because of which each B cell can express Ig from only one of the two inherited parental alleles. This process is called allelic exclusion, and it ensures that each cell can express receptors of a single specificity. A second signal triggers recombination at the Ig light chain locus, first κ and then λ. Whichever functional light chain is produced associates with the μ chain to form the complete membrane-associated IgM antigen receptor. This receptor again delivers signals that promote survival and proliferation, thus preserving and expanding cells that express complete antigen receptors (the second checkpoint during maturation). Signals from the antigen receptor shut off production of the recombinase enzyme and further recombination at unrecombined light chain loci. As a result, each B cell produces either one κ or λ light chain from one of the inherited parental alleles. The presence of two sets of light chain genes simply increases the chance of completing successful gene recombination and receptor expression. The IgM-expressing B lymphocyte is the *immature B cell*. Its further maturation may occur in the bone marrow or after it leaves the bone marrow and enters peripheral lymphoid tissues. The final maturation step involves coexpression of IgD with IgM, which occurs because the recombined V(D)J heavy chain RNA may be spliced onto the Cμ RNA or the Cδ RNA, giving rise to a μ or δ mRNA, respectively. We know that the ability of B cells to respond to antigens develops together with the coexpression of IgM and IgD, but why both classes of receptor are needed is not known. The IgM+ IgD+ cell is the *mature B cell*, able to respond to antigen in peripheral lymphoid tissues.

The B cell repertoire is further shaped by negative selection. In this process, if an immature B cell binds an antigen in the bone marrow with high affinity, further maturation is stopped. The B cell either dies by apoptosis, or it may reactivate the recombinase enzyme, generate a second light chain, and change the specificity of the antigen receptor (a process called receptor editing). The antigens most commonly found in the bone marrow are self antigens that are abundantly expressed throughout the body (i.e., are ubiquitous), such as blood proteins, and membrane molecules common to all cells. Therefore, negative selection eliminates potentially dangerous cells that can recognize and react against ubiquitous self antigens.

The process of Ig gene recombination is random and cannot be inherently biased toward recognition of microbes, yet the receptors that are produced are able to recognize the antigens of the large number and variety of microbes that the immune system must defend against. It is likely that the repertoire of B lymphocytes is generated randomly, selected positively for expression of intact receptors, and selected negatively against strong recognition of self antigens. What is left after these selection processes is the collection of mature B cells able to recognize all the microbial antigens one may encounter.

Maturation and Selection of T Lymphocytes

The process of T lymphocyte maturation has some unique features, which are largely related to the specificity of different subsets of T cells for peptides displayed by different classes of MHC molecules. T cell progenitors migrate from the bone marrow to the thymus, where the entire process of maturation occurs (Fig. 4-13). The most immature progenitors are called *pro-T cells* or *double-negative T cells* because they do not express CD4 or CD8. These cells expand in number mainly under the influence of IL-7 produced in the thymus. Some of the progeny of double-negative cells undergo TCR β gene recombination, mediated by the V(D)J recombinase. (The γδ T cells undergo similar recombination involving the TCR γ and δ loci, but they appear to be a distinct lineage, and they will not be discussed further.) If the β chain protein is synthesized, it is expressed on the surface in association with an invariant protein called pre-Tα, to form the pre-TCR complex of *pre-T cells*. If the complete β chain is not produced in a pro-T cell, that cell dies. The pre-TCR complex delivers intracellular signals in response to assembly alone or the recognition of some unknown ligand. These signals promote survival, proliferation, allelic exclusion at the TCR β chain locus, and TCR α chain gene recombination, much like the signals from the pre-BCR complex in developing B cells. Failure to express the α chain and the complete TCR again results in death of the cell. The surviving cells express both the CD4 and CD8 coreceptors, and these cells are called *double-positive T cells* (or double-positive thymocytes). Different clones of double-positive T cells express different αβ TCRs. If the TCR of a T cell recognizes an MHC molecule in the thymus, which has to be a self MHC molecule displaying a self peptide, that T cell is selected to survive. T cells that do not recognize an MHC molecule in the thymus die by apoptosis; these T cells would not be useful because they would be incapable of seeing MHC-displayed cell-associated antigens in that individual. This preservation of self MHC-restricted (i.e., useful) T cells is the process of positive selection. During this process, T cells whose TCRs recognize class I MHC–peptide complexes preserve the expression of CD8, the coreceptor that binds to class I MHC, and lose expression of CD4, the coreceptor specific for class II MHC molecules. Conversely, if a T cell recognizes class II MHC–peptide complexes, that cell maintains expression of CD4 and loses expression of CD8. Thus, what emerges are *single-positive T cells*, which are either CD8+ class I MHC restricted or CD4+ class II MHC restricted. During this process, the T cells also become functionally segregated: the CD8+ T cells are capable

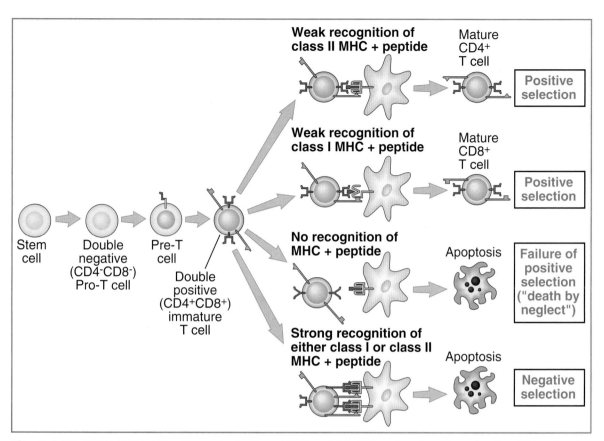

Figure 4–13   Steps in the maturation and selection of MHC-restricted T lymphocytes. The maturation of T lymphocytes in the thymus proceeds through sequential steps that are often defined by the expression of the CD4 and CD8 coreceptors. The TCR β chain is first expressed at the double-negative pre-T cell stage, and the complete TCR is expressed in double-positive cells. Maturation culminates in the development of CD4+ and CD8+ single-positive T cells. As in B cells, failure to express antigen receptors at any stage leads to death of the cells by apoptosis.

of becoming CTLs on activation, and the CD4+ cells are helper cells. How the functional segregation accompanies coreceptor expression is not known.

Immature, double-positive T cells whose receptors strongly recognize MHC-peptide complexes in the thymus undergo apoptosis. This is the process of **negative selection,** and it serves to eliminate T lymphocytes that could react in a harmful way against self proteins that are present in the thymus, and presumably throughout the body. It may seem surprising that both positive selection and negative selection are mediated by recognition of the same set of self MHC–self peptide complexes in the thymus. (Note that the thymus can only contain self MHC molecules

and self peptides; microbial peptides are concentrated in peripheral lymphoid tissues and tend not to enter the thymus.) The likely explanation for these distinct outcomes is that if the antigen receptor of a T cell recognizes a self MHC–self peptide complex with low avidity, the result is positive selection, but high-avidity recognition leads to negative selection. High-avidity recognition happens if the self peptide is abundant in the thymus (and therefore everywhere in the body) and if the T cell expresses a TCR that has a high affinity for that self peptide. These are the situations in which antigen recognition could lead to harmful immune responses against the self antigen, and so the T cell has to be eliminated. Low-avidity recognition of self is unlikely to be harmful. As in the case of B cells, the ability to recognize foreign antigens seems to rely on chance: T cells that weakly recognize self antigens in the thymus may strongly recognize and respond to foreign microbial antigens in the periphery.

SUMMARY

▶ In the adaptive immune system, the molecules responsible for specific recognition of antigens are antibodies and T cell antigen receptors.

▶ Antibodies (also called immunoglobulins, or Ig) may be produced as membrane receptors of B lymphocytes and as proteins secreted by antigen-stimulated B cells that have differentiated into antibody-secreting cells. Secreted antibodies are the effector molecules of humoral immunity, capable of neutralizing microbes and microbial toxins and eliminating them by activating various effector mechanisms.

▶ T cell antigen receptors (TCRs) are membrane receptors and are not secreted.

▶ The core structure of antibodies consists of two heavy chains and two light chains forming a disulfide-linked complex. Each chain consists of a variable (V) region, which is the portion that recognizes antigen, and a constant (C) region, which provides structural stability and, in heavy chains, performs the effector functions of antibodies.

▶ T cell receptors consist of an α chain and a β chain. Each chain contains one V region and one C region, and both chains participate in the recognition of antigens, which for most T cells are peptides displayed by MHC molecules.

▶ The V regions of Ig and TCR molecules contain hypervariable segments, also called complementarity-determining regions, which are the regions of contact with antigens.

▶ The genes that encode antigen receptors consist of multiple segments that are separate in the germline and are brought together during the maturation of lymphocytes. In B cells, the Ig gene segments undergo recombination as the cells mature in the bone marrow, and in T cells the TCR gene segments undergo recombination during maturation in the thymus.

▶ Receptors of different specificities are generated in part by different combinations of V, D, and J gene segments. The process of recombination introduces variability in the nucleotide sequences at the sites of recombination by adding or removing nucleotides from the junctions. The result of this introduced variability is the development of a diverse repertoire of lymphocytes, in which clones of cells with different antigen specificities express receptors that differ in sequence and recognition, and most of the differences are concentrated at the regions of gene recombination.

▶ During their maturation, lymphocytes undergo alternating cycles of proliferation and antigen receptor expression and traverse several checkpoints at which they are selected such that only cells with complete functional antigen receptors are preserved and expanded. In addition, T lymphocytes are positively selected to recognize peptide antigens displayed by self MHC molecules.

▶ Immature lymphocytes that strongly recognize self antigens are negatively selected and prevented from completing their maturation, thus eliminating cells with the potential of reacting in harmful ways against self tissues.

⇄ Review Questions

1 What are the functionally distinct domains (regions) of antibody and T cell receptor molecules? What features of the amino acid sequences in these regions are important for their functions?

2 What are the differences in the types of antigens recognized by antibodies and T cell receptors?

3 What mechanisms contribute to the diversity of antibody and TCR molecules? Which of these mechanisms contributes the most to the diversity?

4 What are some of the checkpoints during lymphocyte maturation that ensure survival of the useful cells?

5 What is the phenomenon of negative selection, and what is its importance?

Cell-Mediated Immune Responses

Activation of T Lymphocytes by Cell-Associated Microbes

5

Cell-mediated immunity is the arm of the adaptive immune response whose role is to combat infections by intracellular microbes. This type of immunity is mediated by T lymphocytes. Two types of infections may lead to microbes finding a haven inside cells, from where they have to be eliminated by cell-mediated immune responses (Fig. 5-1). First, microbes are ingested by phagocytes as part of the early defense mechanisms of innate immunity, but some of these microbes have evolved to resist the microbicidal activities of phagocytes. Many pathogenic intracellular bacteria and protozoa are able to survive, and even replicate, in the vesicles of phagocytes. Some of these phagocytosed microbes may enter the cytoplasm of infected cells and multiply in this compartment, using the nutrients of the infected cells. Cytoplasmic microbes are protected from microbicidal mechanisms, because these mechanisms are confined to vesicular compartments (where they cannot damage the host cells). Second, viruses may bind to receptors on a wide variety of cells and are able to infect and replicate in the cytoplasm of these cells. These cells often do not possess intrinsic mechanisms for destroying the viruses. Some viruses cause latent infections, in which the viral DNA is integrated in the host genome and viral proteins, but not infectious viral particles, are produced in the infected cells. The elimination of microbes that are able to live in phagocytic vesicles or in the cytoplasm of infected cells is the main function of T lymphocytes in

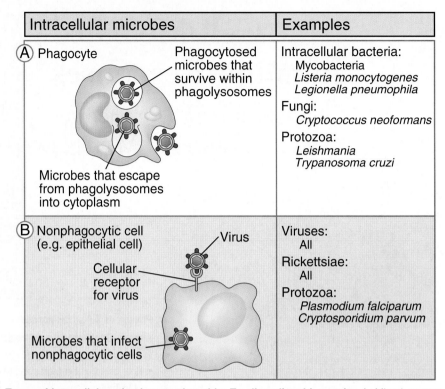

Intracellular microbes	Examples

(A) Phagocyte — Phagocytosed microbes that survive within phagolysosomes — Microbes that escape from phagolysosomes into cytoplasm	Intracellular bacteria:
	    Mycobacteria
	    Listeria monocytogenes
	    Legionella pneumophila
	Fungi:
	    Cryptococcus neoformans
	Protozoa:
	    Leishmania
	    Trypanosoma cruzi

(B) Nonphagocytic cell (e.g. epithelial cell) — Virus — Cellular receptor for virus — Microbes that infect nonphagocytic cells	Viruses:
	    All
	Rickettsiae:
	    All
	Protozoa:
	    Plasmodium falciparum
	    Cryptosporidium parvum

Figure 5–1   Types of intracellular microbes combated by T cell-mediated immunity. A. Microbes may be ingested by phagocytes and survive within vesicles (phagolysosomes) or escape into the cytoplasm where they are not susceptible to the microbicidal mechanisms of the phagocytes. B. Viruses may bind to receptors on many cell types, including nonphagocytic cells, and replicate in the cytoplasm of the infected cells. Some viruses establish latent infections, in which viral proteins are produced in infected cells (not shown).

adaptive immunity. CD4$^+$ helper T lymphocytes also help B cells to produce antibodies. A common feature of all these reactions is that to perform their functions T lymphocytes have to interact with other cells, which may be phagocytes, infected host cells, or B lymphocytes. Recall that the specificity of T cells for peptides displayed by major histocompatibility complex (MHC) molecules ensures that the T cells can only see and respond to antigens associated with other cells (see Chapters 3 and 4). This chapter discusses the way in which T lymphocytes are activated by recognition of cell-associated antigens and other stimuli. The following questions are addressed:

- What signals are needed to activate T lymphocytes, and what cellular receptors are used to sense and respond to these signals?

- How are the few naive T cells specific for any microbe converted into the large number of effector T cells endowed with the ability to eliminate the microbe?

- What molecules are produced by T lymphocytes that mediate their communications with other cells, such as macrophages and B lymphocytes?

After the description of how T cells recognize and respond to the antigens of cell-associated microbes, in Chapter 6 a discussion is presented of how these T cells function to eliminate the microbes.

Phases of T Cell Responses

The responses of T lymphocytes to cell-associated microbial antigens consist of a series of sequential

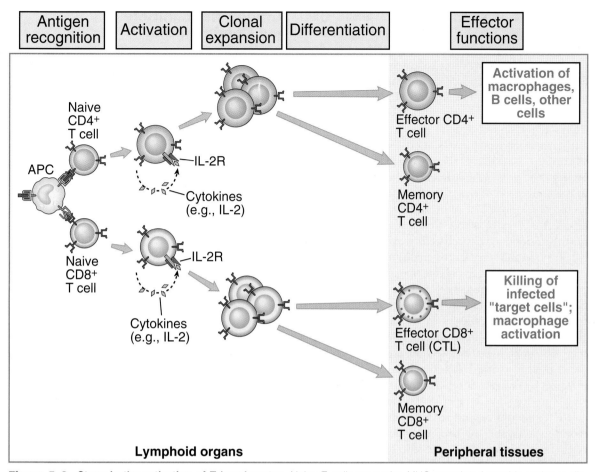

Figure 5–2 Steps in the activation of T lymphocytes. Naive T cells recognize MHC-associated peptide antigens displayed on APCs and other signals (not shown). The T cells respond by producing cytokines, such as IL-2, and expressing receptors for these cytokines, leading to an autocrine pathway of cell proliferation. The result is clonal expansion of the T cells. Some of the progeny differentiate into effector cells, which serve various functions in cell-mediated immunity, and memory cells, which survive for long periods. (The effector functions of T lymphocytes are described in Chapter 6.)

steps that result in an increase in the number of antigen-specific T cells and the conversion of naive T cells to effector cells (Fig. 5-2). As we have discussed in previous chapters, naive T lymphocytes constantly recirculate through peripheral lymphoid organs searching for foreign protein antigens. Naive T cells express antigen receptors and other molecules that make up the machinery of antigen recognition, but naive lymphocytes are incapable of performing the effector functions required for eliminating microbes. To perform these functions, the naive T cells have to be stimulated to differentiate into effector cells, and this process is initiated by antigen recognition. The protein antigens of microbes are transported from the portals of entry of the microbes to the same peripheral lymphoid organs where naive T cells reside. In these organs, the antigens are processed and displayed by MHC molecules on professional antigen-presenting cells (APCs) (see Chapter 3). Thus, naive T lymphocytes first encounter protein antigens in the peripheral lymphoid organs. At the same time as the T cells are seeing antigen, they receive additional signals from microbes or from innate immune reactions to the microbes.

In response to this combination of stimuli, the antigen-specific T cells begin to secrete proteins called **cytokines,** whose multiple functions in cell-mediated immunity are described later in this chapter. Some cytokines function together with antigen and microbe-derived second signals to stimulate the proliferation of the antigen-specific T cells. The result of this proliferation is a rapid increase in the number of antigen-specific lymphocytes, a process called **clonal expansion.** A fraction of these activated lymphocytes undergo the process of **differentiation,** which results in the conversion of naive T cells, whose function is to recognize microbial antigens, into a population of effector T cells, whose function is to eliminate microbes. Some effector T cells may remain in the lymph node and function to eradicate infected cells in the lymph node or to provide signals to B cells that promote antibody responses against the microbes. Some effector T cells leave the lymphoid organs where they differentiated from naive T cells, enter the circulation, and migrate to any site of infection, where they can eradicate the infection (see Chapter 6). Other progeny of the T cells that have proliferated in response to antigen develop into **memory T cells,** which are long lived, functionally inactive, and circulate for months or years ready to rapidly respond to repeat exposures to the same microbe. As effector T cells eliminate the infectious agent, the stimuli that triggered T cell expansion and differentiation are also eliminated. As a result, the greatly expanded clone of antigen-specific lymphocytes dies, thus returning the system to its basal resting state. This sequence of events is common to CD4+ T lymphocytes and CD8+ T lymphocytes, although, as will be seen later, there are important differences in the properties and effector functions of CD4+ and CD8+ cells.

With this background we proceed to a description of the individual steps in T cell responses. The process of activation of T lymphocytes also involves biochemical signals that are generated by antigen recognition and are translated into the biologic responses of the lymphocytes. This chapter ends with a brief discussion of the biochemistry of T lymphocyte activation.

Antigen Recognition and Costimulation

The initiation of T cell responses requires multiple receptors on the T cells recognizing ligands on APCs: the TCR recognizes MHC-associated peptide antigens, CD4 or CD8 coreceptors recognize the MHC molecules, adhesion molecules strengthen the binding of T cells to APCs, and receptors for costimulators recognize second signals provided by the APCs (Fig. 5-3). The molecules other than antigen receptors that are involved in T cell responses to antigens are often called **accessory molecules** of T lymphocytes. Accessory molecules are invariant among all T cells. Their functions fall into three categories: recognition, signaling, and adhesion. Different accessory molecules bind to different ligands, and each of these interactions plays a distinct and complementary role in the process of T cell activation.

Recognition of MHC-Associated Peptides

The T cell receptor for antigen (the TCR) and the CD4 or CD8 coreceptor together recognize the complex of peptide antigens and MHC molecules on

Figure 5-3 Ligand-receptor pairs involved in T cell activation. A. The major surface molecules of CD4+ T cells involved in the activation of these cells (the receptors), and the molecules on APCs (the ligands) recognized by the receptors are shown. CD8+ T cells use most of the same molecules, except that the TCR recognizes peptide-class I MHC complexes, and the coreceptor is CD8, which recognizes class I. Immunoreceptor tyrosine-based activation motifs (ITAMs) are the regions of signaling proteins that are phosphorylated on tyrosine residues and become docking sites for other signaling molecules (see Fig. 5-14). CD3 is composed of three polypeptide chains. B. The important properties are summarized of the major "accessory" molecules of T cells, so called because they participate in responses to antigens but are not the receptors for antigen. CTLA-4 (CD152) is a T cell receptor for B7 molecules that delivers inhibitory signals; its role in shutting off T cell responses is described in Chapter 9. VLA molecules are integrins involved in leukocyte binding to endothelium (see Fig. 6-2, Chapter 6).

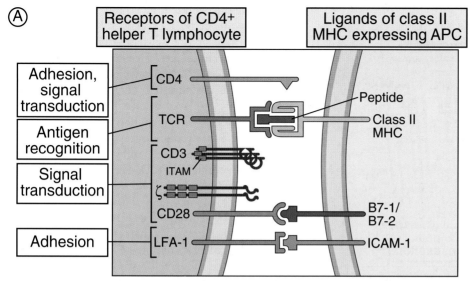

T cell accessory molecule	Function	Ligand	
		Name	Expressed on
CD3	Signal transduction by TCR complex	None	
ζ	Signal transduction by TCR complex	None	
CD4	Adhesion and signal transduction	Class II MHC	Antigen-presenting cells
CD8	Adhesion and signal transduction	Class I MHC	Antigen-presenting cells, CTL target cells
CD28	Signal transduction (costimulation)	B7-1/B7-2	Antigen-presenting cells
CTLA-4	Signal transduction (negative regulation)	B7-1/B7-2	Antigen-presenting cells
LFA-1	Adhesion	ICAM-1	Antigen-presenting cells, endothelium
VLA-4	Adhesion	VCAM-1	Endothelium

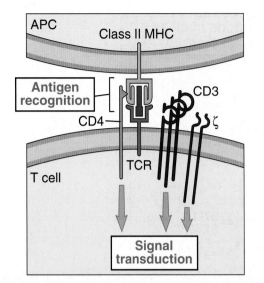

Figure 5–4   Antigen recognition and signal transduction during T cell activation. Different T cell molecules recognize antigen and deliver the signal to the interior of the cell as a result of antigen recognition. Note that two or more TCRs need to be cross-linked to initiate signals, but only a single TCR is shown for simplicity. The CD3 and ζ proteins are noncovalently attached to the TCR α and β chains by interactions between charged amino acids in the transmembrane domains of these proteins (not shown). The figure illustrates a CD4+ T cell; the same interactions are involved in the activation of CD8+ T cells, except that the coreceptor is CD8 and the TCR recognizes a peptide-class I MHC complex.

APCs, and this recognition provides the first, or initiating, signal for T cell activation (Fig. 5-4). As we discussed in Chapter 3, when protein antigens are ingested by APCs from the extracellular milieu into vesicles, these antigens are processed into peptides that are displayed by class II MHC molecules. In contrast, protein antigens that are present in the cytoplasm are processed into peptides that are displayed by class I molecules. The TCR consists of an α chain and a β chain, both of which participate in antigen recognition (see Chapter 4). The TCR of a peptide antigen-specific T cell recognizes the displayed peptide and simultaneously recognizes residues of the MHC molecule that are located around the peptide-binding cleft. Every mature MHC-restricted T cell expresses either CD4 or CD8, which are called coreceptors because they function with the TCR to bind MHC molecules. At the same time as the TCR is recognizing the peptide-MHC complex, CD4 or CD8 recognizes the class II or class I MHC molecule, respectively, at a site separate from the peptide-binding cleft. Thus, CD4+ T cells, which function as cytokine-producing helper cells, recognize microbial antigens that are ingested from the extracellular milieu and are displayed by class II MHC molecules, and CD8+ T cells, which function as cytolytic T lymphocytes (CTLs), recognize peptides derived from cytoplasmic microbes displayed by class I molecules. The specificity of CD4 and CD8 for different classes of MHC molecules and the distinct pathways of processing of vesicular and cytosolic antigens ensure that the "correct" T cells respond to different microbes (see Fig. 3-15, Chapter 3). Two or more TCRs and coreceptors need to be engaged simultaneously to initiate the T cell response, because only if multiple TCRs and coreceptors are brought together can appropriate biochemical signaling cascades be activated (discussed later in the chapter). Therefore, any one T cell can respond only if it encounters an array of peptide-MHC complexes on an APC. Also, each T cell needs to engage antigen (i.e., MHC-associated peptides) for a long period, at least for several minutes, or multiple times to generate enough biochemical signals to initiate a response. Once these conditions are achieved, the T cell begins its activation program.

The biochemical signals that lead to T cell activation are triggered by a set of proteins that are linked to the TCR to form the TCR complex and by the CD4 or CD8 coreceptor (see Fig. 5-4). Different T cells must possess antigen receptors that are variable enough to recognize diverse antigens and other molecules that serve the conserved signaling roles and do not need to be variable. In lymphocytes, these two types of functions, antigen recognition and signaling, are segregated into different sets of molecules. The TCR recognizes antigens, but it is not able to transmit biochemical signals to the interior of the cell. The TCR is noncovalently associated with a complex of three proteins that make up CD3 and with a homodimer of another signaling protein called the ζ chain. The TCR, CD3, and ζ chain make up the TCR complex. In the TCR complex, the function of antigen recognition is performed by the variable TCR α and β chains whereas the conserved signaling function is performed by the attached CD3 and ζ proteins. The mechanisms of signal transduction by these proteins of the TCR complex are discussed later in the chapter.

A small subset of T cells expresses TCRs made up of γ and δ chains, which are structurally similar to the α and β chains of the TCRs that are present in most T cells. γδ T cells are often found at epithelial surfaces and are believed to defend the host against pathogens that are commonly encountered at epithelia. Most γδ T cells do not recognize MHC-associated peptides; instead, they recognize lipids and other molecules that may be common to many microbes.

T cells can also be activated by molecules that bind to the TCRs of many or all clones of T cells, regardless of the peptide-MHC specificity of the TCR. These polyclonal activators of T cells include antibodies specific for the TCR or associated CD3 proteins, polymeric carbohydrate-binding proteins such as phytohemagglutinin, and certain microbial proteins called superantigens. Polyclonal activators are often used as experimental tools to study T cell activation responses and in clinical settings to test for T cell function or to prepare metaphase spreads for chromosomal analyses. Microbial superantigens may cause serious disease by causing activation and excessive cytokine release from many T cells.

Role of Adhesion Molecules in T Cell Activation

Adhesion molecules on T cells recognize their ligands on APCs and stabilize the binding of the T cells to the APCs. Most TCRs bind the peptide-MHC complexes for which they are specific with low affinity. A possible reason for this weak recognition is that T cells are positively selected during their maturation by weak recognition of self antigens, and their ability to recognize foreign microbial peptides is fortuitous and not predetermined (see Chapter 4). (Recall that this type of selection is inevitable considering that the thymus, where T cells mature, cannot possibly contain the entire universe of microbial peptides, and the antigens that maturing T cells can encounter in the thymus are self antigens.) It is, therefore, not surprising that T cells recognize foreign antigens weakly. To induce a productive response, the binding of T cells to APCs must be stabilized for a sufficiently long period that the necessary signaling threshold is achieved. This stabilization function is performed by adhesion molecules on the T cells whose ligands are expressed on APCs. The most important of these adhesion molecules belong to the family of heterodimeric (two-chain) proteins called **integrins.** The major T cell integrin involved in binding to APCs is leukocyte function–associated antigen-1 (LFA-1), whose ligand on APCs is called intercellular adhesion molecule-1 (ICAM-1).

Integrins play an important role in enhancing T cell responses to microbial antigens in two ways (Fig. 5-5). On resting naive T cells, which are cells that have not previously recognized and been activated by antigen, the LFA-1 integrin is in a low-affinity state. If a T cell is exposed to chemokines produced as part of the innate immune response to infection, that T cell's LFA-1 molecules are converted to a high-affinity state and cluster together within minutes. As a result, T cells bind strongly to APCs at sites of infection. Antigen recognition by a T cell also increases the affinity of that cell's LFA-1. Therefore, once a T cell sees antigen, it increases the strength of its binding to the APC presenting that antigen, providing a positive feedback loop. Thus, integrin-mediated adhesion is critical for the ability of T cells to bind to APCs displaying microbial antigens.

Integrins also play an important role in directing the migration of effector T cells from the circulation to sites of infection. This process is discussed in Chapter 6.

Role of Costimulation in T Cell Activation

The full activation of T cells is dependent on the recognition of costimulators on APCs (Fig. 5-6). We have previously referred to costimulators as "second signals" for T cell activation (see Chapters 2 and 3). The name "costimulator" derives from the fact that these molecules provide stimuli to T cells that function together with stimulation by antigen. The best defined costimulators for T cells are two related proteins called B7-1 (CD80) and B7-2 (CD86), both of which are expressed on professional APCs and whose expression is greatly increased when the APCs

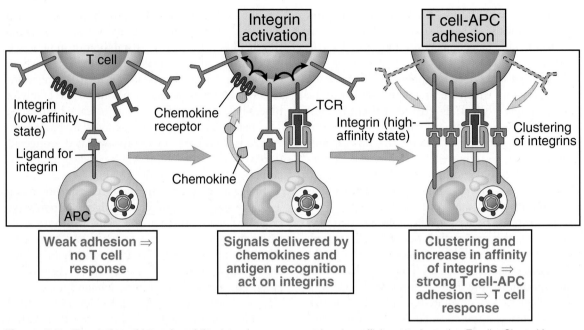

Figure 5–5   Regulation of integrin avidity. Integrins are present in a low-affinity state in resting T cells. Chemokines produced by APCs and signals induced by the TCR when it recognizes antigen both act on integrins and lead to their clustering and to conformational changes that increase the affinity of the integrins for their ligands. As a result, the integrins bind with high avidity to their ligands on APCs, and thus promote T cell activation.

encounter microbes. These B7 proteins are recognized by a receptor called CD28, which is expressed on virtually all T cells. Signals from CD28 on T cells binding to B7 on APCs work together with signals generated by binding of the TCR and coreceptor to peptide-MHC complexes on the same APCs. CD28-mediated signaling is essential for initiating the responses of naive T cells; and in the absence of CD28-B7 interactions, engagement of the TCR alone is unable to activate the T cells and may even lead to long-lived T cell unresponsiveness. (The importance of this type of unresponsiveness for preventing immune reactions to self antigens will be discussed in Chapter 9.) The requirement for costimulation ensures that naive T lymphocytes are activated fully by microbial antigens, because, as stated previously, microbes stimulate the expression of B7 costimulators on APCs. The APCs express several other molecules that are structurally similar to B7-1 and B7-2 and may also function as costimulators or as negative regulators of T cell responses. These different B7-like mol-

ecules may be particularly important in activation or regulation of effector T cells.

Another set of molecules that participate in increasing costimulatory signals for T cells are CD40 ligand (CD154) on the T cells and CD40 on APCs. These molecules do not directly enhance T cell activation. Instead, CD40L expressed on an antigen-stimulated T cell binds to CD40 on APCs and activates the APCs to express more B7 costimulators and to secrete cytokines, such as IL-12, that enhance T cell differentiation. Thus, the CD40L-CD40 interaction promotes T cell activation by making APCs better APCs.

The role of costimulation in T cell activation explains an old observation that we have mentioned in earlier chapters. Protein antigens, such as those used as vaccines, fail to elicit T cell–dependent immune responses unless these antigens are administered with substances that activate macrophages and other APCs. Such substances are called **adjuvants,** and they function mainly by inducing

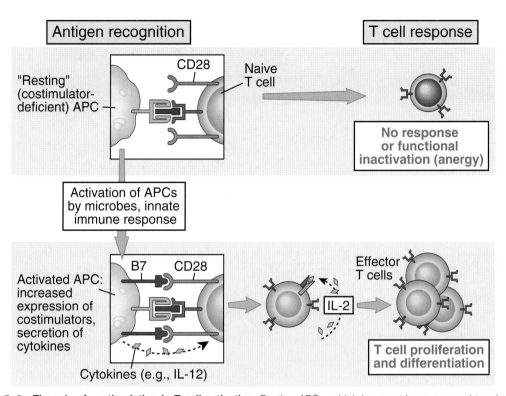

Figure 5-6   The role of costimulation in T cell activation. Resting APCs, which have not been exposed to microbes or adjuvants, may present peptide antigens but they do not express costimulators and are unable to activate naive T cells. Naive T cells that have recognized antigen without costimulation may become unresponsive to subsequent exposure to antigen, even if costimulators are present, and this state of unresponsiveness is called *anergy*. Microbes, and cytokines produced during innate immune responses to microbes, induce the expression of costimulators, such as B7 molecules, on the APCs. The B7 costimulators are recognized by the CD28 receptor on naive T cells, providing "signal 2," and in conjunction with antigen recognition ("signal 1"), this recognition initiates T cell responses.

the expression of costimulators on APCs and by stimulating the APCs to secrete cytokines that activate T cells. Most adjuvants are products of microbes (e.g., killed mycobacteria) or substances that mimic microbes. Thus, adjuvants convert inert protein antigens into mimics of pathogenic microbes.

Understanding the nature and biology of costimulators is an evolving story, and much remains to be learned about the structure and functions of this family of proteins. These issues are of practical importance because enhancing the expression of costimulators may be useful for stimulating T cell responses (e.g., against tumors), and blocking costimulators may be a strategy for inhibiting unwanted responses.

Clinical trials of agents that block B7:CD28 and CD40:CD40L interactions are now ongoing in transplant recipients to reduce or prevent graft rejection (see Chapter 10).

The activation of CD8+ T cells is stimulated by recognition of class I MHC–associated peptides and requires costimulation and/or helper T cells (Fig. 5-7). CD8+ T cells recognize peptides that may be produced from cytoplasmic proteins, such as viral proteins, in any nucleated cell. The development of CD8+ CTLs in some viral infections requires the concomitant activation of CD4+ helper T cells. It is believed that in such infections, infected cells are ingested by host APCs, mainly dendritic cells, and the viral antigens are "cross-presented" by the APCs (see

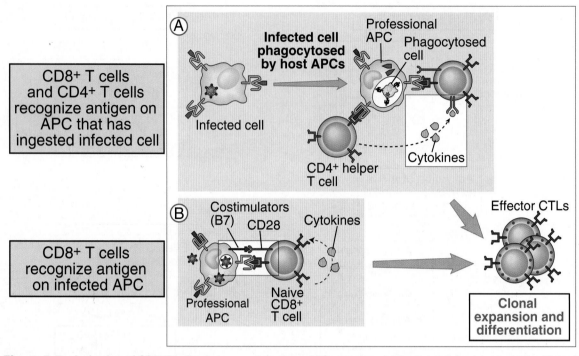

Figure 5–7   Activation of CD8⁺ T cells. A. In some infections, APCs may ingest infected cells and present microbial antigens to CD8⁺ T cells and to CD4⁺ helper T cells. The helper T cells then produce cytokines that stimulate the expansion and differentiation of the CD8⁺ T cells. It is also thought that helper cells may activate APCs to make them competent at stimulating CD8⁺ T cells (not shown). B. CD8⁺ T cell recognizes class I MHC–associated peptides and receives costimulatory signals if a professional APC harbors a cytoplasmic microbe.

Fig. 3-5, Chapter 3). The same APC may present viral antigens from the cytosol in complexes with class I MHC molecules and from vesicles in complex with class II MHC molecules. Thus, both CD8⁺ T cells and CD4⁺ T cells specific for viral antigens are activated near one another. The CD4⁺ T cells may produce cytokines or membrane molecules that help to activate the CD8⁺ T cells; thus, the clonal expansion of CD8⁺ and their differentiation into effector and memory CTLs may be dependent on help provided by CD4⁺ T cells. This is a likely explanation for the defective CTL responses to many viruses in patients infected with the human immunodeficiency virus (HIV), which kills CD4⁺ but not CD8⁺ T cells. CTL responses to some viruses do not appear to require help from CD4⁺ T cells for reasons that are not known.

Now that the stimuli that are required to activate naive T lymphocytes have been described, the next question to be addressed is how the T cells respond to these stimuli.

Responses of T Lymphocytes to Antigens and Costimulation

The recognition of antigen and costimulators by T cells initiates an orchestrated set of responses that culminate in the expansion of the antigen-specific clones of lymphocytes and the differentiation of the naive T cells into effector cells and memory cells (see Fig. 5-2). Many of the responses of T cells are mediated by cytokines that are secreted by the T cells and act on the T cells themselves and on many other cells involved in immune defenses. In the following section each component of the biologic responses of T cells is discussed.

Secretion of Cytokines and Expression of Cytokine Receptors

In response to antigen and costimulators, T lymphocytes, especially CD4$^+$ T cells, rapidly secrete several different cytokines that have diverse activities (Fig. 5-8). Cytokines are a large group of proteins that function as mediators of immunity and inflammation. In innate immune responses, cytokines are produced mainly by macrophages (see Chapter 2); and in adaptive immunity, cytokines are secreted by T cells. These proteins share some important properties, although different cytokines have distinct activities and play different roles in immune responses.

The first cytokine to be produced by CD4$^+$ T cells, within 1 to 2 hours after activation, is interleukin-2 (IL-2). (The term *interleukin* refers to the fact that many of these proteins are produced by leukocytes and act on leukocytes.) Activation also rapidly enhances the ability of T cells to bind and respond to IL-2, by regulating the expression of the IL-2 receptor (Fig. 5-9). The high-affinity receptor for IL-2 is a three-chain molecule. Naive T cells express two signaling chains of this receptor but do not express the chain that enables the receptor to bind IL-2 with high affinity.

Figure 5-8 Properties of the major cytokines produced by CD4$^+$ helper T lymphocytes. A. The general properties of all cytokines and the mechanisms responsible for these properties are summarized. B. The biologic actions of selected cytokines involved in T cell–mediated immunity are summarized. TGF-β functions mainly as an inhibitor of immune responses; its role is discussed in Chapter 9. The cytokines of innate immunity are shown in Figure 2-11.

Ⓐ General properties of cytokines

Property	Mechanism
Produced transiently in response to antigen	TCR signal and costimulation induce cytokine gene transcription
Usually acts on same cell that produces the cytokine (autocrine) or nearby cells (paracrine)	T cell activation induces expression of both cytokines and high-affinity receptors for cytokines
Pleiotropism: each cytokine has multiple biologic actions	Many different cell types may express receptors for a particular cytokine
Redundancy: multiple cytokines may share the same or similar biologic activities	Many cytokines use same conserved signaling pathways

Ⓑ Biologic actions of selected T cell cytokines

Cytokine	Principal action	Cellular source(s)
Interleukin-2 (IL-2)	T cell growth stimulation	CD4+ and CD8+ T cells
IL-4	B cell switching to IgE	CD4+ T cells, mast cells
IL-5	Activation of eosinophils	CD4+ T cells, mast cells
Interferon-γ (IFN-γ)	Activation of macrophages	CD4+ and CD8+ T cells, natural killer cells
TGF-β	Inhibition of T cell activation	CD4+ T cells; many other cell types

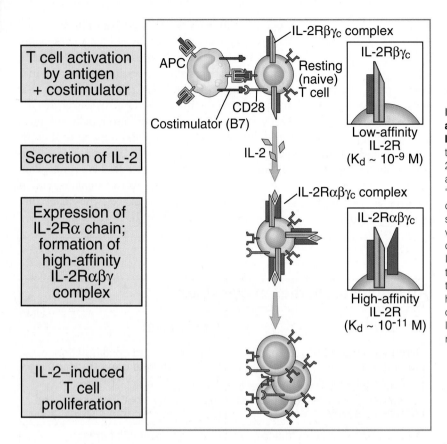

T cell activation
by antigen
+ costimulator

Secretion of IL-2

Expression of
IL-2Rα chain;
formation of
high-affinity
IL-2Rαβγ
complex

IL-2–induced
T cell
proliferation

Figure 5–9 The role of IL-2 and IL-2 receptors in T cell proliferation. Naive T cells express the low-affinity IL-2 receptor (IL-2R) complex, made up of the β and γ_c chains ("γ_c" refers to the "common γ" chain because it is a component of the receptors for several other cytokines). On activation by antigen recognition and costimulation, the cells produce IL-2 and express the α chain of the IL-2R, which associates with the β and γ_c chains to form the high-affinity IL-2 receptor. Binding of IL-2 to its receptor initiates proliferation of the T cells that recognized the antigen.

Within hours after activation by antigens and co-stimulators, the T cells produce the third chain of the receptor and now the complete IL-2 receptor is able to bind IL-2 strongly. Thus, IL-2 produced by an antigen-stimulated T cell preferentially binds to and acts on the same T cell. The principal action of IL-2 is to stimulate proliferation of T cells; for this reason IL-2 is also called T cell growth factor. IL-2 stimulates T cells to enter the cell cycle and begin to divide, resulting in an increase in the number of the antigen-specific T cells. Differentiated effector CD4+ T cells produce many other cytokines, and the functions of some of the major ones are described later.

CD8+ T lymphocytes that recognize antigen and costimulators do not appear to secrete large amounts of IL-2, yet, as we shall see later, these lymphocytes proliferate prodigiously during immune responses. It is possible that antigen recognition is able to drive the proliferation of CD8+ T cells without a requirement

for much IL-2. Alternatively, as we mentioned earlier, in some cases, CD8+ T activation may require help from CD4+ T cells that are activated nearby to provide IL-2.

Clonal Expansion

Within 1 or 2 days after activation, T lymphocytes begin to proliferate, resulting in expansion of antigen-specific clones. This expansion quickly provides a large pool of antigen-specific lymphocytes from which effector cells can be generated to combat infection. The magnitude of clonal expansion is remarkable, especially for CD8+ T cells. For instance, before infection, the number of CD8+ T cells specific for any one microbial protein antigen is about 1 in 10^5 or 10^6 lymphocytes in the body. At the peak of some viral infections, which may be within a week after the infection, as many as 10% to 20% of all the lymphocytes in the lymphoid organs may be specific for that virus. This means that the antigen-specific clones have increased by more than 10,000-fold, with an estimated doubling time of about 6 hours. Several features of this clonal expansion are surprising. First, this enormous expansion of T cells specific for a microbe is not accompanied by a detectable increase in "bystander" cells that do not recognize that microbe. Second, even in infections with complex microbes that contain many protein antigens, the majority of the expanded clones are specific for only a few, and often less than five, immunodominant peptides of that microbe. The expansion of CD4+ T cells appears to be much less, probably on the order of 100-fold to 1000-fold. This difference in the magnitude of clonal expansion of CD8+ T cells and CD4+ T cells may reflect differences in their functions. CD8+ CTLs are effector cells that themselves kill infected cells, and many CTLs may be needed to kill large numbers of infected cells. In contrast, CD4+ effector cells secrete cytokines that activate other effector cells, as described later, and a small number of cytokine producers may be all that is needed.

Differentiation of Naive T Cells into Effector Cells

The progeny of antigen-stimulated proliferating T cells begin to differentiate into effector cells that function to eradicate infections. This process of differentiation is the result of changes in gene expression (e.g., the activation of genes encoding cytokines [in CD4+ and CD8+ T cells] or cytolytic proteins [in CD8+ CTLs]). It begins in concert with clonal expansion, and differentiated effector cells appear within 3 or 4 days after exposure to microbes. These cells leave the peripheral lymphoid organs and migrate to the site of infection. Here the effector cells again encounter the microbial antigens that stimulated their development. On recognition of antigen, the effector cells respond in ways that serve to eradicate the infection. Effector cells of the CD4+ and CD8+ populations perform different functions, and their patterns of differentiation are similarly distinct.

CD4+ helper T cells differentiate into effector cells that respond to antigen by producing surface molecules and cytokines that function mainly to activate macrophages and B lymphocytes (Fig. 5-10). The most important cell surface protein involved in the effector function of CD4+ T cells is CD40 ligand (CD40L). The CD40L gene becomes transcriptionally active in CD4+ T cells in response to antigen recognition and costimulation, and the result is that CD40L is expressed on helper T cells after activation. It binds to its receptor, CD40, which is expressed mainly on macrophages, B lymphocytes, and dendritic cells. Engagement of CD40 activates these cells, and thus CD40L is an important participant in the activation of macrophages and B lymphocytes by helper T cells (see Chapters 6 and 7). As discussed earlier, the interaction of CD40L on T cells with CD40 on dendritic cells stimulates the expression of costimulators on these APCs and the production of T cell–activating cytokines, thus providing a positive feedback (amplification) mechanism for APC-induced T cell activation.

The analysis of cytokine production by helper T cells has answered a long-standing question in immunology. It has been known for many years that the immune system responds very differently to different microbes. For instance, intracellular microbes such as mycobacteria are ingested by phagocytes but resist intracellular killing. The adaptive immune response to such microbes results in the activation of the phagocytes to kill the ingested microbes. In striking contrast, helminthic parasites are too large to be phagocytosed, and the immune response to helminths is dominated by the production of IgE antibodies and the activation of eosinophils. IgE antibody coats (opsonizes) the helminths, and the eosinophils use their IgE-specific Fc receptors to bind to and destroy the helminths. Both types of immune responses are dependent on CD4+ helper T cells, but for many years it was not clear how the CD4+ helper cells are able to stimulate such distinct immune effector mechanisms. This puzzle was answered by the discovery that there are different types of CD4+ effector T cells that perform distinct functions, as described below.

CD4+ helper T cells may differentiate into subsets of effector cells that produce distinct sets of cytokines that perform different functions. The best defined of these subsets are called T_H1 cells and T_H2 cells (for type 1 helper T cells and type 2 helper T

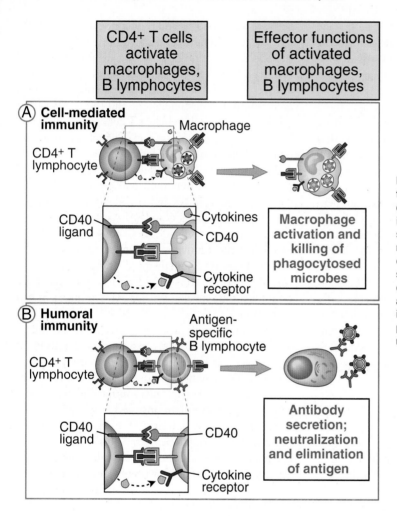

Figure 5–10 The molecules involved in the effector functions of CD4⁺ helper T cells. CD4⁺ T cells that have differentiated into effector cells express CD40L and secrete cytokines. CD40L binds to CD40 on macrophages or B lymphocytes, and cytokines bind to their receptors on the same cells. The combination of signals delivered by CD40 and cytokine receptors activates macrophages in cell-mediated immunity (A) and activates B cells to produce antibodies in humoral immune responses (B).

cells) (Fig. 5-11). The most important cytokine produced by T_H1 cells is **interferon-γ** (IFN-γ), so called because it was discovered as a cytokine that inhibited (or interfered with) viral infection. IFN-γ is a potent activator of macrophages. It also stimulates the production of antibody isotypes that promote the phagocytosis of microbes, because these antibodies bind directly to phagocyte Fc receptors, and they activate complement, generating products that bind to phagocyte complement receptors. (These functions of antibodies are described in Chapter 8.) Therefore, T_H1 cells stimulate phagocyte-mediated ingestion and killing of microbes, the key component of cell-mediated immunity. IFN-γ also stimulates the expres-

sion of class II MHC molecules and B7 costimulators on APCs, especially macrophages, and this action of IFN-γ may serve to amplify T cell responses. T_H2 cells, on the other hand, produce IL-4, which stimulates the production of IgE antibodies, and IL-5, which activates eosinophils. Therefore, T_H2 cells stimulate phagocyte-independent, eosinophil-mediated immunity, which is especially effective against helminthic parasites. Some of the cytokines produced by T_H2 cells, such as IL-4, IL-10, and IL-13, inhibit macrophage activation and suppress T_H1 cell-mediated immunity. Therefore, the efficacy of cell-mediated immune responses against a microbe may be determined by a balance between the activation of

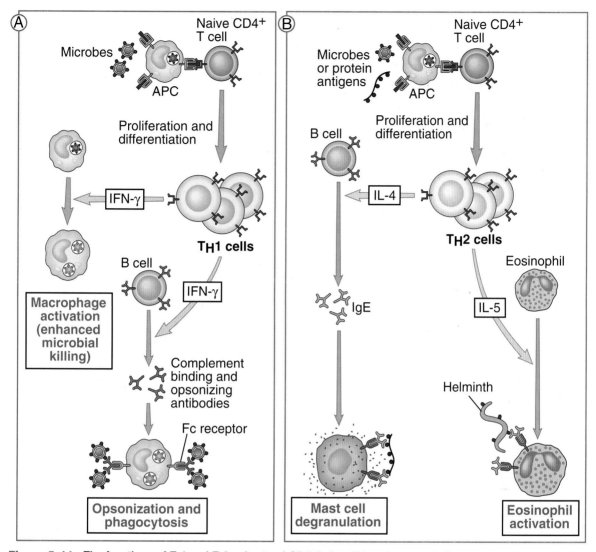

Figure 5–11 **The functions of T$_H$1 and T$_H$2 subsets of CD4$^+$ helper T lymphocytes.** A. T$_H$1 cells produce the cytokine IFN-γ, which activates phagocytes to kill ingested microbes and stimulates the production of antibodies that promote the ingestion of microbes by the phagocytes. B. T$_H$2 cells specific for microbial or nonmicrobial protein antigens produce the cytokines IL-4, which stimulates the production of IgE antibody, and IL-5, which activates eosinophils. IgE participates in the activation of mast cells by protein antigens and coats helminths for destruction by eosinophils. *Continued*

T$_H$1 and T$_H$2 cells in response to that microbe. We will return to this concept and its importance in infectious diseases in Chapter 6. It is likely that many differentiated CD4$^+$ T cells produce various mixtures of cytokines, stimulate multiple effector mechanisms, and cannot be readily classified into T$_H$1 and T$_H$2 subsets.

The development of T$_H$1 and T$_H$2 cells is not a random process but is regulated by the stimuli that naive CD4$^+$ T cells receive when they encounter microbial antigens (Fig. 5-12). Macrophages and dendritic cells respond to many bacteria and viruses by producing a cytokine called IL-12. When naive T cells recognize the antigens of these microbes, which

© Property	T_H1 subset	T_H2 subset

Cytokines produced
    IFN-γ, IL-2, TNF
    IL-4, IL-5, IL-13
    IL-10
    IL-3, GM-CSF
	+++
	-
	+/-
	++
		-
		+++
		++
		++

Cytokine receptor expression
    IL-12R β chain
    IL-18R
	++
	++
		-
		-

Chemokine receptor expression
    CCR3, CCR4
    CXCR3, CCR5
	+/-
	++
		++
		+/-

Ligands for E- and P- selectin	++	+/-
Antibody isotypes stimulated	IgG2a (mouse)	IgE; IgG1 (mouse)/ IgG4 (humans)
Macrophage activation	+++	-

Figure 5–11, Cont'd C. The main differences between T_H1 and T_H2 subsets of helper T cells are summarized. Note that many helper T cells are not readily classified into these distinct and polarized subsets. The chemokine receptors are called CCR or CXCR because they bind chemokines classified into CC or CXC chemokines based on whether key cysteines are adjacent or separated by one amino acid. Different chemokine receptors control the migration of different types of cells. These, in combination with the selectins, determine whether T_H1 or T_H2 cells dominate in different inflammatory reactions in various tissues.

are being presented by the same APCs, the T cells are also exposed to IL-12. IL-12 promotes the differentiation of the T cells into the T_H1 subset, which then produce IFN-γ to activate macrophages to kill the microbes. This sequence illustrates an important principle that has been mentioned in earlier chapters, that the innate immune response— in this case, IL-12 production by APCs—influences the nature of the subsequent adaptive immune response, driving it toward T_H1 cells. If the infectious microbe does not elicit IL-12 production by APCs, as may be the case with helminths, the T cells themselves produce IL-4, which induces the differentiation of these cells towards the T_H2 subset. The balance between T_H1 and T_H2 differentiation may be influenced by types of dendritic cells that initially respond

to particular infections. Several subsets of dendritic cells have been identified that differ in the classes of microbes they respond to and the cytokines they secrete when activated by the microbes and, therefore, in the types of effector T cells (T_H1 or T_H2) that they induce.

The differentiation of CD4$^+$ helper T cells into T_H1 and T_H2 subsets is an excellent example of the specialization of adaptive immunity, illustrating how immune responses to different types of microbes are designed to be most effective against these microbes. Furthermore, once T_H1 or T_H2 cells develop from antigen-stimulated helper T cells, each subset produces cytokines that enhance the differentiation of T cells toward that subset and inhibits development of the reciprocal population. This "cross-regulation"

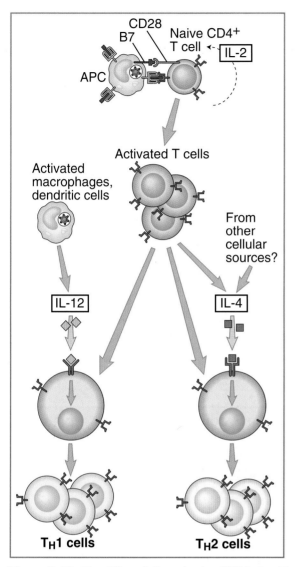

Figure 5–12 The differentiation of naive CD4+ helper T cells into T$_H$1 and T$_H$2 effector cells. After their activation by antigen and costimulators, naive helper T cells may differentiate into T$_H$1 and T$_H$2 cells under the influence of cytokines. IL-12 produced by microbe-activated macrophages and dendritic cells stimulates differentiation of CD4+ T cells into T$_H$1 effectors. In the absence of IL-12, the T cells themselves (and perhaps other cells) produce IL-4, which stimulates their differentiation into T$_H$2 effectors.

may lead to increasing polarization of the response in one direction or the other.

CD8+ T lymphocytes activated by antigen and costimulators differentiate into CTLs that are able to kill infected cells expressing the antigen. Effector CTLs kill infected cells by secreting proteins that create pores in the membranes of the infected cells and induce DNA fragmentation and apoptotic death of these cells. The differentiation of naive CD8+ T cells into effector CTLs is accompanied by the synthesis of the molecules that kill infected cells. The mechanisms of CTL-mediated killing are discussed in more detail in Chapter 6.

Development of Memory T Lymphocytes

A fraction of antigen-activated T lymphocytes differentiates into long-lived memory T cells. Memory cells survive even after the infection is eradicated and antigen as well as the innate immune reaction to the infectious pathogen are no longer present. These memory T cells can be found in lymphoid tissues, in mucosal barriers, and in the circulation. We do not know what keeps memory cells alive or what factors determine whether the progeny of antigen-stimulated lymphocytes will differentiate into effector cells or memory cells. Memory T cells do not continue to produce cytokines or kill infected cells, but they may do so rapidly on encountering the antigen that they recognize. Thus, memory cells are a pool of lymphocytes waiting for the infection to return.

Decline of the Immune Response

The entire process of T cell clonal expansion and differentiation occurs in the peripheral lymphoid organs. Effector cells and memory cells leave these tissues and enter the circulation, able to locate infection anywhere in the body (see Chapter 6). As the infection is cleared and the stimuli for lymphocyte activation disappear, many of the cells that had proliferated in response to antigen are deprived of survival factors. As a result, these cells die by a process of apoptosis (programmed cell death). The response subsides within 1 or 2 weeks after the infection is eradicated, and the only sign that a T cell–mediated immune response had occurred is the pool of surviving memory lymphocytes.

The generation of a useful T cell response has to overcome several problems, and T cells have evolved numerous mechanisms to achieve this goal. First, naive T cells have to find the antigen. The problem of locating antigen is solved by APCs that capture the antigen and concentrate it in the specialized lymphoid organs through which naive T cells recirculate. Second, the correct type of T lymphocytes (i.e., CD4+ helper T cells or CD8+ CTLs) must respond to antigens from the extracellular and intracellular compartments. This selectivity is determined by the specificity of the CD4 and CD8 coreceptors for class II and class I MHC molecules, and the segregation of extracellular (vesicular) and intracellular (cytoplasmic) protein antigens for display by class II and class I MHC molecules, respectively. Third, T cells must interact with antigen-bearing APCs for long enough to be activated. Adhesion molecules that stabilize T cell binding to APCs ensure sufficiently long T cell–APC contacts. Fourth, T cells should respond to microbial antigens but not to harmless proteins. This preference for microbes is maintained because T cell activation requires costimulators that are induced on APCs by microbes. Finally, antigen recognition by a small number of T cells has to be converted into a response that is large enough to be effective. This conversion is maximized by several amplification mechanisms that are induced by microbes and by activated T cells themselves and lead to enhanced T cell activation.

As we have seen in this chapter, the biology of T cell activation is quite well understood. On the other hand, we still have only an incomplete understanding of the biochemical links between recognition of antigen and costimulators and the biologic responses of the lymphocytes. In the final section of the chapter the current views of signal transduction by the TCR complex are summarized, taking into account that this remains an area of investigation with many unanswered questions.

Biochemical Pathways of T Cell Activation

On recognition of antigens and costimulators, T cells express proteins that are involved in proliferation, differentiation, and effector functions of the cells (Fig. 5-13). Naive T cells that have not encountered antigen (so-called resting cells) have a low level of protein synthesis. Within minutes of antigen recognition, new gene transcription and protein synthesis are seen in the activated T cells. The functions of many of these newly expressed proteins have been mentioned earlier.

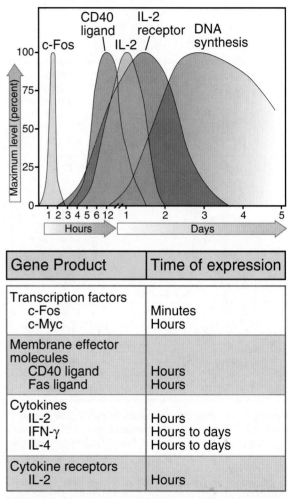

Gene Product	Time of expression
Transcription factors	
c-Fos	Minutes
c-Myc	Hours
Membrane effector molecules	
CD40 ligand	Hours
Fas ligand	Hours
Cytokines	
IL-2	Hours
IFN-γ	Hours to days
IL-4	Hours to days
Cytokine receptors	
IL-2	Hours

Figure 5–13 Proteins produced by antigen-stimulated T cells. Antigen recognition by T cells results in the synthesis and expression of a variety of proteins, examples of which are shown. The kinetics of production of these proteins are approximations and may vary in different T cells and with different types of stimuli. The possible effects of costimulation on the patterns or kinetics of gene expression are not shown.

The biochemical pathways that link antigen recognition with T cell responses consist of the activation of enzymes, recruitment of adapter proteins, and production of active transcription factors (Fig. 5-14). These biochemical pathways are initiated by cross-linking of the TCR, and they occur at or near the TCR complex. Multiple TCRs and coreceptors are brought together when they bind MHC-peptide complexes on APCs. In addition, there is an orderly redistribution of other proteins in both the APC and

T cell membranes at the point of cell:cell contact; these proteins are involved in adhesion and signaling and are important for optimal induction of activating signals in the T cell. This region of contact between the APC and T cell, including the redistributed membrane proteins, is called the immunologic synapse. The clustering of CD4 or CD8 coreceptors activates a tyrosine protein kinase called Lck that is attached to the cytoplasmic tails of these coreceptors. As we discussed in Chapter 4 and earlier in this chapter,

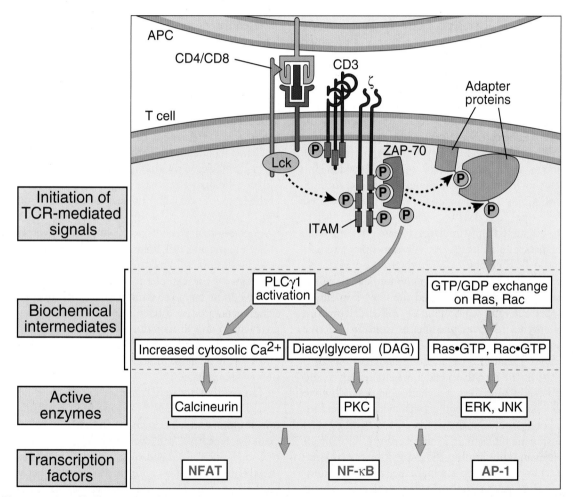

Figure 5–14 Signal transduction pathways in T lymphocytes. Antigen recognition by T cells induces early signaling events, which include tyrosine phosphorylation of molecules of the TCR complex and the recruitment of adapter proteins to the site of T cell antigen recognition. These early events lead to the activation of several biochemical intermediates, which in turn activate transcription factors that stimulate transcription of genes whose products mediate the responses of the T cells. The possible effects of costimulation on these signaling pathways are not shown. PLCγ1 refers to the γ1 isoform of phosphatidylinositol-specific phospholipase C.

several transmembrane signaling proteins are associated with the TCR, including the CD3 and ζ chains. CD3 and ζ contain tyrosine-rich motifs, called immunoreceptor tyrosine-based activation motifs (ITAMs), that are critical for signaling. Once it is activated, Lck phosphorylates tyrosine residues contained within the ITAMs of the ζ and CD3 proteins. The phosphorylated ITAMs of the ζ chain become docking sites for a tyrosine kinase called ZAP-70 (ζ-associated protein of 70 kD), which is also phosphorylated by Lck and thereby made enzymatically active. The active ZAP-70 then phosphorylates various adapter proteins and enzymes, which assemble near the TCR complex and mediate additional signaling events. Two major signaling pathways linked to ζ chain phosphorylation and ZAP-70 are the calcium-NFAT pathway and the Ras/Rac-MAP kinase pathway.

Nuclear factor of activated T cells (NFAT) is a transcription factor whose activation is dependent on Ca^{2+} ions. The calcium-NFAT pathway is initiated by ZAP-70–mediated phosphorylation and activation of an enzyme called phospholipase C (PLC), which catalyzes the hydrolysis of plasma membrane inositol phospholipids. One byproduct of PLC-mediated phospholipid breakdown, called inositol 1,4,5-triphosphate (IP_3), stimulates release of Ca^{2+} ions from intracellular stores. At the same time, signals from the TCR complex lead to the influx of extracellular Ca^{2+} into the cell. Cytoplasmic Ca^{2+} binds a protein called calmodulin, and the Ca^{2+}-calmodulin complex activates a phosphatase called calcineurin. This enzyme removes phosphates from an inactive cytosolic transcription factor called nuclear factor of activated T cells. Once dephosphorylated, NFAT is able to migrate into the nucleus, where it binds to and activates the promoters of several genes, including the genes encoding the T cell growth factor interleukin-2 and components of the IL-2 receptor. A drug called **cyclosporine** binds to and inhibits the activity of calcineurin and thus inhibits the production of cytokines by T cells. This agent is widely used as an immunosuppressive drug to prevent graft rejection; its advent has been one of the major factors in the success of organ transplantation in the past decade (see Chapter 10).

The Ras/Rac-MAP kinase pathways include the guanosine triphosphate (GTP) binding Ras and Rac proteins, which are biologically active when bound to GTP, several adapter proteins, and a cascade of enzymes that eventually activate one of a family of mitogen-activated protein (MAP) kinases. The pathways are initiated by ZAP-70–dependent phosphorylation and accumulation of adapter proteins at the plasma membrane, leading to the recruitment of Ras or Rac and their activation by exchange of GTP and guanosine diphosphate (GDP). Both Ras-GTP and Rac-GTP initiate different enzyme cascades, leading to the activation of distinct MAP kinases. The terminal MAP kinases in these pathways, called extracellular signal regulated kinase (ERK) and c-Jun amino(N)-terminal kinase (JNK), promote the expression of a protein called c-Fos and the phosphorylation of another protein called c-Jun. C-Fos and phosphorylated c-Jun combine to form the active transcription factor AP-1 (activating protein-1), which enhances the transcription of several T cell genes.

Other biochemical events involved in TCR signaling include activation of the serine-threonine kinase called protein kinase C (PKC) and activation of the transcription factor nuclear factor-κB (NF-κB). PKC is activated by diacylglycerol, which, like IP_3, is generated by phospholipase C–mediated hydrolysis of membrane inositol lipids. A T cell-specific PKC isoform, PKC-θ, is linked to activation of NF-κB. NF-κB exists in the cytoplasm of resting T cells in an inactive form, bound to an inhibitor called IκB. TCR signals generated by antigen recognition lead to phosphorylation and dissociation of the bound inhibitor of NF-κB. As a result, NF-κB is released and able to move to the nucleus, where it activates the transcription of several genes.

The various transcription factors we have mentioned, including NFAT, AP-1, and NF-κB, stimulate transcription and subsequent production of cytokines, cytokine receptors, cell cycle inducers, and effector molecules such as CD40L (see Fig. 5-13). All these signals are initiated by antigen recognition, because binding of the TCR and coreceptors to antigen (peptide-MHC complexes) is necessary to assemble the signaling molecules and initiate their enzymatic activity.

It was stated earlier that recognition of costimulators, such as B7 molecules, by their receptor (i.e.,

CD28) is essential for full T cell responses. The signals transduced by CD28 on binding to B7 costimulators are even less defined than are TCR-triggered signals. It is possible that CD28 engagement amplifies TCR signals or that CD28 initiates a distinct set of signals that complement TCR signals. These possibilities, of course, are not mutually exclusive.

SUMMARY

▶ T lymphocytes are the cells of cell-mediated immunity, the arm of the adaptive immune system that combats intracellular microbes, which may be microbes that are ingested by phagocytes and live within these cells or microbes that infect nonphagocytic cells.

▶ The responses of T lymphocytes consist of sequential phases: recognition of cell-associated microbes by naive T cells, expansion of the antigen-specific clones by proliferation, and differentiation of some of the progeny into effector cells and memory cells.

▶ T cells use their antigen receptors to recognize peptide antigens displayed by MHC molecules on antigen-presenting cells (which accounts for the specificity of the ensuing response) and polymorphic residues of the MHC molecules (accounting for the MHC restriction of T cell responses).

▶ Antigen recognition by the TCR triggers signals that are delivered to the interior of the cells by molecules associated with the TCR (the CD3 and ζ chains) and by the coreceptors, CD4 or CD8, which recognize class II or class I MHC molecules, respectively.

▶ The binding of T cells to antigen-presenting cells is enhanced by adhesion molecules, notably the integrins, whose affinity for their ligands is increased by chemokines produced in response to microbes and by antigen recognition by the TCR.

▶ APCs exposed to microbes or to cytokines produced as part of the innate immune reactions to microbes express costimulators that are recognized by receptors on T cells and deliver necessary "second signals" for T cell activation.

▶ In response to antigen recognition and costimulation, T cells secrete cytokines, some of which induce proliferation of the antigen-stimulated T cells and others mediate the effector functions of T cells.

▶ CD4$^+$ helper T cells may differentiate into subsets of effector cells that produce restricted sets of cytokines and perform different functions. T_H1 cells, which produce IFN-γ, activate phagocytes to eliminate ingested microbes and stimulate the production of opsonizing and complement-binding antibodies. T_H2 cells, which produce IL-4 and IL-5, stimulate IgE production and activate eosinophils, which function mainly in defense against helminths.

▶ CD8$^+$ T cells recognize peptides of intracellular (cytoplasmic) protein antigens and may require help from CD4$^+$ T cells to differentiate into effector CTLs. The function of CTLs is to kill cells producing cytoplasmic microbial antigens.

▶ The biochemical signals triggered in T cells by antigen recognition result in the activation of various transcription factors that stimulate the expression of genes encoding cytokines, cytokine receptors, and other molecules involved in T cell responses.

⇄ Review Questions

1 What are the components of the TCR complex? Which of these components are responsible for antigen recognition and which for signal transduction?

2 What are some of the accessory molecules that T cells use to initiate their responses to antigens, and what are the functions of these molecules?

3 What is costimulation? What is the physiologic significance of costimulation? What are some of the ligand-receptor pairs that are involved in costimulation?

4 What is the principal growth factor for T cells? Why do antigen-specific T cells expand more than other ("bystander") T cells on exposure to an antigen?

5 What are the major subsets of CD4$^+$ helper T cells, and how do they differ?

6 What signals are required to induce the responses of CD8$^+$ T cells?

7 Summarize the links between antigen recognition, the major biochemical signaling pathways in T cells, and the production of transcription factors.

Effector Mechanisms of Cell-Mediated Immunity

Eradication of Intracellular Microbes

6

The specialized immune mechanisms that function to eradicate intracellular microbes constitute cell-mediated immunity. The effector phase of cell-mediated immunity is carried out by T lymphocytes, and antibodies play no role in eradicating infections by microbes that are living inside host cells. The phases of cell-mediated immunity consist of the activation of naive T cells to proliferate and to differentiate into effector cells and the elimination of cell-associated microbes by the actions of these effector T cells. In Chapter 3 the function of major histocompatibility complex (MHC) molecules in displaying the antigens of intracellular microbes for recognition by T lymphocytes was described, and in Chapter 5 the way in which naive T cells recognize these antigens in lymphoid organs and develop into effector cells was discussed. In this chapter, the following questions are addressed:

- How do effector T lymphocytes locate intracellular microbes at any site in the body?
- How do effector T cells eradicate infections by these microbes?

Types of Cell-Mediated Immunity

There are two types of cell-mediated immune reactions designed to eliminate different types of intracellular microbes: CD4+ T cells activate phagocytes to destroy microbes

105

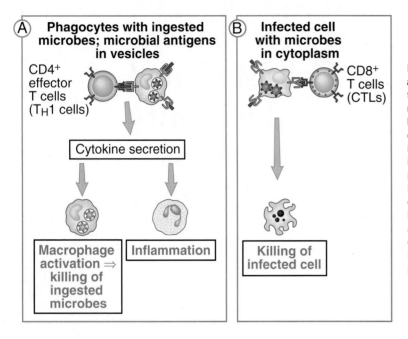

Figure 6–1   Cell-mediated immunity against intracellular microbes. A. Effector T cells of the CD4+ TH1 subset recognize the antigens of microbes ingested by phagocytes and activate the phagocytes to kill the microbes and induce inflammation. Phagocyte activation and inflammation are responses to cytokines produced by the T cells (discussed later). CD8+ T lymphocytes also produce cytokines that elicit the same reactions, but CD8+ T cells recognize microbial antigens in the cytoplasm of infected cells (not shown). B. CD8+ CTLs kill infected cells with microbes in the cytoplasm. CTLs, cytolytic T lymphocytes.

residing in the vesicles of these phagocytes, and CD8+ T cells kill any cell containing microbes or microbial proteins in the cytoplasm, thus eliminating the reservoir of infection (Fig. 6-1). This separation of the effector functions of T lymphocytes is not absolute. Some CD4+ T cells are capable of killing infected macrophages, and CD8+ T cells activate macrophages to eliminate phagocytosed microbes. Nevertheless, phagocyte activation, which is the principal function of CD4+ T cells in cell-mediated immunity, and CD8+ mediated killing of infected cells are fundamentally different immune reactions and are described separately.

Microbial infections may occur anywhere in the body, and some infectious pathogens are able to infect and live within host cells. Pathogenic microbes that infect and survive inside host cells include (1) many bacteria and some protozoa that are ingested by phagocytes but resist the killing mechanisms of these phagocytes and live in vesicles or cytoplasm and (2) viruses that infect phagocytic and nonphagocytic cells and live in the cytoplasm of these cells (see Fig. 5-1, Chapter 5). Effector T cells whose function is to eradicate these microbes are generated from naive T cells that were stimulated by microbial antigens in lymph nodes and spleen (see Chapter 5). The differentiated effector T cells then migrate to the site of infection. Phagocytes at these sites that have ingested the

microbes into intracellular vesicles display peptide fragments of microbial proteins attached to class II MHC molecules for recognition by effector T cells of the CD4+ subset. Peptide antigens derived from microbes living in the cytoplasm of infected cells are displayed by class I MHC molecules for recognition by CD8+ effector T cells. Antigen recognition by the effector T cells then activates these cells to perform their task of eliminating the infectious pathogens. Thus, in cell-mediated immunity, T cells recognize protein antigens at two stages: naive T cells recognize antigens in lymphoid tissues and respond by proliferating and by differentiating into effector cells, and effector T cells recognize the same antigens anywhere in the body and respond by eliminating these microbes (Fig. 6-2).

In the remainder of this chapter, we will describe first how differentiated effector T cells locate microbes in tissues and then how CD4+ and CD8+ cells eliminate these microbes.

Migration of Effector T Lymphocytes to Sites of Infection

Effector T cells migrate to sites of infection because these lymphocytes express high levels of adhesion

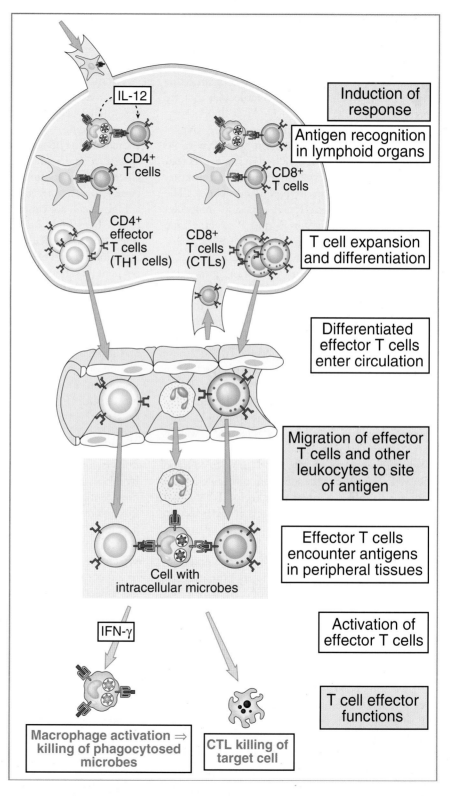

Figure 6–2 The induction and effector phases of cell-mediated immunity. Induction of response: CD4+ T cells and CD8+ T cells recognize peptides that are derived from protein antigens and presented by professional antigen-presenting cells in peripheral lymphoid organs. The T lymphocytes are stimulated to proliferate and differentiate, and effector cells enter the circulation.

Migration of effector T cells and other leukocytes to the site of antigen: Effector T cells and other leukocytes migrate through blood vessels in peripheral tissues by binding to endothelial cells that have been activated by cytokines produced in response to infection in these tissues.

molecules that bind to ligands that are expressed on endothelium on exposure to microbes and because chemoattractant cytokines are produced at the infection site. The process of differentiation of naive T lymphocytes into effector cells is accompanied by changes in the profiles of adhesion molecules that are expressed on these cells (Fig. 6-3). After their activation, T lymphocytes are able to migrate out of the lymph nodes. T cell activation also leads to an increase in the expression of adhesion molecules that bind to molecules expressed on microbe- or cytokine-stimulated endothelium in peripheral tissues. The most important of these T cell adhesion molecules are glycoprotein ligands for E- and P-selectins and the high-affinity forms of the integrins LFA-1 (LFA, leukocyte function–associated antigen) and VLA-4 (VLA referring to very late activation molecules, because they appear later than LFA-1 during the course of T cell activation). Meanwhile, at the site of infection, one of the innate immune responses to the infection is the secretion of cytokines by macrophages responding to the pathogen. Two of these macrophage-derived cytokines, tumor necrosis factor (TNF) and interleukin-1 (IL-1), act on the endothelial cells of small blood vessels adjacent to the infection site. TNF and IL-1 stimulate the endothelial cells to increase expression of E- and P-selectins as well as ligands for integrins, especially ICAM-1 (intercellular adhesion molecule-1, the ligand for LFA-1) and VCAM-1 (vascular cell adhesion molecule-1, the ligand for the VLA-4 integrin). Effector T cells that are passing through the blood vessels at the infection site bind weakly to the selectins and roll along the endothelial surface. When the integrins of these effector T cells encounter their ligands on the endothelium, the T cells bind firmly to the endothelium and begin the process of migrating out of the blood vessels to the site of infection. Essentially the same molecular interactions are responsible for the migration of other leukocytes, such as neutrophils and monocytes, to sites of infection (see Chapter 2, Fig. 2-5). On activation, T cells not only increase the expression of the adhesion molecules that enable them to bind to vessels at sites of infection but also lose expression of L-selectin, a molecule that mediates naive T cell migration into lymph nodes. Therefore, activated T cells tend to stay out of normal lymph nodes. This, of course, makes sense, because naive T cells need to enter lymph nodes to locate microbes and protein antigens and initiate immune responses, but the cells do not need to do this after they have been activated.

At the same time as effector T lymphocytes are being arrested on the endothelium, macrophages and endothelial cells respond to the infectious microbes by producing another set of cytokines, the chemokines. The principal function of chemokines is to attract and stimulate the motility of leukocytes. Chemokines are often displayed on endothelial cells bound to cell surface proteoglycans, thus providing a high local concentration near the site of infection. Chemokines are produced at the extravascular infection site by leukocytes that are reacting to the infectious microbe, and this creates a concentration gradient of chemokines toward the infection. The endothelial cell–associated chemokines act on loosely adherent T cells to increase the affinity of their integrins for endothelial ligands (see Fig. 5-5, Chapter 5). The chemokines also act on firmly adherent T cells and stimulate the motility of these cells, and the concentration gradient draws the T cells through the vessel wall into the site of infection. Thus, circulating effector T lymphocytes migrate, or "home," to sites of infection and become concentrated at these sites.

The homing of effector T cells to a site of infection is independent of antigen recognition, but lymphocytes that recognize microbial antigens are preferentially retained at the site (Fig. 6-4). Because the homing of effector T cells to sites of infection is dependent on adhesion molecules and chemokines, and not on antigen recognition, all effector T cells present in the blood that were generated in response to different microbial infections can enter the site of any infection. This nonselective migration presumably maximizes the ability of effector lymphocytes to search out the microbes they can specifically recognize and eliminate. However, the same lack of selectivity creates a problem: how are lymphocytes specific for a microbe focused on to that microbe for long enough to perform their function? A likely answer is that an effector T lymphocyte that has left the circulation and entered a tissue specifically recognizes microbial antigen, and the cell is again activated. One consequence of activation is an increase in the

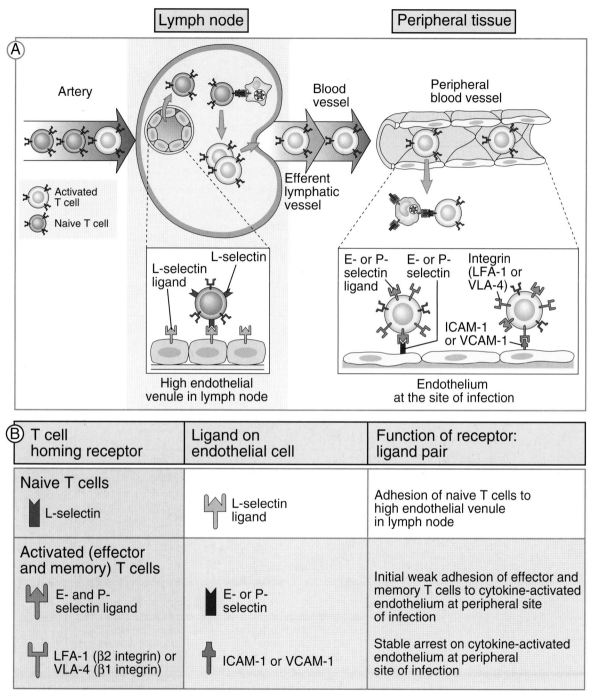

Figure 6–3   Migration of naive and effector T lymphocytes. A. Naive T lymphocytes home to lymph nodes as a result of L-selectin binding to its ligand on high endothelial venules (HEVs), which are present only in lymph nodes. Activated T lymphocytes, including effector cells, home to sites of infection in peripheral tissues, and this migration is mediated by E-selectin and P-selectin and integrins. In addition, different chemokines that are produced in lymph nodes and sites of infection also participate in the recruitment of T cells to these sites (not shown). B. The functions of the principal T cell homing receptors and their ligands are shown.

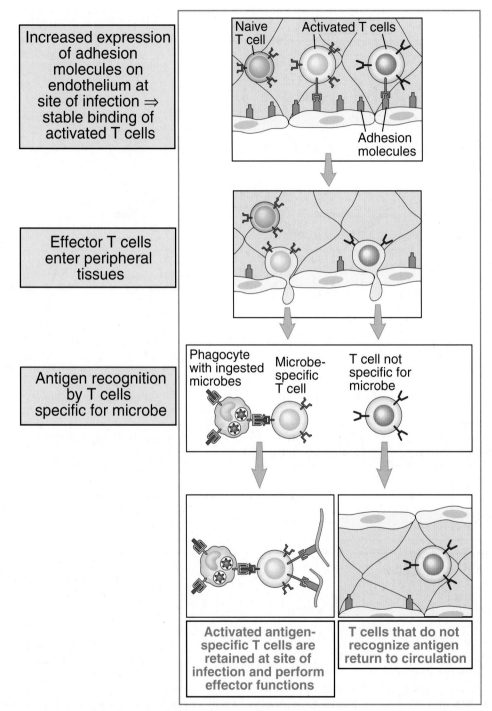

Figure 6–4 **Migration and retention of effector T cells at sites of infection.** Effector T cells migrate to sites of infection by using receptors to bind to ligands that are induced on endothelium by cytokines produced during innate immune reactions to microbes. T cells that recognize microbial antigens in extravascular tissues are retained at these sites by integrin-mediated adhesion to the extracellular matrix. These antigen-specific T cells perform their effector function of eradicating the infection, whereas T cells that do not see antigen return via lymphatic vessels to the circulation.

expression and binding affinity of VLA integrins on the T cells. Some of these integrins specifically bind to molecules present in the extracellular matrix, such as hyaluronic acid and fibronectin. Therefore, the antigen-stimulated lymphocytes adhere firmly to the tissue near the antigen and the cells stay long enough to respond to the microbe and eradicate the infection. Lymphocytes that enter the tissue but do not recognize an antigen are not activated to adhere. They enter lymphatic vessels draining the tissue and return to the circulation, prepared to home to another site of infection in search of the microbial antigen for which they are specific.

The net result of this sequence of cell migration and retention is that effector T lymphocytes, which were produced in the peripheral lymphoid organs in response to an infection, are able to locate that infectious microbe at any site in the body. These effector lymphocytes are activated by the microbe and respond in ways that eliminate the microbe. In contrast to the activation of naive T cells, which requires antigen presentation and costimulation by professional antigen-presenting cells (APCs), differentiated effector cells are activated by antigen recognition and appear to be less dependent on costimulation than are naive cells. Because of this difference, the proliferation and differentiation of naive T cells are confined to lymphoid organs where professional APCs display antigens, but the functions of effector T cells may be directed at any host cell displaying microbial antigens, not just professional APCs.

Although both CD4$^+$ helper T lymphocytes and CD8$^+$ cytolytic T lymphocytes (CTLs) produce cytokines that participate in eliminating infections, CTLs also employ a distinct mechanism to directly kill infected cells. Therefore, we will discuss the effector mechanisms of these lymphocyte classes individually and conclude by describing how the two classes of lymphocytes may cooperate to get rid of intracellular microbes.

Effector Functions of CD4$^+$ T Lymphocytes

Cell-mediated immunity was discovered as a form of immunity to an intracellular bacterial infection that could be transferred from immune animals to naive animals by cells (now known to be T lymphocytes) but not by serum antibodies (Fig. 6-5). It was known from the earliest studies that the specificity of cell-mediated immunity against different microbes was a function of the lymphocytes, but the elimination of the microbes was a function of activated macrophages. The roles of T lymphocytes and phagocytes in cell-mediated immunity are now well understood.

In cell-mediated immunity, CD4$^+$ T lymphocytes of the T_H1 subset activate macrophages that have phagocytosed microbes, resulting in increased microbicidal activities of the phagocytes and killing of the ingested microbes. The ability of T cells to activate macrophages is dependent on antigen recognition, accounting for the specificity of the reaction. Essentially, the same reaction may be elicited by injecting a microbial protein into the skin of an individual who has been immunized against the microbe by prior infection or vaccination. This reaction is called **delayed-type hypersensitivity (DTH),** because it occurs 24 to 48 hours after an immunized individual is challenged with a microbial protein (i.e., the reaction is delayed) and because it reflects an increased sensitivity to antigen challenge. The delay occurs because it takes 24 to 48 hours for circulating effector T lymphocytes to home to the site of antigen challenge, respond to the antigen at this site, and induce a detectable reaction. DTH reactions are manifested by infiltrates of T cells and monocytes into the tissues, edema and fibrin deposition caused by increased vascular permeability in response to cytokines produced by CD4$^+$ T cells, and tissue damage induced by the products of macrophages activated by T cells (Fig. 6-6). DTH reactions are often used to determine if individuals have been previously exposed to and have responded to an antigen. For instance, a DTH reaction to a mycobacterial antigen (called PPD, for purified protein derivative) is an indicator of a T cell response to the mycobacteria. This is the basis for the PPD skin test, which is frequently used to detect past or active mycobacterial infection.

The following section describes how T lymphocytes activate macrophages and how the macrophages eliminate phagocytosed microbes.

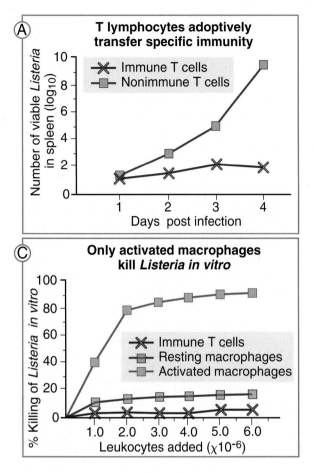

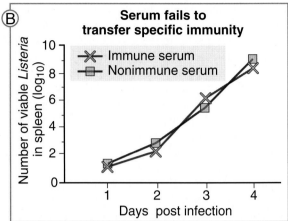

Figure 6–5 Cell-mediated immunity to an intracellular bacterium, *Listeria monocytogenes*. In this experiment, lymphocytes or serum (a source of antibodies) was taken from a mouse that had previously been exposed to a sublethal dose of *Listeria* bacteria (immune mouse) and transferred to a normal (naive) mouse, and the recipient of the "adoptive transfer" was challenged with the bacteria. The numbers of bacteria were measured in the spleen of the recipient mouse to determine if the transfer had conferred immunity. Protection against bacterial challenge (seen by reduced recovery of live bacteria) was induced by the transfer of immune lymphoid cells, now known to be T cells (A), but not by the transfer of serum (B). The bacteria were killed *in vitro* by activated macrophages but not by T cells (C). Therefore, protection is dependent on antigen-specific T lymphocytes, but bacterial killing is the function of activated macrophages.

T Cell–Mediated Macrophage Activation

Effector T lymphocytes of the T_H1 subset that recognize macrophage-associated antigens activate the macrophages by CD40 ligand–CD40 interactions and by secreting the macrophage-activating cytokine interferon-γ (IFN-γ) (Fig. 6-7). As we discussed in Chapter 3, macrophages ingest microbes into intracellular vesicles, called phagosomes, that fuse with lysosomes to form phagolysosomes. The microbial proteins in these vesicles are processed, and a few microbial peptides are displayed by class II MHC molecules on the surface of the macrophages. Effector CD4$^+$ T cells specific for these peptides recognize the class II–associated peptides. The T cells respond by expressing on their surface the effector molecule CD40 ligand (CD40L, or CD154), which binds to the CD40 receptor that is expressed on macrophages. At the same time, the effector T cells, being of the T_H1 subset, secrete the macrophage-activating cytokine IFN-γ, which binds to its receptors on macrophages. Binding of IFN-γ to its receptor functions together with engagement of CD40 to trigger biochemical signaling pathways that lead to the production of several transcription factors. These transcription factors turn on the transcription of genes that encode lysosomal proteases and enzymes that stimulate the synthesis of microbicidal reactive oxygen intermediates and nitric oxide. The requirement for the membrane-associated CD40L–CD40 interaction ensures that macrophages that are in direct contact with T cells are the ones

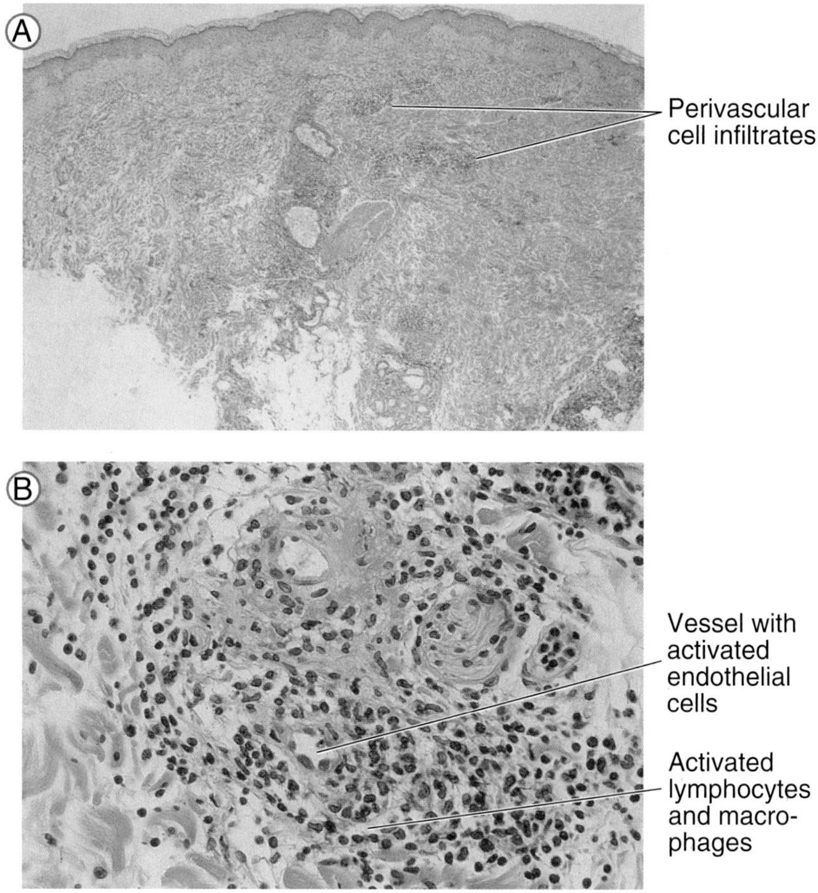

Figure 6–6 **The morphology of a delayed-type hypersensitivity (DTH) reaction.** In an individual previously exposed to an antigen, skin challenge with that antigen elicits a DTH reaction. Histopathologic examination of the reaction shows perivascular mononuclear cell infiltrates in the dermis (A). At higher magnification, the infiltrate is seen to consist of activated lymphocytes and macrophages surrounding small blood vessels in which the endothelial cells are activated (B). (Courtesy of Dr. J. Faix, Department of Pathology, Stanford University School of Medicine, Palo Alto, CA.)

Perivascular cell infiltrates

Vessel with activated endothelial cells

Activated lymphocytes and macrophages

that are activated best. The macrophages that contact T cells are also the macrophages that are presenting antigens of phagocytosed microbes, and these are the phagocytes that need to be activated. The secreted IFN-γ enhances macrophage activation and amplifies the response.

The interaction between macrophages and T lymphocytes is an excellent example of bidirectional interactions between cells of the innate and adaptive immune systems (i.e., macrophages and T lymphocytes) (Fig. 6-8). Macrophages that have phagocytosed microbes produce the cytokine IL-12. IL-12 stimulates the differentiation of naive CD4⁺ T cells to the T_H1 subset, which produces IFN-γ on encountering macrophage-associated microbial antigens; IL-12 also increases the amount of IFN-γ pro-

duced by these T cells. The IFN-γ then activates the phagocytes to kill the ingested microbes, thus completing the circle.

CD4⁺ T lymphocytes perform functions in addition to macrophage activation in cell-mediated immune reactions. Antigen-stimulated CD4⁺ T cells secrete cytokines such as TNF, which act on vascular endothelium to increase the expression of adhesion molecules and production of chemokines. As a result, more T cells and other leukocytes, including blood neutrophils and monocytes, are recruited into the site of infection. Thus, the T cell response is amplified, and additional phagocytes are called in to assist in eradicating the infection. This T cell–stimulated cellular infiltration, and an accompanying vascular reaction, are typical of inflammation. Inflammation is a compo-

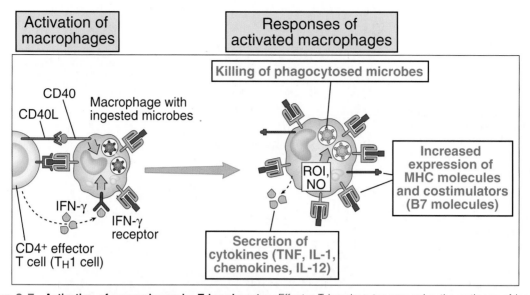

Figure 6–7 **Activation of macrophages by T lymphocytes.** Effector T lymphocytes recognize the antigens of ingested microbes on macrophages. In response to this recognition, the T lymphocytes express CD40L, which engages CD40 on the macrophages, and the T cells secrete IFN-γ, which binds to IFN-γ receptors on the macrophages. This combination of signals activates the macrophages to produce microbicidal substances that kill the ingested microbes. Activated macrophages also secrete cytokines that induce inflammation (TNF, IL-1, chemokines) and activate T cells (IL-12), and they express more MHC molecules and costimulators, which enhance T cell responses. The illustration shows a CD4+ T cell recognizing class II MHC–associated peptides and activating the macrophage, but the same reaction may be elicited by a CD8+ T cell that recognizes class I MHC–displayed peptides derived from cytoplasmic microbial antigens.

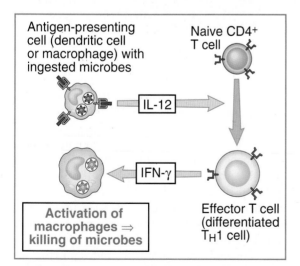

Figure 6–8 **Cytokine-mediated interactions between T lymphocytes and macrophages in cell-mediated immunity.** Macrophages that encounter microbes secrete the cytokine IL-12, which stimulates naive CD4+ T cells to differentiate into IFN-γ–secreting TH1 cells and enhances IFN-γ production. IFN-γ activates the macrophages to kill ingested microbes.

nent of T cell–mediated reactions, such as DTH, and is also seen in innate immune reactions to microbes (see Chapter 2). In addition to their role in helping macrophages eradicate phagocytosed microbes, CD4+ T cells help CD8+ T cells to differentiate into active CTLs and help B lymphocytes to differentiate into antibody-producing cells (see Chapters 5 and 7).

CD8+ T lymphocytes that recognize class I MHC–associated microbial peptides on macrophages are also able to activate macrophages to kill intracellular microbes. Recall that class I MHC–associated peptides are produced from cytoplasmic proteins, which may be derived from phagocytosed microbes (and, of course, from infection of nonphagocytic cells). Some microbes are ingested by macrophages into vesicles, and the microbes or their proteins pass through the membranes of the vesicles into the cytoplasm, where they are processed into class I MHC–binding peptides. In such infections, CD8+ T cells also function to activate the macrophages, by essentially the same mechanism as that used by CD4+ cells, namely, CD40L- and IFN-γ–mediated activation. Macrophage activation is not useful for defense against microbes, such as viruses, that live and replicate only in the cytoplasm, because the microbicidal mechanisms of macrophages are largely limited to vesicles. Obviously, macrophage activation is also of little value for eliminating viral infections of cells other than these phagocytes.

Elimination of Microbes by Activated Macrophages

Macrophage activation leads to the expression of enzymes that catalyze the production of microbicidal substances in phagosomes and phagolysosomes (see Fig. 6-7). We described the microbicidal mechanisms of activated phagocytes in Chapter 2, when we discussed the role of phagocytes in innate immunity (see Fig. 2-7, Chapter 2). To reiterate the key points, the major microbicidal substances produced in the lysosomes of macrophages are reactive oxygen intermediates (ROIs), nitric oxide (NO), and proteolytic enzymes. These mechanisms are activated in innate immunity when macrophages encounter microbes. As described previously, effector T_H1 cells are potent activators of the same microbicidal mechanisms in cell-mediated immunity. Cell-mediated immunity is critical for host defense in two situations: when macrophages are not activated by the microbes themselves (i.e., when innate immunity is ineffective) and when pathogenic microbes have evolved to resist the defense mechanisms of innate immunity. In these situations, the additional macrophage activation by T cells changes the balance between microbes and host defense in favor of the macrophages, thus serving to eradicate intracellular infections.

The substances that are toxic to microbes may injure normal tissues if they are released into the extracellular milieu, because these substances do not distinguish between microbes and host cells. This is the reason for tissue injury (a reflection of "hypersensitivity") in DTH reactions, which often accompany protective cell-mediated immunity. It is also the reason why prolonged macrophage activation in chronic cell-mediated immune reactions is associated with considerable injury to adjacent normal tissues. For instance, in mycobacterial infections, which are difficult to eradicate, much of the pathology is caused by a sustained T cell and macrophage response that attempts to wall off the bacteria. Histologically, such chronic cell-mediated immune responses often appear as granulomas, which are collections of activated lymphocytes and macrophages with fibrosis and tissue necrosis around the microbe.

Activated macrophages serve several roles, in addition to killing microbes, that are important in cell-mediated immunity (see Fig. 6-8 and Fig. 2-8, Chapter 2). Activated macrophages secrete cytokines, including TNF, IL-1, and chemokines, which stimulate the recruitment of neutrophils, monocytes, and effector T lymphocytes to the site of infection. Macrophages produce other cytokines, such as platelet-derived growth factor, that stimulate the growth and activities of fibroblasts and endothelial cells, helping to repair tissue after the infection is cleared. Macrophage activation also leads to the increased expression of class II MHC molecules and costimulators on these cells, thus enhancing their antigen-presenting function, which promotes T cell activation and amplifies the cell-mediated immune reaction.

Role of T_H2 Cells in Cell-Mediated Immunity

The T_H2 subset of CD4+ T lymphocytes stimulates eosinophil-rich inflammation and also functions to limit the injurious consequences of macrophage activation. When differentiated T_H2 cells recognize antigens, the cells produce the cytokines IL-4 and IL-5 (and also IL-10, which is produced by many other cell populations). IL-4 stimulates the production of IgE antibody, and IL-5 activates eosinophils. This reaction is important for defense against helminthic infections, because eosinophils bind to IgE-coated helminths and the helminths are killed by the granule proteins of eosinophils.

Several cytokines produced by T_H2 cells, including IL-4, IL-10, and IL-13, also inhibit macrophage activation. Because of this action, T_H2 cells may serve to terminate T_H1-mediated DTH reactions and thus limit the tissue injury that often accompanies T_H1 cell–mediated protective immunity. The relative activation of T_H1 and T_H2 cells in response to an infectious microbe may determine the outcome of the infection (Fig. 6-9). For instance, the protozoan

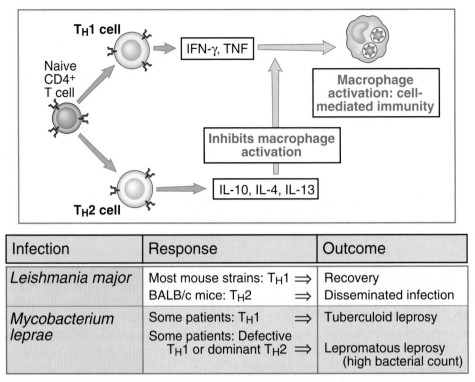

Infection	Response	Outcome
Leishmania major	Most mouse strains: $T_H1 \Rightarrow$ BALB/c mice: $T_H2 \quad\Rightarrow$	Recovery Disseminated infection
Mycobacterium leprae	Some patients: $T_H1 \quad\Rightarrow$ Some patients: Defective T_H1 or dominant $T_H2 \Rightarrow$	Tuberculoid leprosy Lepromatous leprosy (high bacterial count)

Figure 6–9   The balance between T_H1 and T_H2 cell activation determines the outcome of intracellular infections. Naive $CD4^+$ T lymphocytes may differentiate into T_H1 cells, which activate phagocytes to kill ingested microbes, and T_H2 cells, which inhibit macrophage activation. The balance between these two subsets may influence the outcome of infections, as illustrated by *Leishmania* infection in mice and leprosy in humans.

parasite *Leishmania major* lives inside macrophages and its elimination requires the activation of the macrophages by *L. major*–specific T_H1 cells. Most inbred strains of mice make an effective T_H1 response to the parasite and are thus able to eradicate the infection. In some inbred mouse strains the response to *L. major* is dominated by T_H2 cells, and these mice succumb to the infection. *Mycobacterium leprae*, the bacterium that causes leprosy, is a pathogen for humans that also lives inside macrophages and may be eliminated by cell-mediated immunity. Some individuals infected with *M. leprae* are unable to eradicate the infection and develop destructive lesions, called lepromatous leprosy. In contrast, other patients develop strong cell-mediated immunity with activated T cells and macrophages around the infection and few surviving bacteria; this form of less destructive disease is called tuberculoid leprosy. Some studies have shown that the tuberculoid form is associated with the activation of *M. leprae*–specific T_H1 cells, whereas the destructive lepromatous form is associated with a defect in T_H1 cell activation and a dominant T_H2 response. The same principle, that the T cell cytokine response to an infectious pathogen is an important determinant of the outcome of the infection, may be true for many other infectious diseases.

As we mentioned earlier, activated macrophages are best at killing microbes that are confined to vesicles, but microbes that directly enter the cytoplasm (e.g., viruses) or escape from phagosomes into the cytoplasm (e.g., some phagocytosed bacteria) are relatively resistant to the microbicidal mechanisms of phagocytes. Eradication of such pathogens requires the second major effector mechanism of cell-mediated immunity, namely, cytolytic T lymphocytes (CTLs).

Effector Functions of CD8⁺ Cytolytic T Lymphocytes

CD8⁺ CTLs recognize class I MHC–associated peptides on infected cells and kill these cells, thus eliminating the reservoir of infection (Fig. 6-10). The sources of class I–associated peptides are protein antigens synthesized in the cytoplasm and protein antigens of phagocytosed microbes that escape from phagocytic vesicles into the cytoplasm (see Chapter 3). Differentiated CD8⁺ CTLs recognize class I MHC–peptide complexes on the surface of infected cells by their T cell receptor (TCR) and by the CD8 coreceptor. (These infected cells are also called "targets" of CTLs, because they are destined to be killed by the CTLs.) Cytolytic T lymphocytes adhere tightly to cells, mainly by virtue of integrins on the CTLs binding to their ligands on the infected cells. The antigen receptors and coreceptors of the CTL cluster at the site of contact with the target cell. The CTLs are activated by antigen recognition and firm adhesion; at this stage in their lives, the CTLs do not require costimulation or T cell help for activation. Therefore, differentiated CTLs are able to kill any infected cell in any tissue.

Antigen recognition by effector CTLs results in the activation of signal transduction pathways that lead to the exocytosis of the contents of the CTL's granules to the region of contact with the targets. CTLs kill target cells mainly as a result of their granule contents creating pores in target cell membranes and introducing into the target cells substances that induce DNA fragmentation and apoptosis. The pore-forming protein of CTL granules is called **perforin.** When perforin is secreted from CTLs, it inserts into the target cell membrane and is induced to polymerize by the high concentration of Ca^{2+} ions present in the extracellular environment. Polymerized perforin forms a pore in the target cell membrane. At the same time the CTLs secrete granule enzymes called **granzymes,** which enter target cells through the perforin pores or by binding to receptors on target cell membranes followed by endocytosis. Granzymes cleave and thereby activate enzymes called caspases that are present in the cytoplasm of the target cells, and the active caspases induce apoptosis. (Caspases

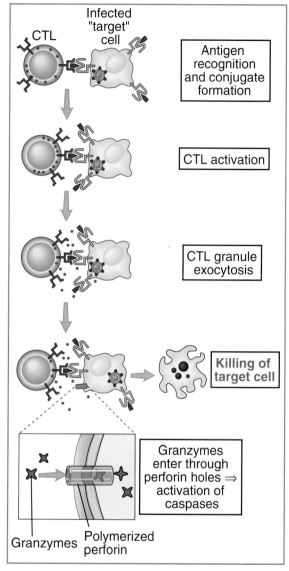

Figure 6–10 Mechanisms of killing of infected cells by CD8⁺ CTLs. CTLs recognize class I MHC–associated peptides of cytoplasmic microbes in infected cells and form tight adhesions ("conjugates") with these cells. Adhesion molecules, such as integrins, stabilize the binding of the CTLs to infected cells (not shown). The CTLs are activated to release ("exocytose") their granule contents toward the infected cell (referred to as "targets" of CTL killing). The granule contents include perforin, which forms pores in the target cell membrane, and granzymes, which enter the target cell through these pores (or by receptor-mediated endocytosis) and induce apoptosis.

are so named because they are cysteine proteases that cleave proteins at aspartic acid residues; their major function is to induce apoptosis.) Activated CTLs also express a membrane protein called Fas ligand, which binds to a death-inducing receptor, called Fas (CD95), on target cells (see Chapter 9, Fig. 9-6). Engagement of Fas activates caspases and induces target cell apoptosis; this pathway of CTL killing does not require granule exocytosis and is probably a minor pathway. The net result of these effector mechanisms of CTLs is that the infected cells are killed. Cells that have undergone apoptosis are rapidly phagocytosed and eliminated. The mechanisms that induce fragmentation of target cell DNA, which is the hallmark of apoptosis, may also break down the DNA of microbes living inside the infected cells. Each CTL can kill a target cell, detach, and go on to kill additional targets.

As we mentioned earlier, CD8+ T lymphocytes also secrete the cytokine IFN-γ, which activates macrophages to destroy phagocytosed microbes and enhance the recruitment of additional leukocytes. Thus, CD8+ CTLs, like CD4+ helper cells, contribute to the elimination of microbes ingested by phagocytes.

Although we have described the effector functions of CD4+ T cells and CD8+ T cells separately, it is clear from our discussion that these types of T lymphocytes function cooperatively to eradicate intracellular microbes (Fig. 6-11). If microbes are phagocytosed and remain sequestered in macrophage vesicles, CD4+ T cells may be enough to eradicate these infections by secreting IFN-γ and activating the microbicidal mechanisms of the macrophages. If, however, the microbes are able to escape from vesicles into the cytoplasm, they become insusceptible to T cell–mediated macrophage activation, and their elimination requires killing of the infected cells by CD8+ CTLs.

Resistance of Pathogenic Microbes to Cell-Mediated Immunity

Different microbes have evolved diverse mechanisms to resist T lymphocyte-mediated host defense (Fig. 6-12). Many intracellular bacteria, such as *Mycobacterium tuberculosis*, *Legionella pneumophila*, and *Listeria monocytogenes*, inhibit the fusion of

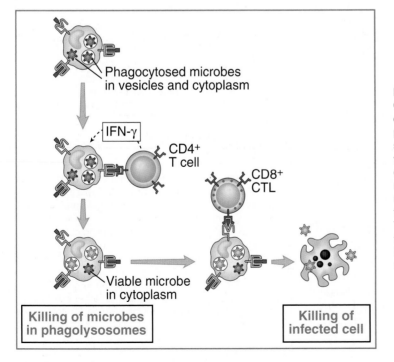

Figure 6–11 Cooperation between CD4+ and CD8+ T cells in the eradication of intracellular infections. In a macrophage infected by an intracellular bacterium, some of the bacteria are sequestered in vesicles (phagosomes) and others may escape into the cytoplasm. CD4+ T cells recognize antigens derived from the vesicular microbes and activate the macrophage to kill the microbes in the vesicles. CD8+ T cells recognize antigens derived from the cytoplasmic bacteria and are needed to kill the infected cell, thus eliminating the reservoir of infection.

Microbe	Mechanism	
Mycobacteria	Inhibition of phagolysosome fusion	Phagosome with ingested mycobacteria / Lysosome with enzymes / Mycobacteria survive within phagosome
Herpes simplex virus (HSV)	Inhibition of antigen presentation: HSV peptide interferes with TAP transporter	Cytosolic protein / Proteasome / ER / TAP / CD8+ CTL — Inhibition of proteasomal activity: EBV, human CMV / Block in TAP transport: HSV / Removal of class I from ER: CMV — Inhibition of antigen presentation
Cytomegalovirus (CMV)	Inhibition of antigen presentation: inhibition of proteasomal activity; removal of class I MHC molecules from endoplasmic reticulum (ER)	
Epstein-Barr virus (EBV)	Inhibition of antigen presentation: inhibition of proteasomal activity	
Epstein-Barr virus (EBV)	Production of IL-10, inhibition of macrophage activation	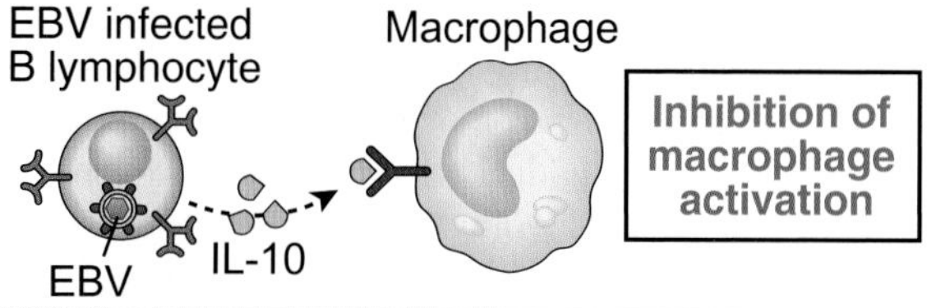 EBV infected B lymphocyte / Macrophage / EBV / IL-10 — Inhibition of macrophage activation
Pox virus	Inhibition of effector cell activation: production of soluble cytokine receptors	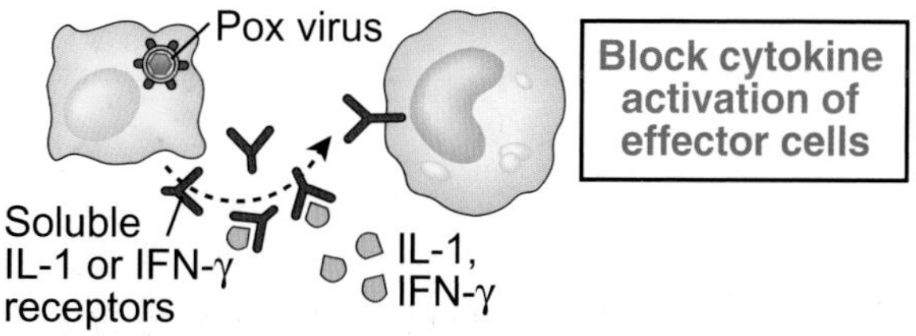 Pox virus / Soluble IL-1 or IFN-γ receptors / IL-1, IFN-γ — Block cytokine activation of effector cells

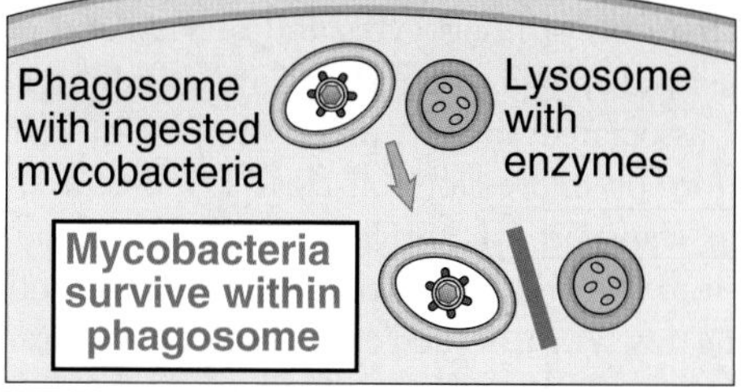

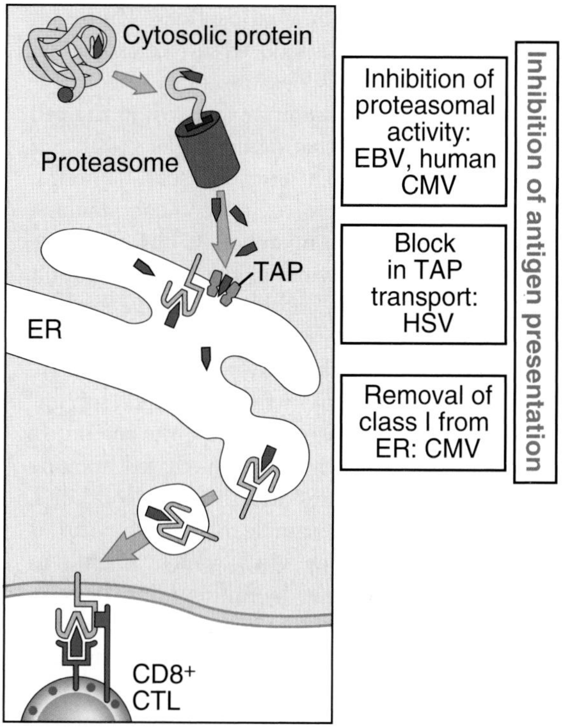

Figure 6–12 Evasion of cell-mediated immunity by microbes. Different bacteria and viruses resist the effector mechanisms of cell-mediated immunity by different mechanisms, selected examples of which are shown in this figure. *TAP*, transporter associated with antigen processing.

phagosomes with lysosomes and create pores in phagosome membranes, escaping into the cytoplasm. Thus, these microbes are able to resist the microbicidal mechanisms of phagocytes and survive and even replicate inside phagocytes. Many viruses inhibit class I MHC–associated antigen processing, by inhibiting production or expression of class I molecules, by blocking transport of antigenic peptides from the cytosol into the endoplasmic reticulum (ER), and by removing newly synthesized class I molecules from the ER. All these viral mechanisms reduce the loading of class I MHC molecules by viral peptides. The result of this defective loading is reduced surface expression of class I MHC molecules, because empty class I molecules are unstable and are not expressed on the cell surface. It is interesting that natural killer (NK) cells are activated by class I–deficient cells (see Chapter 2). Thus, host defenses evolve to combat immune evasion mechanisms of microbes: CTLs recognize class I MHC–associated viral peptides, viruses inhibit class I MHC expression, and NK cells have evolved to recognize the absence of class I MHC molecules. Other viruses produce inhibitory cytokines, or soluble ("decoy") cytokine receptors that bind and "sop up" cytokines such as IFN-γ, thus reducing the amount of cytokines available to trigger cell-mediated immune reactions. Yet other viruses directly infect and kill T lymphocytes; the best example of such a virus is human immunodeficiency virus, which is able to survive in infected persons by killing CD4$^+$ T cells. The outcome of infections is influenced by the strength of host defenses and the ability of pathogens to resist these defenses. The same principle is evident when the effector mechanisms of humoral immunity are considered.

One approach for tilting the balance between the host and microbes in favor of protective immunity is to vaccinate individuals to enhance immune responses. The principles of vaccination strategies are described at the end of Chapter 8, after the discussion of humoral immunity.

SUMMARY

▶ Cell-mediated immunity is the arm of adaptive immunity that eradicates infections by intracellular microbes. Cell-mediated immune reactions are of two types: CD4$^+$ T cells activate macrophages to kill ingested microbes that are able to survive in the vesicles of the phagocytes, and CD8$^+$ CTLs kill cells harboring microbes in their cytoplasm, thus eliminating reservoirs of infection.

▶ Effector T cells are generated in peripheral lymphoid organs, mainly lymph nodes draining sites of microbe entry, by the activation of naive T lymphocytes. The effector T cells are able to migrate to any site of infection.

▶ The migration of effector T cells is controlled by adhesion molecules, which are induced on these cells after activation and bind to their ligands, which are induced on endothelial cells by microbes and by cytokines produced during innate immune responses to microbes. The migration of T cells is independent of antigen, but cells that recognize microbial antigens in tissues are retained at these sites.

▶ Effector cells of the T$_H$1 subset of CD4$^+$ T cells recognize the antigens of microbes that have been ingested by macrophages. These T cells express CD40 ligand and secrete IFN-γ, which function cooperatively to activate macrophages.

▶ Activated macrophages produce substances, including reactive oxygen intermediates, nitric oxide, and lysosomal enzymes, that kill ingested microbes. Macrophages also produce cytokines that induce inflammation and other cytokines that promote fibrosis and tissue repair.

▶ Effector CD4$^+$ T cells of the T$_H$2 subset stimulate eosinophilic inflammation and inhibit macrophage activation. Eosinophils are important in host defense against helminthic parasites. The balance between activation of T$_H$1 and T$_H$2 cells determines the outcomes of many infections, with T$_H$1 cells promoting and T$_H$2 cells suppressing defense against intracellular microbes.

▶ CD8$^+$ T cells differentiate into CTLs that kill infected cells, mainly by inducing DNA fragmentation and apoptosis. CD4$^+$ and CD8$^+$ T cells often function cooperatively to eradicate intracellular infections.

▶ Many pathogenic microbes have evolved mechanisms to resist cell-mediated immunity. These mechanisms include inhibiting phagolysosome fusion, escaping from the vesicles of phagocytes, inhibiting the assembly of class I MHC–peptide complexes, and producing inhibitory cytokines or decoy cytokine receptors.

Review Questions

1 What are the types of T lymphocyte–mediated immune reactions that eliminate microbes that are sequestered in the vesicles of phagocytes and microbes that live in the cytoplasm of infected host cells?

2 Why do differentiated effector T cells (which have been activated by antigen) migrate preferentially to tissues that are sites of infection and not to lymph nodes?

3 What are the mechanisms by which T cells activate macrophages, and what are the responses of macrophages that result in the killing of ingested microbes?

4 What are the roles of T_H1 and T_H2 cells in defense against intracellular microbes and helminthic parasites?

5 How do CD8$^+$ CTLs kill cells infected with viruses?

6 What are some of the mechanisms by which intracellular microbes resist the effector mechanisms of cell-mediated immunity?

Humoral Immune Responses

7

Activation of B Lymphocytes and Production of Antibodies

Humoral immunity is mediated by antibodies and is the arm of the adaptive immune response that functions to neutralize and eliminate extracellular microbes and microbial toxins. Humoral immunity is more important than cellular immunity in defending against microbes with capsules rich in polysaccharides and lipids, and against polysaccharide and lipid toxins. The reason for this is that B cells respond to, and produce antibodies specific for, many types of molecules, but T cells, the mediators of cellular immunity, recognize and respond only to protein antigens. Antibodies are produced by B lymphocytes and their progeny. Naive B lymphocytes recognize antigens but do not secrete antibodies, and activation of these cells stimulates their differentiation into antibody-secreting effector cells. In this chapter, the process and mechanisms of B cell activation and antibody production are described, with the focus on the following questions:

- How are receptor-expressing B lymphocytes activated and converted to antibody-secreting cells?

- How is the process of B cell activation regulated so that the most useful types of antibodies are produced in response to different types of microbes?

Chapter 8 describes how the antibodies that are produced during humoral immune responses function to defend individuals against microbes and toxins.

Phases and Types of Humoral Immune Responses

Naive B lymphocytes express two classes of membrane-bound antibodies, IgM and IgD, that function as the receptors for antigens. These naive B cells are activated by antigens and by other signals that are discussed later in the chapter. The activation of B lymphocytes results in the proliferation of antigen-specific cells, also called clonal expansion, and their differentiation into effector cells that actively secrete antibodies (Fig. 7-1). The secreted antibodies have the same specificity as the naive B cell membrane receptors that recognized antigen to initiate the response. During their differentiation, some B cells may begin to produce antibodies of different heavy chain classes (or isotypes), which mediate different effector functions and are specialized to combat different types of microbes. This process is called **heavy chain class (isotype) switching.** Repeated exposure to a protein antigen results in the production of antibodies with increasing affinity for the antigen. This process is called **affinity maturation,** and it leads to the production of antibodies with improved capacity to bind to and neutralize microbes and their toxins.

Antibody responses to different antigens are classified as T-dependent or T-independent, based

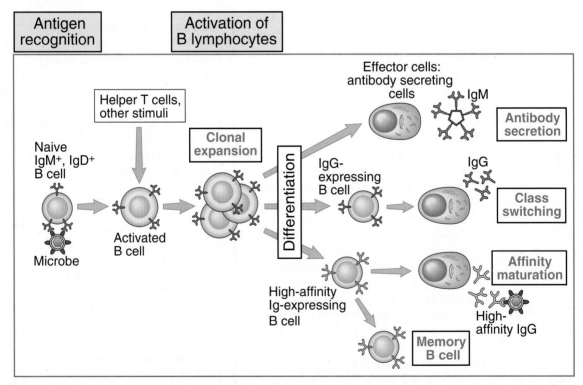

Figure 7–1   Phases of humoral immune responses. Naive B lymphocytes recognize antigens, and under the influence of helper T cells and other stimuli (not shown), the B cells are activated to proliferate, giving rise to clonal expansion, and to differentiate into antibody-secreting effector cells. Some of the activated B cells undergo heavy chain class switching and affinity maturation, and some become long-lived memory cells.

on the requirement for T cell help. B lymphocytes recognize and are activated by a wide variety of antigens, including proteins, polysaccharides, lipids, and small chemicals. Protein antigens are processed in antigen-presenting cells and recognized by helper T lymphocytes, which play an important role in B cell activation and are powerful inducers of heavy chain class switching and affinity maturation. (The term *helper* T lymphocytes came from the discovery that some T cells stimulate, or help, B lymphocytes to produce antibodies.) In the absence of T cell help, protein antigens elicit weak or no antibody responses. Therefore, protein antigens, and the antibody responses to these antigens, are called "T-dependent." Polysaccharides, lipids, and other nonprotein antigens stimulate antibody production without the involvement of helper T cells. Therefore, these nonprotein antigens, and the antibody responses to them, are called "T-independent." The antibodies produced in response to T-independent antigens show relatively little heavy chain class switching and affinity maturation. We know a great deal about the role of helper T cells in antibody production, and much of this chapter is devoted to antibody responses to T-dependent protein antigens. Responses to T-independent antigens are discussed further at the end of the chapter.

Antibody responses to the first and subsequent exposures to an antigen, called primary and secondary responses, differ quantitatively and qualitatively (Fig. 7-2). The amounts of antibody produced after the first encounter with an antigen (i.e., primary responses) are smaller than the amounts of antibody produced on repeated immunization (i.e., secondary responses). With protein antigens, secondary responses also show increased heavy chain class switching and affinity maturation, because repeated stimulation by an antigen leads to increases in the numbers of helper T lymphocytes.

With this introduction, the discussion proceeds to the stimuli that activate B lymphocytes, how naive B cells differentiate into antibody-secreting cells, and the processes of heavy chain class switching and affinity maturation. The activation of naive B lymphocytes is initiated by the recognition of antigen. Therefore, the discussion begins with a description of how B cells recognize and respond to these antigens.

Stimulation of B Lymphocytes by Antigen

Humoral immune responses are initiated when antigen-specific B lymphocytes in the lymphoid follicles of the spleen, lymph nodes, and mucosal lymphoid tissues recognize antigens. Some of the antigens of microbes that enter tissues or are present in the blood are transported to and concentrated in the B cell–rich follicles of the peripheral lymphoid organs; the mechanisms responsible for this uptake of antigen into the B cell zones are not well defined. B lymphocytes specific for an antigen use their membrane-bound immunoglobulin (Ig) receptors to recognize the antigen in its native conformation (i.e., without a need for processing). The recognition of antigen triggers signaling pathways that initiate B cell activation. As for T lymphocytes, B cell activation also requires second signals, many of which are produced during innate immune reactions to microbes. In the following section, the signals for B cell activation are described, followed by discussion of the functional consequences of these signals.

Antigen-Induced Signaling in B Cells

Antigen-induced clustering of membrane Ig receptors triggers biochemical signals that are transduced by receptor-associated signaling molecules (Fig. 7-3). The process of B lymphocyte activation is, in principle, similar to the activation of T cells (see Chapter 5). In B cells, Ig receptor–mediated signal transduction requires the bringing together (cross-linking) of two or more receptor molecules. Receptor cross-linking occurs when two or more antigen molecules in an aggregate, or repeating epitopes of one antigen molecule, bind to adjacent Ig molecules in the membrane of a B cell. Polysaccharides, lipids, and other nonprotein antigens often contain multiple identical epitopes in each molecule and are therefore able to bind to numerous Ig receptors on a B cell at the same time.

Signals initiated by antigen receptor cross-linking are transduced by receptor-associated proteins. Membrane IgM and IgD, the antigen receptors of naive B lymphocytes, are highly variable proteins with short

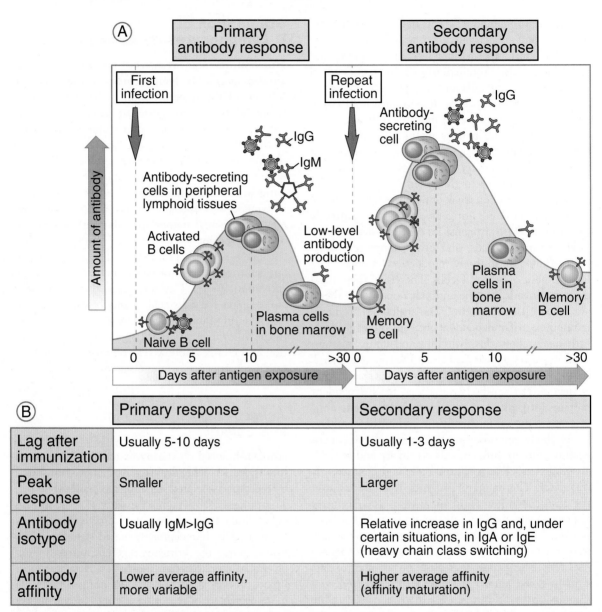

B	Primary response	Secondary response
Lag after immunization	Usually 5-10 days	Usually 1-3 days
Peak response	Smaller	Larger
Antibody isotype	Usually IgM>IgG	Relative increase in IgG and, under certain situations, in IgA or IgE (heavy chain class switching)
Antibody affinity	Lower average affinity, more variable	Higher average affinity (affinity maturation)

Figure 7–2 Features of primary and secondary antibody responses. Primary and secondary antibody responses differ in several respects, illustrated schematically in panel A and summarized in panel B. In a primary response, naive B cells in peripheral lymphoid tissues are activated to proliferate and differentiate into antibody-secreting cells and memory cells. Some antibody-secreting plasma cells may migrate to and survive in the bone marrow for long periods. In a secondary response, memory B cells are activated to produce larger amounts of antibodies, often with more heavy chain class switching and affinity maturation. Many of the features of secondary responses (e.g., heavy chain class switching and affinity maturation) are seen mainly in responses to protein antigens, because these changes in B cells are stimulated by helper T cells and only proteins activate T cells. The kinetics of the responses may vary with different antigens and types of immunization.

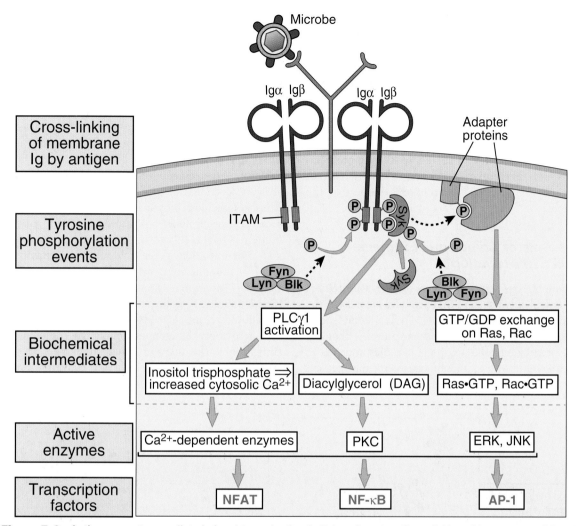

Figure 7–3 Antigen receptor–mediated signal transduction in B lymphocytes. Cross-linking of Ig receptors of B cells by antigen triggers biochemical signals that are transduced by the Ig-associated proteins Igα and Igβ. These signals induce early tyrosine phosphorylation events, activation of various biochemical intermediates and enzymes, and activation of transcription factors. Similar signaling events are seen in T cells after antigen recognition. Note that signaling requires cross-linking of at least two Ig receptors by antigens, but only a single receptor is shown for simplicity.

cytoplasmic domains. These membrane receptors recognize antigens but do not themselves transduce signals. The receptors are noncovalently attached to two proteins, called Igα and Igβ, to form the **B cell receptor (BCR) complex** (analogous to the T cell receptor [TCR] complex of T lymphocytes). The cytoplasmic domains of Igα and Igβ contain conserved immunoreceptor tyrosine-based activation motifs (ITAMs), which are found in signaling subunits of many other activating receptors in the immune system (e.g., the CD3 and ζ proteins of the TCR complex; see Chapter 5). When two or more antigen receptors of a B cell are clustered, the tyrosines in the ITAMs of Igα and Igβ are phosphorylated by kinases associated with the BCR complex. These phosphotyrosines become docking sites for adapter proteins that themselves get phosphorylated and then recruit a number of signaling molecules. The components of receptor-induced signaling cascades are not as well understood in B cells as they are in T lymphocytes, but the signaling events are essentially similar in the two lymphocyte populations (see Chapter 5, Fig. 5-14). The net result of receptor-induced signaling in B cells is the activation of transcription factors that turn on genes whose protein products are involved in B cell proliferation and differentiation. Some of the important proteins are described later in this section of the chapter.

The Role of Complement Proteins in B Cell Activation

B lymphocytes express a receptor for a protein of the complement system that provides signals for the activation of the cells (Fig. 7-4). The complement system is a collection of plasma proteins that are activated by microbes and by antibodies attached to microbes and whose function as effector mechanisms

of host defense is well known (see Chapter 8). When the complement system is activated by a microbe, the microbe becomes coated with breakdown products of the most abundant complement protein, C3. One of these breakdown products is a fragment called C3d. B lymphocytes express a receptor, called the type 2 complement receptor (CR2, or CD21), that binds C3d. B cells that are specific for a microbe's antigens recognize the antigen by their Ig receptors and simultaneously recognize the bound C3d by the CR2 receptor. Engagement of CR2 greatly enhances antigen-dependent activation responses of B cells. Thus, complement proteins provide second signals for B cell activation, functioning in concert with antigen (which is "signal 1") to initiate B cell proliferation and differentiation. This role of complement in humoral immune responses again illustrates an idea we have mentioned previously, that microbes or innate immune responses to microbes provide signals in addition to antigen that are necessary for lymphocyte activation. In humoral immunity, complement activation is the relevant innate immune response and C3d is the second signal for B lymphocytes,

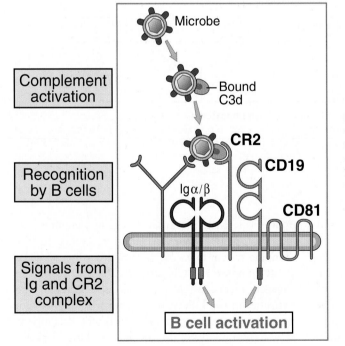

Figure 7-4   The role of the complement protein C3d in B cell activation. Activation of complement by microbes leads to the binding of a complement breakdown product, C3d, to the microbes. The B cell simultaneously recognizes a microbial antigen (by the Ig receptor) and bound C3d (by the CR2 receptor). CR2 is attached to a complex of proteins (CD19, CD81) that are involved in delivering activating signals to the B cell.

analogous to the costimulators of antigen-presenting cells for T lymphocytes.

Functional Consequences of Antigen-Mediated B Cell Activation

The consequences of B cell activation by antigen (and second signals) are to initiate B cell proliferation and differentiation and to prepare the B cells to interact with helper T lymphocytes (if the antigen is a protein) (Fig. 7-5). The activated B lymphocytes enter the cell cycle and begin to proliferate, resulting in expansion of the antigen-specific clones. The magnitude of B cell clonal expansion is not well defined. The cells may also begin to synthesize more IgM and to produce some of this IgM in a secreted form. Thus, antigen stimulation induces the early phase of the humoral immune response. This response is greatest when the antigen is multivalent, cross-links many antigen receptors, and activates complement strongly, all of which are typically seen with polysaccharides and other T-independent antigens (which are discussed in detail later in the chapter).

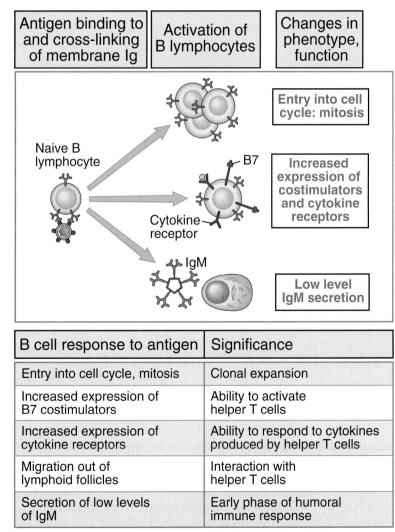

Figure 7–5 Functional consequences of Ig-mediated B cell activation. The activation of B cells by antigen in lymphoid organs initiates the process of B cell proliferation and IgM secretion and "prepares" the B cell to activate helper T cells and respond to T cell help by increasing the expression of costimulators and receptors for T cell cytokines and by stimulating migration of the B cells toward the T cell–rich zones of the lymphoid organs.

B cell response to antigen	Significance
Entry into cell cycle, mitosis	Clonal expansion
Increased expression of B7 costimulators	Ability to activate helper T cells
Increased expression of cytokine receptors	Ability to respond to cytokines produced by helper T cells
Migration out of lymphoid follicles	Interaction with helper T cells
Secretion of low levels of IgM	Early phase of humoral immune response

Most soluble protein antigens do not contain multiple identical epitopes, are not capable of cross-linking many receptors on B cells, and will therefore stimulate weak responses on their own. Antigen stimulation induces at least three other changes in B lymphocytes that enhance the ability of these B cells to interact with helper T lymphocytes. B cell activation leads to increased expression of B7 costimulators, which provide second signals for T cell activation, and the expression of receptors for cytokines, which are the secreted mediators of helper T cell functions. Activated B cells also reduce their expression of receptors for chemokines that are produced in lymphoid follicles and whose function is to keep the B cells in these follicles. As a result, the activated B cells migrate out of the follicles and toward the anatomic compartment where helper T cells are concentrated.

So far we have described how B lymphocytes recognize antigens and receive the signals that initiate humoral immune responses. As stated at the outset, antibody responses to protein antigens require the participation of helper T cells. In the next section the interactions of helper T cells with B lymphocytes are described.

The Function of Helper T Lymphocytes in Humoral Immune Responses to Protein Antigens

For a protein antigen to stimulate an antibody response, B lymphocytes and helper T lymphocytes specific for that antigen must come together in lymphoid organs and interact in a way that stimulates B cell proliferation and differentiation. We know this process works very efficiently, because protein antigens elicit excellent antibody responses within 3 to 7 days of antigen exposure. The efficiency of the process raises many questions. How do B cells and T cells specific for epitopes of the same antigen find one another, considering that both types of lymphocytes specific for any one antigen are rare, probably less than 1 in 100,000 of all the lymphocytes in the body? How do helper T cells specific for an antigen interact with B cells specific for the same antigen and not with irrelevant B cells? What signals are delivered by helper T cells that stimulate not only the secretion of antibody

but also the special features of the antibody response to proteins, namely, heavy chain class switching and affinity maturation? As is apparent in the discussion that follows, the answers to these questions are now well understood.

Activation and Migration of Helper T Cells

Helper T cells that have been activated to differentiate into effector cells interact with antigen-stimulated B lymphocytes at the edges of lymphoid follicles in the peripheral lymphoid organs (Fig. 7-6). Naive CD4+ helper T lymphocytes are stimulated to proliferate and differentiate into cytokine-producing effector cells as a result of recognizing antigens on professional antigen-presenting cells (APCs) in the lymphoid organs. The process of T cell activation was described in Chapter 5. To reiterate the important points, the initial activation of T cells requires antigen recognition and costimulation. Therefore, T cell activation is induced best by microbial antigens and by protein antigens that are administered with adjuvants, which stimulate the expression of costimulators on professional APCs. Also, the antigens that stimulate CD4+ helper T cells are derived from extracellular microbes and proteins that are processed and displayed bound to class II major histocompatibility complex (MHC) molecules of APCs in the T cell–rich zones of peripheral lymphoid tissues. Here, the CD4+ T cells that recognize the antigens may differentiate into effector cells capable of producing various cytokines; the T_H1 and T_H2 subsets described in Chapter 5 are examples of such differentiated effector cells. Differentiated effector T cells begin to migrate out of their normal sites of residence. As discussed in Chapter 6, some of these T lymphocytes enter the circulation, find microbial antigens at distant sites, and eradicate the microbes by the reactions of cell-mediated immunity. Other differentiated helper T cells migrate toward the edges of lymphoid follicles at the same time that antigen-stimulated B lymphocytes within the follicles are beginning to migrate outward. This directed migration of the B and T cells toward one another depends on changes in the expression of certain chemokine receptors on the activated lymphocytes and the production of the

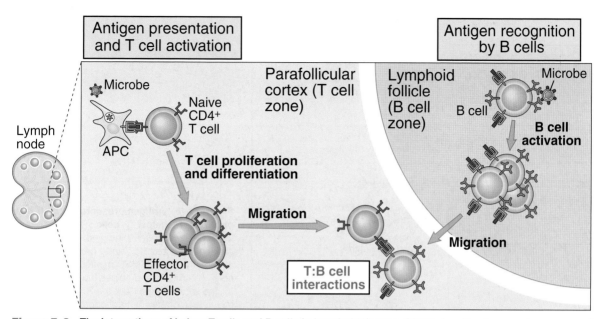

Figure 7–6   **The interactions of helper T cells and B cells in lymphoid tissues.** CD4[+] helper T cells recognize processed protein antigens displayed by professional APCs and are activated to proliferate and differentiate into effector cells. These effector T cells begin to migrate toward lymphoid follicles. Naive B lymphocytes, which reside in the follicles, recognize antigens in this site and are activated to migrate out of the follicles. The two cell populations come together at the edges of the follicles and interact.

chemokines that bind to these receptors in the follicles and T cell zones of the lymph node. The B and T cells encounter one another at the edges of lymphoid follicles, and the next step in their interaction occurs here.

Presentation of Antigens by B Lymphocytes to Helper T Cells

B lymphocytes that bind protein antigens by their specific antigen receptors endocytose these antigens, process them in endosomal vesicles, and display class II MHC–associated peptides for recognition by CD4[+] helper T cells (Fig. 7-7). The membrane Ig of B cells is a high-affinity receptor that enables a B cell to specifically bind a particular antigen even when the extracellular concentration of the antigen is very low. In addition, antigen bound by membrane Ig is endocytosed very efficiently and is delivered to the intracellular endosomal vesicles where proteins are processed into peptides that bind to class II MHC molecules (see Chapter 3). Therefore, B lymphocytes

are very efficient APCs for the antigens they specifically recognize. Note that any one B cell may bind a conformational epitope of a protein antigen, internalize and process the protein, and display multiple peptides of that protein for T cell recognition. Therefore, B cells and T cells recognize different epitopes of the same protein antigen. Because B cells present the antigen for which they have specific receptors, and helper T cells specifically recognize peptides derived from the same antigen, the ensuing interaction remains antigen specific. As we mentioned earlier, antigen-activated B lymphocytes also express costimulators, such as B7 molecules, that stimulate the helper T cells that recognize antigen displayed by the B cells.

Mechanisms of Helper T Cell–Mediated Activation of B Lymphocytes

Helper T lymphocytes that recognize antigen presented by B cells activate the B cells by expressing

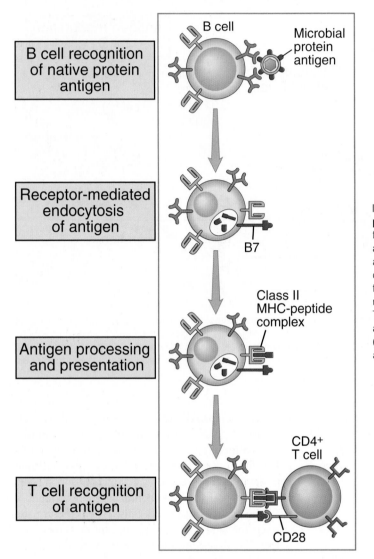

B cell recognition of native protein antigen

Receptor-mediated endocytosis of antigen

Antigen processing and presentation

T cell recognition of antigen

Figure 7–7   Antigen presentation by B lymphocytes to helper T cells. B cells specific for a protein antigen bind and internalize that antigen, process it, and present peptides attached to class II MHC molecules to helper T cells. The B cells and helper T cells are specific for the same antigen, but the B cells recognize native (conformational) epitopes and the helper T cells recognize peptide fragments of the antigen. B cells also express costimulators (e.g., B7 molecules) that play a role in T cell activation.

CD40 ligand (CD40L) and by secreting cytokines (Fig. 7-8). The process of helper T cell–mediated B lymphocyte activation is analogous to the process of T cell–mediated macrophage activation in cell-mediated immunity (see Chapter 6). CD40L on activated helper T cells binds to CD40 expressed on B lymphocytes. Engagement of CD40 delivers signals to the B cells that stimulate proliferation (clonal expansion) and the synthesis and secretion of antibodies. At the same time, cytokines produced by the helper T cells bind to cytokine receptors on B lymphocytes

and stimulate more B cell proliferation and Ig production. The requirement for the CD40L-CD40 interaction ensures that only T and B lymphocytes in physical contact engage in productive interactions. As we described previously, the antigen-specific lymphocytes are the ones that physically interact, thus ensuring that the antigen-specific B cells are also the ones that are activated. Helper T cell signals also stimulate heavy chain class switching and affinity maturation, which are typically seen in antibody responses to T-dependent protein antigens.

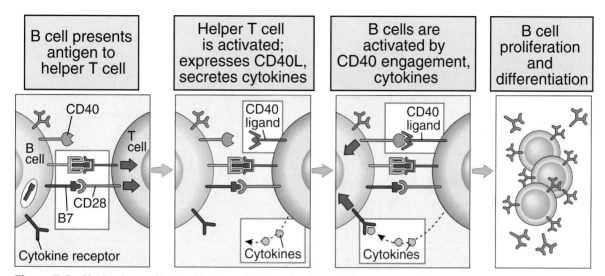

Figure 7–8 Mechanisms of helper T cell–mediated activation of B lymphocytes. Helper T cells recognize peptide antigens presented by B cells and costimulators (e.g., B7 molecules) on the B cells. The helper T cells are activated to express CD40L and secrete cytokines, both of which bind to their receptors on the same B cells and activate the B cells.

Heavy Chain Class (Isotype) Switching

Helper T cells stimulate the progeny of IgM + IgD expressing B lymphocytes to produce antibodies of different heavy chain classes (isotypes) (Fig. 7-9). The importance of class switching is that it enables humoral immune responses to different microbes to adapt in order to optimally combat these microbes. For instance, an important defense mechanism against the extracellular stages of most bacteria and viruses is to coat (opsonize) these microbes with antibodies and cause them to be phagocytosed by neutrophils and macrophages. This reaction is best mediated by antibody classes, such as IgG1 and IgG3 (in humans), that bind to high-affinity phagocyte Fc receptors specific for the γ heavy chain (see Chapter 8). In contrast, helminths are best eliminated by eosinophils, and therefore defense against these parasites involves coating them with antibodies to which eosinophils bind. The antibody class that is able to do this is IgE, because eosinophils have high-affinity receptors for the Fc portion of the ε heavy chain. Thus, effective host defense requires that the immune system should make different antibody isotypes in

response to different microbes, even though all naive B lymphocytes specific for all these microbes express the same antigen receptors, which are of the IgM and IgD isotypes. The process of heavy chain class switching provides this plasticity in humoral immune responses.

Heavy chain class switching is initiated by CD40L-mediated signals, and switching to different classes is stimulated by different cytokines. The signals delivered by CD40L and cytokines act on activated B cells and induce switching in some of the progeny of these cells. In the absence of CD40 or CD40L, B cells secrete only IgM and fail to switch to other isotypes, indicating the essential role of this ligand-receptor pair in class switching. A disease called the **X-linked hyper-IgM syndrome** is caused by inactivating mutations in the CD40L gene, which is located in the X chromosome. In this disease, much of the serum antibody is IgM, because of defective heavy chain class switching. Patients also suffer from defective cell-mediated immunity against intracellular microbes, because CD40L is important for T cell–mediated immunity (see Chapter 6). Cytokines influence which heavy chain class an individual B cell and its progeny will switch to.

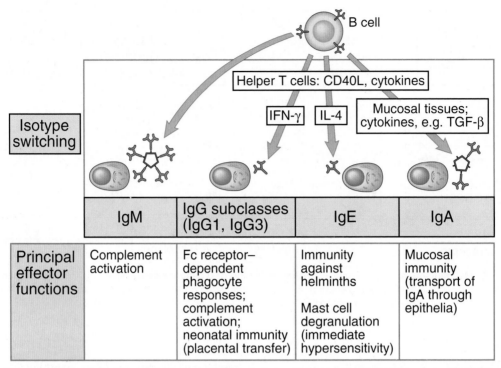

Figure 7-9   Ig heavy chain class (isotype) switching. Antigen-stimulated B lymphocytes may differentiate into IgM antibody–secreting cells, or, under the influence of CD40L and cytokines, some of the B cells may differentiate into cells that produce different Ig heavy chain classes. The principal effector functions of some of these classes are listed; all classes may function to neutralize microbes and toxins. IFN, interferon; IL, interleukin; TGF, transforming growth factor.

The molecular basis of heavy chain class switching is understood quite precisely (Fig. 7-10). IgM-producing B cells, which have not undergone switching, contain in their Ig heavy chain locus a rearranged VDJ gene adjacent to the first constant region cluster, which is Cμ. The heavy chain mRNA is produced by splicing of VDJ RNA to Cμ RNA, and this mRNA is translated to produce the μ heavy chain, which combines with a light chain to give rise to IgM antibody. Thus, the first antibody produced by B cells is IgM. Signals from CD40 and cytokine receptors stimulate transcription through one of the constant regions that is downstream of Cμ. In the intron 5′ of each constant region (except Cδ) is a conserved nucleotide sequence called the switch region. When a downstream constant region becomes transcriptionally active, the switch region 3′ of Cμ recombines with the switch region 5′ of that downstream constant region, and all the intervening DNA is deleted. The

enzyme activation–induced deaminase plays a key role in these events. This process is called **switch recombination.** It brings the rearranged VDJ adjacent to a downstream C region. The result is that the B cell begins to produce a new heavy chain class (which is determined by the C region of the antibody) with the same specificity as the original B cell (since specificity is determined by the rearranged VDJ).

Cytokines produced by helper T cells determine which heavy chain class is produced by influencing which heavy chain constant region gene participates in switch recombination (see Fig. 7-9). For instance, the production of opsonizing antibodies, which bind to phagocyte Fc receptors, is stimulated by interferon (IFN)-γ , the signature cytokine of T_H1 cells. These opsonizing antibodies promote phagocytosis, a prelude to microbe killing by phagocytes. IFN-γ is also a phagocyte-activating cytokine, and it stimulates the microbicidal activities of phagocytes. Thus, the

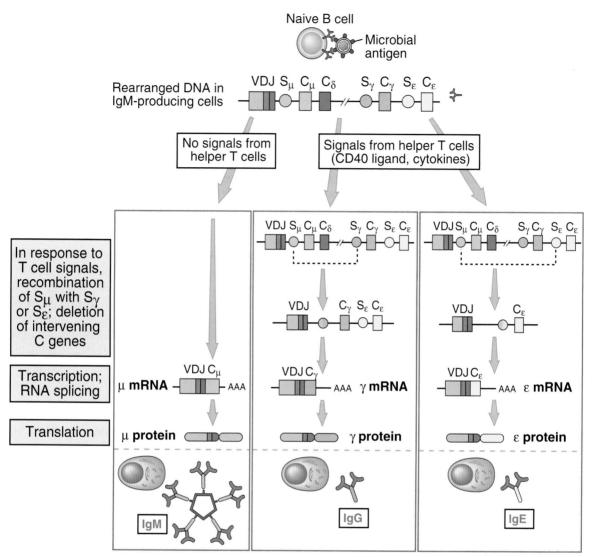

Figure 7–10   Mechanism of Ig heavy chain class switching. In an IgM-secreting B cell (left panel), the primary transcript of the rearranged VDJ heavy chain gene is spliced onto the μ RNA to produce the μ heavy chain and IgM antibody, because the μ gene is closest to the VDJ gene. Signals from helper T cells (CD40 ligation and cytokines) may induce recombination of switch (S) regions such that the rearranged VDJ gene is moved close to a C gene downstream of Cμ. (Switch recombination is shown by dashed lines.) Subsequently, the VDJ primary RNA is spliced onto the RNA from the downstream C gene, producing a heavy chain with a new constant region and, therefore, a new class of Ig. The two right panels illustrate how the progeny of an activated B cell may switch to produce two different antibody classes, IgG and IgE. (Exons encoding γ chain subtype heavy chains and α chain heavy chains are not shown for simplicity.)

actions of IFN-γ on B cells complement the actions of this cytokine on phagocytes. Many bacteria and viruses stimulate T_H1 responses, which activate the effector mechanisms that are best at eliminating these microbes. In contrast, switching to the IgE class is stimulated by interleukin (IL)-4, the signature cytokine of T_H2 cells. IgE functions to eliminate helminths, acting in concert with eosinophils, which are activated by the second T_H2 cytokine, IL-5. Predictably, helminths induce strong T_H2 responses. Thus, the nature of the helper T cell response to a microbe guides the subsequent antibody response, making it optimal for combating that microbe. These are excellent examples of how different components of the immune system are regulated coordinately and function together in defense against different types of microbes, and how helper T cells may function as the "master" controllers of immune responses.

The nature of antibody classes produced is also influenced by the site of immune responses. For instance, IgA antibody is the major isotype produced in mucosal lymphoid tissues. This is probably because mucosal tissues contain large numbers of B cells able to switch to IgA and helper T cells whose cytokines stimulate switching to IgA. IgA is the principal antibody class that can be actively secreted through mucosal epithelia (see Chapter 8), and this is presumably why mucosal lymphoid tissues are the major sites of IgA production.

Affinity Maturation

Affinity maturation is the process by which the affinity of antibodies produced in response to a protein antigen increases with prolonged or repeated exposure to that antigen. Because of affinity maturation, the ability of antibodies to bind to a microbe or microbial antigen increases if the infection is persistent or recurrent. The molecular mechanism of affinity maturation was defined when individual (monoclonal) antibodies were isolated at different stages of an immune response to a protein antigen and analyzed for their affinities for the antigen. It was found that the affinity of the antibody increased with prolonged or repeated antigen exposure. This increase in affinity is due to point mutations in the V regions, and particularly in the antigen-binding hypervari-

able regions, of the antibodies produced (Fig. 7-11). Affinity maturation is seen only in responses to helper T cell–dependent protein antigens, suggesting that helper cells are critical in the process. These findings raise two intriguing questions: how do B cells undergo Ig gene mutations, and how are the high-affinity (i.e., most useful) B cells selected to become progressively more numerous?

Affinity maturation occurs in the germinal centers of lymphoid follicles and is the result of somatic hypermutation of Ig genes in dividing B cells followed by the selection of high-affinity B cells by antigen displayed by follicular dendritic cells (Fig. 7-12). Some of the progeny of activated B lymphocytes enter lymphoid follicles and form germinal centers. Within these germinal centers, the B cells proliferate rapidly, with a doubling time of approximately 6 hours, so that one cell may produce about 5000 progeny within a week. (The name "germinal center" came from the morphologic observation that some follicles contain lightly stained centers, and the light staining is a result of the large numbers of dividing cells, many of which are also dying.) During this proliferation, the Ig genes of the B cells become susceptible to point mutations by a process involving the enzyme activation–induced deaminase. The frequency of Ig gene mutations is estimated to be one in 10^3 base pairs per cell per division, which is a thousandfold more than the mutation rate in most genes. For this reason, Ig mutation is called **somatic hypermutation.** This extensive mutation results in the generation of different B cell clones whose Ig molecules may bind with widely varying affinities to the antigen that initiated the response.

Germinal center B cells die by apoptosis unless they are rescued by antigen recognition. At the same time as somatic hypermutation of Ig genes is going on in germinal centers, the antibody that was secreted earlier during the immune response binds residual antigen. The antigen-antibody complexes that are formed may activate complement. These complexes are displayed by cells, called **follicular dendritic cells,** that reside in the germinal center and express receptors for the Fc portions of antibodies and for complement products, both of which help to display the antigen-antibody complexes. Thus, B cells that have undergone somatic hypermutation are given a chance

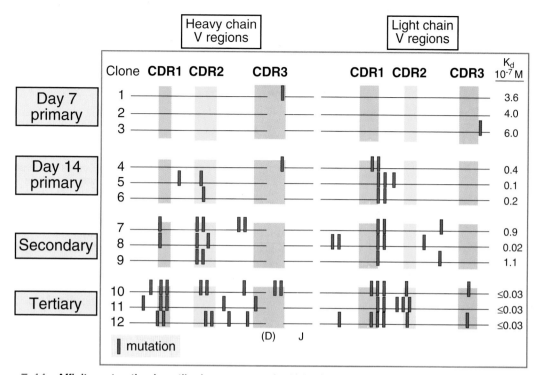

Figure 7–11   Affinity maturation in antibody responses. Analysis of several individual antibodies produced by different clones of B cells against one antigen at different stages of primary, secondary, and tertiary immune responses shows that with time and repeated immunization the antibodies that are produced contain increasing numbers of mutations in their antigen-binding regions (the complementarity-determining regions [CDRs]). The antibodies also show increasing affinities for the antigen, as revealed by the lower dissociation constants (K_d). These results imply that the mutations are responsible for the increased affinities of the antibodies for the immunizing antigen. Secondary and tertiary responses refer to responses to the second and third immunizations with the same antigen. (Adapted from Berek C, and C Milstein. Mutation drift and repertoire shift in the maturation of the immune response. Immunol Rev 96:23-41, 1987; with permission.)

to bind antigen on follicular dendritic cells and be rescued from death. As the immune response develops, or with repeated immunization, the amount of antibody produced increases. As a result, the amount of available antigen decreases. The B cells that are selected to survive must be able to bind antigen at lower and lower concentrations, and therefore these are cells whose antigen receptors are of higher and higher affinity. The selected B cells leave the germinal center and secrete antibodies, resulting in increasing affinity of the antibodies produced as the response develops.

The various stages of antibody responses to T cell–dependent protein antigens occur sequentially and in different anatomic compartments of lymphoid organs (Fig. 7-13). Mature, naive B lymphocytes recognize antigens in lymphoid follicles and migrate out to encounter helper T cells at the edges of the follicles. This interface of the B cell–rich zones and the T cell–rich zones is the site where B cell proliferation and differentiation into antibody-secreting cells begin. The antibody-secreting cells that develop as a consequence of this interaction reside in lymphoid organs, usually outside the B cell–rich follicles, and the secreted antibodies enter the blood. Some antibody-secreting plasma cells migrate to the bone marrow, where they may live for months or years, continuing to produce antibodies even after the antigen is eliminated. It is estimated that more than half the antibodies in the blood of a normal adult are produced by these long-lived antibody-secreting cells, and thus

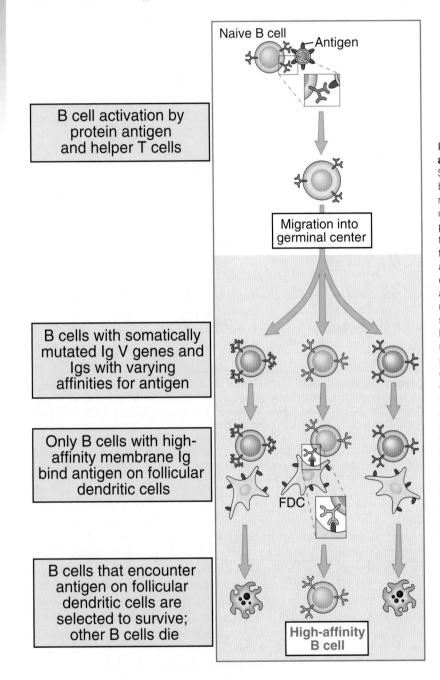

B cell activation by protein antigen and helper T cells

Naive B cell — Antigen

Migration into germinal center

B cells with somatically mutated Ig V genes and Igs with varying affinities for antigen

Only B cells with high-affinity membrane Ig bind antigen on follicular dendritic cells

FDC

B cells that encounter antigen on follicular dendritic cells are selected to survive; other B cells die

High-affinity B cell

Figure 7–12 Selection of high-affinity B cells in germinal centers. Some of the B cells that are activated by antigen, with help from T cells, migrate into follicles to form germinal centers, where they undergo rapid proliferation and accumulate mutations in their Ig V genes. The mutations generate B cells with different affinities for the antigen. Follicular dendritic cells (FDCs) display the antigen, and only B cells that recognize the antigen are selected to survive. FDCs display antigens by binding immune complexes to Fc receptors or by binding immune complexes with attached C3b and C3d complement proteins to C3 receptors (not shown). As more antibody is produced, the amount of available antigen decreases, so the B cells that are selected have to express receptors with higher affinities to bind the antigen. FDCs express CD40L (not shown), and germinal centers contain a few T cells that also express CD40L. CD40L may be the molecule that delivers survival signals to the B cells that recognize antigen on the FDCs.

circulating antibodies reflect each individual's history of antigen exposure. These antibodies provide a level of immediate protection if the antigen (microbe or toxin) reenters the body. Heavy chain class switching is also initiated outside the follicles. Affinity maturation, and perhaps additional class switching, occurs in germinal centers that are formed in follicles. All these events may be seen within a week after exposure to antigen. A fraction of the activated B cells, which are often the progeny of class-switched

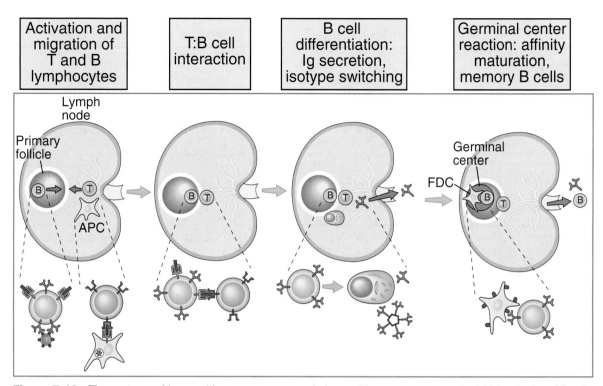

Figure 7–13   The anatomy of humoral immune responses. In humoral immune responses, the initial activation of B cells and helper T cells occurs in different anatomic compartments of peripheral lymphoid organs. Naive B cells recognize antigens in follicles, and helper T cells recognize antigens in T cell–rich zones outside the follicles. The two cell types interact at the edges of the follicles. The differentiation of B cells into antibody-secreting cells occurs mainly outside lymphoid follicles. Affinity maturation occurs in germinal centers, and heavy chain class switching may occur outside follicles and in germinal centers. Some antibody-secreting plasma cells migrate to the bone marrow and continue to produce antibody even after the antigen is eliminated (not shown). Memory B cells develop mainly in the germinal centers and enter the circulation. The illustration shows these reactions in a lymph node, but essentially the same pattern is seen in the spleen.

high-affinity B cells, do not differentiate into active antibody secretors but instead become **memory cells.** Memory B cells do not secrete antibodies, but they circulate in the blood and survive for months or years in the absence of additional antigen exposure, ready to respond rapidly if the antigen is reintroduced.

Antibody Responses to T-Independent Antigens

Polysaccharides, lipids, and other nonprotein antigens elicit antibody responses without the participation of helper T cells. Recall that these nonprotein antigens cannot bind to MHC molecules, and therefore they cannot be seen by T cells (see Chapter 3).

Many bacteria contain polysaccharide-rich capsules, and defense against these bacteria is mediated primarily by antibodies that bind to capsular polysaccharides and target the bacteria for phagocytosis. Despite the importance of antibody responses against such T-independent antigens, very little is known about how these responses are induced. What is known is that antibody responses to T-independent antigens differ in many respects from responses to proteins, and most of these differences are attributable to the roles of helper T cells in antibody responses to proteins (Fig. 7-14). It is thought that because polysaccharide and lipid antigens often contain multivalent arrays of the same epitope, these antigens are able to cross-link many antigen receptors on a specific B cell. This

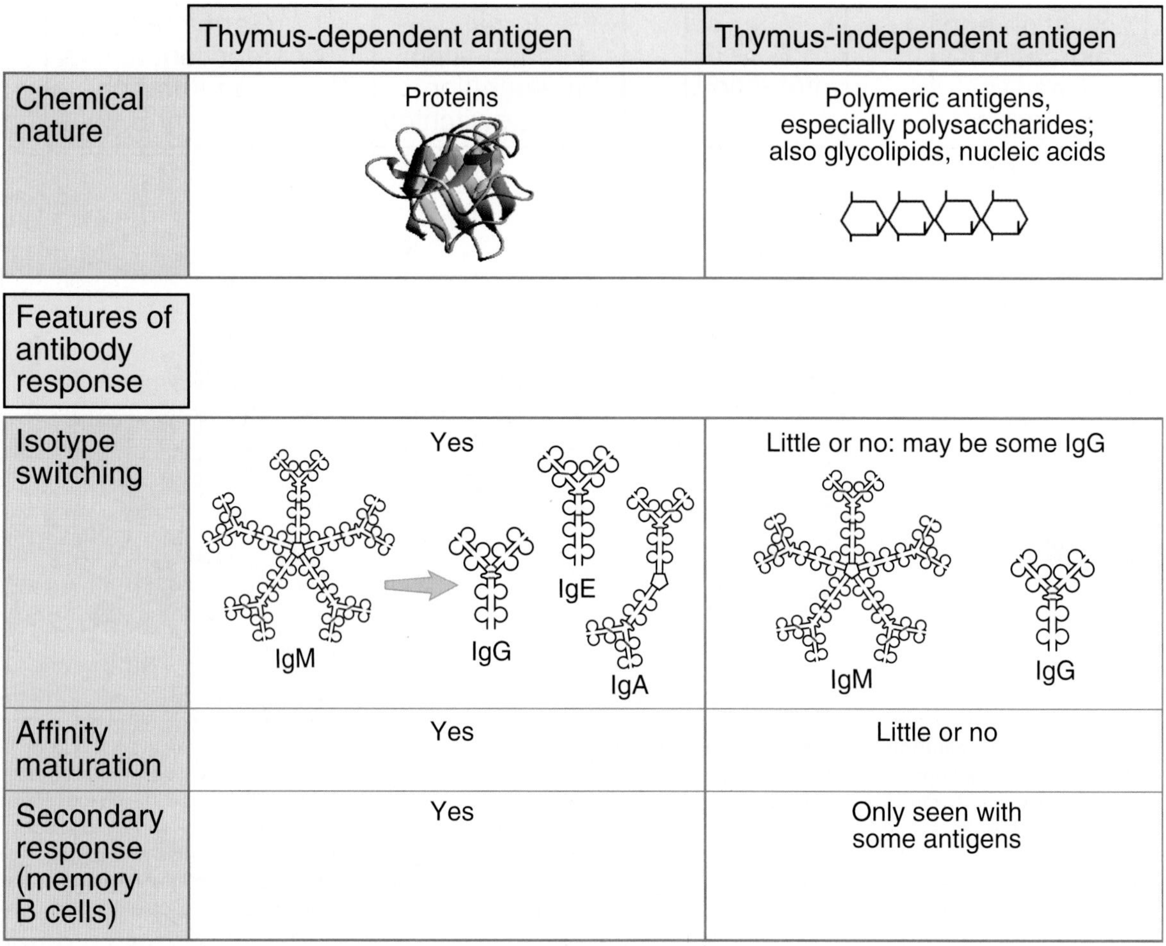

	Thymus-dependent antigen	Thymus-independent antigen
Chemical nature	Proteins	Polymeric antigens, especially polysaccharides; also glycolipids, nucleic acids
Features of antibody response		
Isotype switching	Yes IgM → IgG, IgE, IgA	Little or no: may be some IgG IgM IgG
Affinity maturation	Yes	Little or no
Secondary response (memory B cells)	Yes	Only seen with some antigens

Figure 7–14   Features of antibody responses to T-dependent and T-independent antigens. T-dependent antigens (proteins) and T-independent antigens (nonproteins) induce antibody responses with different characteristics, largely reflecting the influence of helper T cells in the responses to protein antigens.

extensive cross-linking may activate the B cells strongly enough to stimulate their proliferation and differentiation without a requirement for T cell help. Naturally occurring protein antigens are usually not multivalent, and this may be why they do not induce full B cell responses by themselves but depend on helper T cells to stimulate antibody production.

Regulation of Humoral Immune Responses: Antibody Feedback

After B lymphocytes differentiate into antibody-secreting cells and memory cells, a fraction of these cells survive for long periods, but most of the activated B cells probably die by a process of programmed cell death. This gradual loss of the activated B cells contributes to the physiologic decline of the humoral immune response. B cells also use a special mechanism for shutting off antibody production. As IgG antibody is produced and circulates throughout the body, the antibody binds to antigen that is still available in the blood and tissues, forming immune complexes. B cells specific for the antigen may bind the antigen part of the immune complex by their Ig receptors. At the same time, the Fc "tail" of the attached IgG antibody may be recognized by an Fc receptor

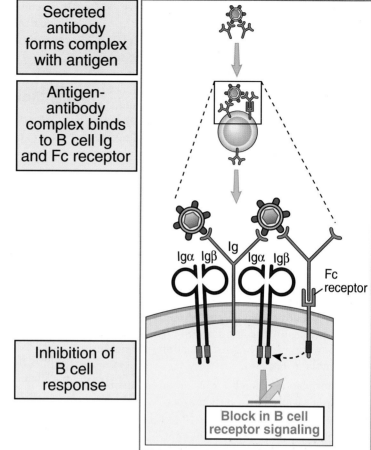

Secreted antibody forms complex with antigen

Antigen-antibody complex binds to B cell Ig and Fc receptor

Igα Igβ   Ig   Igα Igβ   Fc receptor

Inhibition of B cell response

Block in B cell receptor signaling

Figure 7–15 The mechanism of antibody feedback. Secreted IgG antibodies form immune complexes (antigen-antibody complexes) with residual antigen. The complexes interact with B cells specific for the antigen, with the membrane Ig antigen receptors recognizing epitopes of the antigen and a certain type of Fc receptor (FcγRII) recognizing the bound antibody. The Fc receptors block activating signals from the antigen receptor, and thus terminate B cell activation. The cytoplasmic domain of B cell FcγRII contains an immunoreceptor tyrosine-based inhibition motif (ITIM) that binds enzymes that inhibit antigen receptor–mediated B cell activation.

expressed on B cells (Fig. 7-15). This Fc receptor delivers negative signals that shut off antigen receptor-induced signals, thus terminating B cell responses. This process, in which antibody bound to antigen inhibits further antibody production, is called **antibody feedback.** It serves to terminate humoral immune responses once sufficient quantities of IgG antibodies have been produced.

SUMMARY

▶ Humoral immunity is mediated by antibodies, which neutralize and help to eliminate extracellular microbes and their toxins.

▶ Humoral immune responses are initiated by the recognition of antigens by specific immunoglobulin

(Ig) receptors of naive B cells. The binding of antigen cross-links Ig receptors of specific B cells, and biochemical signals are delivered to the inside of the B cells by Ig-associated signaling proteins. A breakdown product of the complement protein C3 is recognized by a receptor on B cells, providing "second signals" for B cell activation. These signals induce B cell clonal expansion, low levels of IgM secretion, and other changes that prepare the B cells to respond to T cell help.

▶ Protein antigens activate CD4+ helper T cells, which stimulate B cell responses. B lymphocytes specific for an antigen bind, internalize, and process that antigen and present class II MHC-displayed peptides to helper T cells also specific for the antigen. The helper T cells express CD40L and secrete cytokines, which function together to stimulate high levels of B cell proliferation and differentiation.

▶ Heavy chain class switching (or isotype switching) is the process by which the isotype, but not the specificity, of the antibodies produced in response to an antigen change as the humoral response proceeds. Isotype switching depends on the combination of CD40L and cytokines. Different cytokines induce switching to different antibody classes, enabling the immune system to respond in the most effective way to different types of microbes.

▶ Affinity maturation is the process by which the affinity of antibodies for protein antigens increases with prolonged or repeated exposure to the antigens. The process occurs when some activated B cells migrate into follicles and form germinal centers. Here the B cells proliferate rapidly and their Ig V genes undergo extensive somatic mutations. The antigen complexed with secreted antibody is displayed by follicular dendritic cells in the germinal centers. B cells that recognize the antigen with high affinity are selected to survive, giving rise to affinity maturation of the antibody response.

▶ Polysaccharides, lipids, and other nonprotein antigens are called T-independent antigens because they induce antibody responses without T cell help. Most T-independent antigens contain multiple identical epitopes that are able to cross-link many Ig receptors on a B cell, providing signals for the B cells that are adequate even in the absence of helper T cell activation. Antibody responses to T-independent antigens show less heavy chain class switching and affinity maturation than do responses to T-dependent protein antigens.

▶ Secreted antibodies form immune complexes with residual antigen and shut off B cell activation by engaging an inhibitory Fc receptor on B cells.

⇄ Review Questions

1 What are the signals that induce B cell responses to (1) protein antigens and (2) polysaccharide antigens?

2 What are some of the differences between primary and secondary antibody responses to a protein antigen?

3 How do helper T cells specific for an antigen interact with B lymphocytes specific for the same antigen? Where in a lymph node do these interactions mainly occur?

4 What are the mechanisms by which helper T cells stimulate B cell proliferation and differentiation? What are the similarities between these mechanisms and the mechanisms of T cell–mediated macrophage activation?

5 What are the signals that induce heavy chain class switching, and what is the importance of this phenomenon for host defense against different microbes?

6 What is affinity maturation? How is it induced, and how are high-affinity B cells selected to survive?

7 What are the characteristics of antibody responses to polysaccharides and lipids? What types of bacteria stimulate mostly these kinds of antibody responses?

Effector Mechanisms of Humoral Immunity

The Elimination of Extracellular Microbes and Toxins

8

Properties of Antibodies That Determine Their Effector Functions

Neutralization of Microbes and Microbial Toxins

Opsonization and Phagocytosis

Antibody-Dependent Cellular Cytotoxicity

Activation of the Complement System

• Pathways of Complement Activation
• Functions of the Complement System
• Regulation of Complement Activation

Functions of Antibodies at Special Anatomic Sites

• Mucosal Immunity
• Neonatal Immunity

Evasion of Humoral Immunity by Microbes

Vaccination

Summary

Humoral immunity is the type of host defense that is mediated by secreted antibodies and is important for protection against extracellular microbes and their toxins. Preventing infection is an important function of the adaptive immune system, and only antibodies mediate this function. Antibodies prevent infections by blocking the ability of microbes to bind to and infect host cells. Antibodies also bind to microbial toxins and prevent them from damaging host cells. In addition, antibodies function to eliminate microbes, toxins, and infected cells from the body. Both antibodies and T lymphocytes participate in the destruction of microbes that have colonized and infected hosts. Antibodies are the only mechanism of adaptive immunity against extracellular microbes, but they cannot reach microbes that live inside cells. However, humoral immunity is vital even for defense against microbes that live and divide inside of cells, such as viruses, because antibodies can bind to these microbes before they enter host cells and thus prevent infection.

Defects in antibody production are associated with increased susceptibility to infections by many bacteria, viruses, and parasites. Most of the effective vaccines that are currently in use work by stimulating the production of antibodies.

This chapter describes how antibodies function in host defense against infections. The following questions are addressed:

- What are the mechanisms used by circulating antibodies to combat different types of infectious agents and their toxins?

- What is the role of the complement system in defense against microbes?

- How do antibodies combat microbes that enter via the gastrointestinal and respiratory tracts?

- How do antibodies protect the fetus and newborn from infections?

Before describing the mechanisms by which antibodies function in host defense, the features of antibody molecules that are important for these functions are summarized.

Properties of Antibodies That Determine Their Effector Functions

Antibodies may function distant from their sites of production. Antibodies are produced after stimulation of B lymphocytes by antigens in peripheral lymphoid organs (i.e., the lymph nodes, the spleen, and mucosal lymphoid tissues). Some of the antigen-stimulated B lymphocytes differentiate into antibody-secreting cells, which synthesize and secrete antibodies of different heavy chain classes (isotypes). These antibodies enter the blood, from where they may reach any peripheral site of infection, and mucosal secretions, where they prevent infections by microbes that try to enter through the epithelia. Thus, antibodies are able to perform their functions throughout the body.

Protective antibodies are produced during the first (primary) response to a microbe and in larger amounts during subsequent (secondary) responses (see Fig. 7-2, Chapter 7). Antibody production begins within the first week after infection or vaccination. Some of the antibody-secreting plasma cells migrate to the bone marrow and live in this tissue, continuing to secrete small amounts of antibodies for months or years. If the microbe again tries to infect the host, the continuously secreted antibodies provide immediate protection. Some antigen-stimulated B lymphocytes differentiate into memory cells, which do not secrete antibodies but lie in wait for the antigen. On subsequent encounter with the microbe, these memory cells rapidly differentiate into antibody-producing cells, providing a large burst of antibody for more effective defense against the infection. A goal of vaccination is to stimulate the development of long-lived antibody-secreting cells and memory cells.

Antibodies use their antigen-binding (Fab) regions to bind to and block the harmful effects of microbes and toxins, and they use their Fc regions to activate diverse effector mechanisms that eliminate these microbes and toxins (Fig. 8-1). This spatial segregation of the antigen recognition and effector functions of antibody molecules was introduced in Chapter 4. Antibodies block the infectivity of microbes and the injurious effects of microbial toxins simply by binding to the microbes and toxins, using their Fab regions to do so. Other functions of antibodies require the participation of various components of host defense, such as phagocytes and the complement system. The Fc portions of immunoglobulin (Ig) molecules, made up of the heavy chain constant regions, contain the binding sites for phagocytes and complement. The effective binding of phagocytes and complement to antibodies occurs only after several Ig molecules recognize and become attached to a microbe or microbial antigen. Therefore, even the Fc-dependent functions of antibodies require antigen recognition by the Fab regions. This feature of antibodies ensures that they activate effector mechanisms only when they need to, that is, when they recognize their target antigens.

Heavy chain class (isotype) switching and affinity maturation enhance the protective functions of antibodies. Class switching and affinity maturation are two changes that occur in the antibodies produced by antigen-stimulated B lymphocytes, especially during responses to protein antigens (see Chapter 7). Heavy chain class switching results in the production of antibodies with distinct Fc regions, capable of different effector functions (see Fig. 8-1). Thus, by switching to different antibody classes in response to

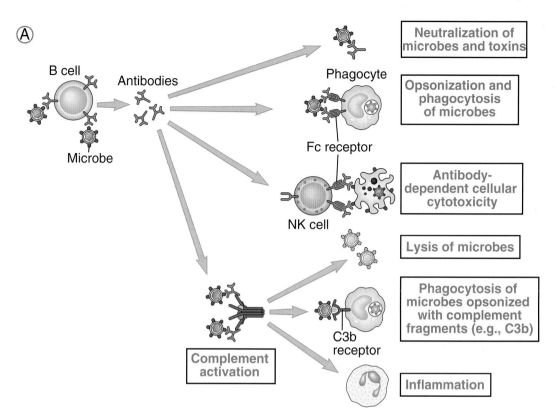

Figure 8–1 is illustrated in the following:

(B) Antibody isotype	Isotype specific effector functions
IgG	Neutralization of microbes and toxins
	Opsonization of antigens for phagocytosis by macrophages and neutrophils
	Activation of the classical pathway of complement
	Antibody-dependent cellular cytotoxicity mediated by NK cells
	Neonatal immunity: transfer of maternal antibody across placenta and gut
	Feedback inhibition of B cell activation
IgM	Activation of the classical pathway of complement
IgA	Mucosal immunity: secretion of IgA into lumens of gastrointestinal and respiratory tracts, neutralization of microbes and toxins
IgE	Antibody-dependent cellular cytotoxicity mediated by eosinophils
	Mast cell degranulation (immediate hypersensitivity reactions)

Figure 8–1 The effector functions of antibodies. Antibodies are produced by the activation of B lymphocytes by antigens and other signals (not shown). Antibodies of different heavy chain classes (isotypes) perform different effector functions, which are illustrated schematically in panel A and summarized in panel B. (Some of the properties of antibodies are listed in Fig. 4-3, Chapter 4.)

various microbes, the humoral immune system is able to recruit host mechanisms that are optimal for combating these microbes. The process of affinity maturation is triggered by prolonged or repeated antigen stimulation, and it leads to the production of antibodies with higher and higher affinities for the antigen. This change increases the ability of antibodies to bind to and neutralize or eliminate microbes, especially if the microbes are persistent or capable of recurrent infections.

With this introduction, the discussion proceeds to the mechanisms used by antibodies to combat infections. Much of the chapter is devoted to effector mechanisms that are not influenced by anatomic considerations; that is, they may be active anywhere in the body. At the end of the chapter, the special features of antibody functions at particular anatomic locations are described.

Neutralization of Microbes and Microbial Toxins

Antibodies bind to and block, or neutralize, the infectivity of microbes and the interactions of microbial toxins with host cells (Fig. 8-2). Most microbes use molecules in their envelopes or cell walls to bind to and gain entry into host cells. Antibodies may attach to these microbial envelope or cell wall molecules and prevent the microbes from infecting and colonizing the host. Neutralization is a very useful defense mechanism because it does not allow an infection to take hold. The most effective vaccines available today work by stimulating the production of neutralizing antibodies, which prevent subsequent infection. Microbes that infect cells may damage these cells, are released, and go on to infect other neighboring cells. Antibodies may find the microbes during their transit from cell to cell and thus limit the spread of infection. If an infectious microbe does colonize the host, its harmful effects may be caused by endotoxins or exotoxins, which often bind to specific receptors on host cells and thus mediate their effects. Antibodies against toxins prevent binding of the toxins to host cells and thus block the harmful effects of the toxins. Emil von Behring's demonstration of this type of humoral immunity mediated by antibodies against diphtheria toxin was the first formal

demonstration of immunity against a microbe and the basis for giving von Behring the first Nobel Prize in Medicine in 1901.

Opsonization and Phagocytosis

Antibodies coat microbes and promote their ingestion by phagocytes (Fig. 8-3). The process of coating particles for subsequent phagocytosis is called **opsonization,** and the molecules that coat microbes and enhance their phagocytosis are called **opsonins.** When several antibody molecules bind to a microbe, an array of Fc regions is formed projecting away from the microbe. If the antibodies belong to certain isotypes (IgG1 and IgG3 in humans), their Fc regions bind to a high-affinity receptor for the Fc regions of γ chains, called FcγRI (CD64), which is expressed on neutrophils and macrophages. As a result, the phagocyte extends its plasma membrane around the opsonized microbe and ingests the microbe into a vesicle called a phagosome, which fuses with lysosomes. The binding of antibody Fc tails to FcγRI also activates the phagocytes, because the FcγRI contains a signaling chain that triggers numerous biochemical pathways in the phagocytes. The activated neutrophil or macrophage produces, in its lysosomes, large amounts of reactive oxygen intermediates, nitric oxide, and proteolytic enzymes, all of which combine to destroy the ingested microbe. Antibody-mediated phagocytosis is the major mechanism of defense against encapsulated bacteria, such as pneumococcus. The polysaccharide-rich capsules of these bacteria protect the organisms from phagocytosis in the absence of antibody, but opsonization by antibody promotes phagocytosis and destruction of the bacteria. The spleen contains large numbers of phagocytes and is an important site of phagocytic clearance of opsonized bacteria. This is why patients who have undergone **splenectomy,** for example, for traumatic rupture of the organ, are susceptible to disseminated infections by encapsulated bacteria.

Antibody-Dependent Cellular Cytotoxicity

Natural killer (NK) cells and other leukocytes may bind to antibody-coated cells and destroy these cells (Fig. 8-4). Natural killer cells express an Fc receptor, called FcγRIII (CD16), that binds to arrays of IgG

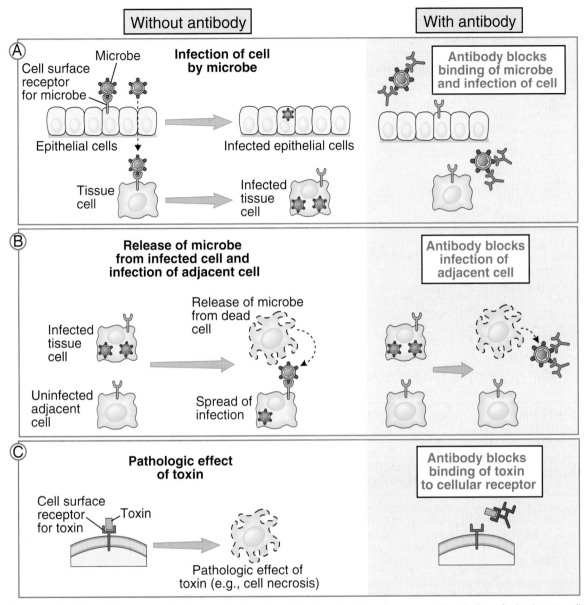

Figure 8–2 Neutralization of microbes and toxins by antibodies. A. Antibodies prevent the binding of microbes to cells and thus block the ability of the microbes to infect host cells. B. Antibodies inhibit the spread of microbes from an infected cell to an adjacent uninfected cell. C. Antibodies block the binding of toxins to cells and thus inhibit the pathologic effects of the toxins.

antibodies attached to a cell. As a result of FcγRIII-mediated signals, the NK cells are activated to discharge their granules, which contain proteins that kill the opsonized targets. This process is called antibody-dependent cellular cytotoxicity (ADCC). It is not known if infected cells commonly express surface molecules that may be recognized by antibodies or in which infections this effector mechanism is active. In fact, it is likely that NK cell–mediated ADCC is not as important as phagocytosis of opsonized microbes in defense against most bacterial and viral infections.

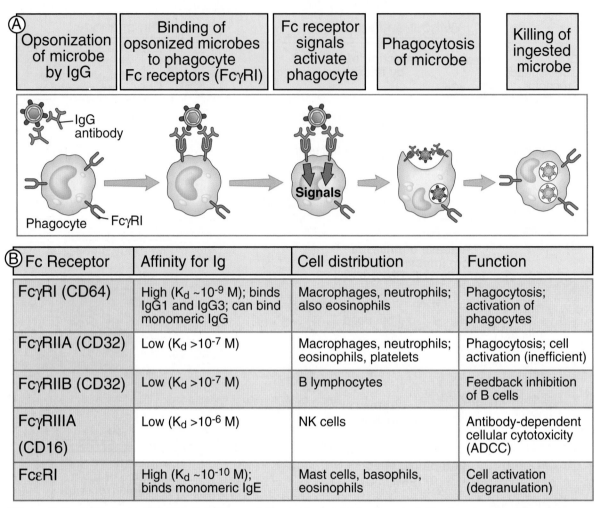

Opsonization of microbe by IgG	Binding of opsonized microbes to phagocyte Fc receptors (FcγRI)	Fc receptor signals activate phagocyte	Phagocytosis of microbe	Killing of ingested microbe

Ⓑ Fc Receptor	Affinity for Ig	Cell distribution	Function
FcγRI (CD64)	High (K_d ~10^{-9} M); binds IgG1 and IgG3; can bind monomeric IgG	Macrophages, neutrophils; also eosinophils	Phagocytosis; activation of phagocytes
FcγRIIA (CD32)	Low (K_d >10^{-7} M)	Macrophages, neutrophils; eosinophils, platelets	Phagocytosis; cell activation (inefficient)
FcγRIIB (CD32)	Low (K_d >10^{-7} M)	B lymphocytes	Feedback inhibition of B cells
FcγRIIIA (CD16)	Low (K_d >10^{-6} M)	NK cells	Antibody-dependent cellular cytotoxicity (ADCC)
FcεRI	High (K_d ~10^{-10} M); binds monomeric IgE	Mast cells, basophils, eosinophils	Cell activation (degranulation)

Figure 8–3   Antibody-mediated opsonization and phagocytosis of microbes. A. Antibodies of certain IgG subclasses bind to microbes and are then recognized by Fc receptors on phagocytes. Signals from the Fc receptors promote the phagocytosis of the opsonized microbes and activate the phagocytes to destroy these microbes. B. The different types of human Fc receptors, and their cellular distribution and functions, are listed.

A special type of ADCC, mediated by eosinophils, plays a role in defense against helminthic infections (see Fig. 8-4). Most helminths are too large to be phagocytosed, and they have thick integuments that make them resistant to many of the microbicidal substances produced by neutrophils and macrophages. The humoral immune response to helminths is dominated by IgE antibodies. The IgE opsonizes the worms, and eosinophils, which express a high-affinity IgE-specific Fc receptor called FcεRI, bind to the opsonized worms. The bound eosinophils are activated to release their granules, which contain proteins that are toxic to helminths. This IgE- and eosinophil-mediated ADCC illustrates how Ig class switching is designed for optimal host defense: B cells respond to helminths by switching to IgE, which is useful against helminths, but B cells respond to most bacteria and viruses by switching to IgG antibodies that promote phagocytosis via FcγRI. As we discussed in Chapters 5 and 7, these patterns of class switching

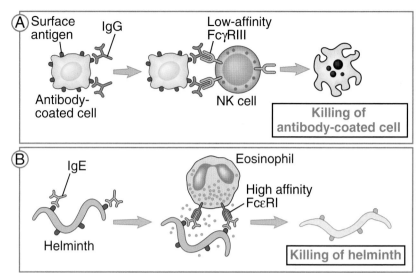

Figure 8–4 Antibody-dependent cellular cytotoxicity (ADCC). A. Antibodies of certain IgG subclasses bind to cells (e.g., infected cells), and the Fc regions of the bound antibodies are recognized by an Fcγ receptor on NK cells. The NK cells are activated and kill the antibody-coated cells. B. IgE antibodies bind to helminthic parasites, and the Fc regions of the bound antibodies are recognized by Fcε receptors on eosinophils. The eosinophils are activated to release their granule contents, which kill the parasites.

are determined by the types of cytokines produced by helper T cells stimulated by the different types of microbes.

Activation of the Complement System

The complement system is a collection of circulating and cell membrane proteins that play important roles in host defense against microbes and in antibody-mediated tissue injury. The term *complement* refers to the ability of these proteins to assist, or complement, the antimicrobial activity of antibodies. The complement system may be activated by microbes in the absence of antibody, as part of the innate immune response to infection, and by antibodies attached to microbes, as part of adaptive immunity (see Fig. 2-11, Chapter 2). There are several features of the complement system that are important for its functions. The activation of complement proteins involves sequential proteolytic cleavage of these proteins and leads to the generation of effector molecules that participate in eliminating microbes in different ways. This cascade of complement protein activation, like all enzymatic cascades, is capable of achieving tremendous amplification, because of which a small number of activated complement molecules early in the cascade may produce a large number of effector mol-

ecules. Activated complement proteins become covalently attached to the cell surfaces where the activation occurs, ensuring that activation is limited to the correct sites. The complement system is tightly regulated by molecules present on normal host cells, and this regulation prevents uncontrolled and potentially harmful complement activation.

In the following section the activation, functions, and regulation of the complement system are described.

Pathways of Complement Activation

There are three major pathways of complement activation, two initiated by microbes in the absence of antibody, called the alternative and lectin pathways and the third initiated by certain isotypes of antibodies attached to antigens, called the classical pathway (Fig. 8-5). There are several proteins in the complement system that interact in a precise sequence. The most abundant complement protein in the plasma, called C3, plays a central role in all three pathways. C3 is spontaneously hydrolyzed in plasma at a low level, but its products are unstable and they are rapidly broken down and lost. The **alternative pathway** is triggered when a breakdown product of C3 hydrolysis, called C3b, is deposited on the surface

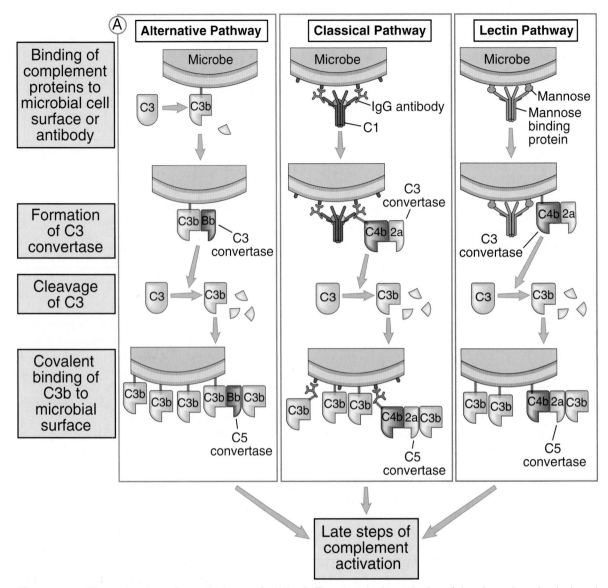

Figure 8–5 The early steps of complement activation. A. The steps in the activation of the alternative, classical, and lectin pathways are shown. Note that the sequence of events is similar in all three pathways, although they differ in their requirement for antibody and in the proteins used.

of a microbe. Here, the C3b forms stable covalent bonds with microbial proteins or polysaccharides and is thus protected from further degradation. (As will be described later, C3b is prevented from binding stably to normal host cells by several regulatory proteins that are present on host cells but absent from

microbes.) The microbe-bound C3b becomes a substrate for the binding of another protein called Factor B, which is broken down by a plasma protease to generate the Bb fragment. This fragment remains attached to the C3b, and the C3bBb complex enzymatically breaks down more C3, functioning as the

ⒷProtein	Serum conc. (μg/mL)	Function
C3	1000-1200	C3b binds to the surface of a microbe where it functions as an opsonin and as a component of C3 and C5 convertases C3a stimulates inflammation
Factor B	200	Bb is a serine protease and the active enzyme of C3 and C5 convertases
Factor D	1-2	Plasma serine protease which cleaves Factor B when it is bound to C3b
Properdin	25	Stabilizes the C3 convertase (C3bBb) on microbial surfaces

ⒸProtein	Serum conc. (μg/mL)	Function
C1 $(C1qr_2s_2)$		Initiates the classical pathway; C1q binds to Fc portion of antibody; C1r and C1s are proteases that lead to C4 and C2 activation
C4	300-600	C4b covalently binds to surface of microbe or cell where antibody is bound and complement is activated C4b binds to C2 for cleavage by C1s C4a stimulates inflammation
C2	20	C2a is a serine protease functioning as an active enzyme of C3 and C5 convertases

Figure 8–5, cont'd B. The important properties of the proteins involved in the early steps of the alternative pathway of complement activation are summarized. C. The important properties of the proteins involved in the early steps of the classical and lectin pathways are summarized. Note that C3, which is listed among the alternative pathway proteins (B), is also the central component of the classical and lectin pathways. Mannose binding protein, but not C1, is the first protein in the lectin pathway.

"alternative pathway C3 convertase." As a result of this convertase activity, many more C3b and C3bBb molecules are produced and become attached to the microbe. Some of the C3bBb molecules bind additional C3b, and the C3bBb3b complex functions as a C5 convertase, to break down the complement protein C5 and initiate the late steps of complement activation.

The **classical pathway** is triggered when IgM or certain subclasses of IgG (IgG1 and IgG3 in humans) bind to antigens (e.g., on a microbial cell surface). As a result of this binding, the Fc regions of the anti-bodies become accessible to complement proteins and two or more Fc regions come close together. When this happens, the C1 complement protein binds to two adjacent Fc regions. The attached C1 becomes enzymatically active, thus resulting in the binding and cleavage of two other proteins, C4 and C2. The resultant C4b2a complex becomes covalently attached to the antibody and to the microbial surface where the antibody is bound. This complex functions as the "classical pathway C3 convertase." It breaks down C3, and the C3b that is generated again becomes attached to the microbe. Some of the C3b binds to the C4b2a complex, and the resultant C4b2a3b complex functions as a C5 convertase.

The **lectin pathway** is initiated in the absence of antibody by the attachment of plasma mannose-binding lectin (MBL) to microbes. MBL is structurally similar to a component of C1 of the classical pathway and serves to activate C4. The subsequent steps are essentially the same as in the classical pathway.

The net result of these early steps of complement activation is that microbes acquire a coat of covalently attached C3b. Note that the alternative and lectin pathways are effector mechanisms of innate immunity and that the classical pathway is a mechanism of adaptive humoral immunity. These pathways differ in how they are initiated, but once they are triggered, their late steps are the same.

The late steps of complement activation (Fig. 8-6) are initiated by the binding of C5 to the C5 convertase, and the proteolysis of C5, generating C5b. The remaining components, C6, C7, C8, and C9, bind sequentially. The final protein in the pathway, C9, polymerizes to form a pore in the cell membrane through which water and ions can enter, causing death of the cell. This poly-C9 is called the membrane attack complex, and its formation is the end result of complement activation.

Functions of the Complement System

The complement system plays an important role in the elimination of microbes during innate and adaptive immune responses. The main effector functions of the complement system are illustrated in Figure 8-7.

Microbes coated with C3b are phagocytosed by virtue of the C3b being recognized by the type 1 complement receptor (CR1, or CD35) expressed on phagocytes. Thus, C3b functions as an opsonin. Opsonization is probably the most important function of complement in defense against microbes. The membrane attack complex can induce osmotic lysis of cells, including microbes. Small peptide fragments of C3, C4, and C5, which are produced by proteolysis, are chemotactic for neutrophils, stimulate the release of inflammatory mediators from various leukocytes, and act on endothelial cells to enhance movement of leukocytes and plasma proteins into tissues. In this way, complement fragments induce inflammatory reactions that also serve to eliminate microbes.

In addition to its antimicrobial effector functions, the complement system provides stimuli for the development of humoral immune responses. When C3 is activated by a microbe, one of its breakdown products, C3d, is recognized by the CR2 receptor on B lymphocytes. Signals delivered by this receptor stimulate B cell responses against the microbe. This process is described in Chapter 7 (see Fig. 7-4) and is an example of an innate immune response to a microbe (complement activation) stimulating an adaptive immune response to the same microbe (B cell activation and antibody production). Complement proteins bound to antigen-antibody complexes are recognized by follicular dendritic cells in germinal centers, allowing the antigens to be displayed for further B cell activation and selection of high-affinity B cells. This complement-dependent antigen display is another way in which the complement system promotes antibody production.

Inherited deficiencies of complement proteins are the cause of human diseases. Deficiency of C3 results in profound susceptibility to infections and is usually fatal in early life. Somewhat surprisingly, deficiencies of the early proteins of the classical pathway, C2 and C4, do not cause immune deficiencies. This observation suggests that the classical and lectin pathways are not absolutely required for defense against infections, and the essential role of C3 in host defense may reflect its involvement in the alternative pathway of complement activation. C2 and C4 deficiencies are associated with an increased incidence of immune complex diseases resembling systemic lupus erythematosus, perhaps because the classical pathway functions to eliminate immune complexes from the circulation. Deficiencies of C9 and membrane attack complex formation result in increased susceptibility to *Neisseria* infections; it is not clear why the membrane attack complex is required for the clearance only of these bacteria.

Regulation of Complement Activation

Mammalian cells express regulatory proteins that inhibit complement activation, thus preventing

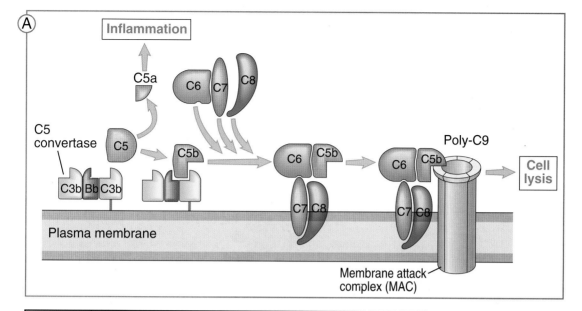

Figure 8–6   The late steps of complement activation. A. The late steps of complement activation start after the formation of the C5 convertase and are identical in the alternative and classical pathways. Products generated in the late steps induce inflammation (C5a) and cell lysis (the membrane attack complex [MAC]). B. The properties of the proteins of the late steps of complement activation are listed.

complement-mediated damage of host cells (Fig. 8-8). Many such regulatory proteins have been described. Decay accelerating factor (DAF) is a membrane protein that disrupts the binding of Factor B to C3b or the binding of C4b2a to C3b, thus terminating complement activation by both the alternative and the classical pathways. Membrane cofactor protein (MCP) serves as a cofactor for the proteolysis of C3b into inactive fragments, a process that is mediated by a plasma enzyme called Factor I. The type 1

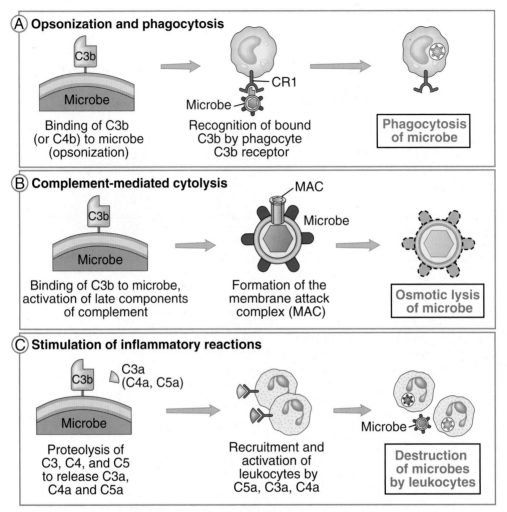

Figure 8–7   The functions of complement. A. C3b opsonizes microbes and is recognized by the type 1 complement receptor (CR1) of phagocytes, resulting in ingestion and intracellular killing of the opsonized microbes. Thus, C3b is an opsonin. CR1 also recognizes C4b, which may serve the same function. Other complement products, such as the inactivated form of C3b (iC3b), also bind to microbes and are recognized by other receptors on phagocytes (e.g., the type 3 complement receptor, a member of the integrin family of proteins). B. The membrane attack complex creates pores in cell membranes and induces osmotic lysis of the cells. C. Small peptides released during complement activation bind to receptors on neutrophils and stimulate inflammatory reactions. The peptides that serve this function are C5a, C3a, and C4a (in decreasing order of potency).

complement receptor (CR1) may serve both functions. A regulatory protein called C1 inhibitor (C1 INH) stops complement activation early, at the stage of C1 activation. Yet other proteins regulate complement activation at the late steps, such as the formation of the membrane attack complex. The presence of these regulatory proteins is an adaptation of mammals. Microbes lack the regulatory proteins and are, therefore, susceptible to complement. Even in mammalian cells the regulation can be overwhelmed by more and more complement activation. Therefore, even mammalian cells can become targets of complement if they

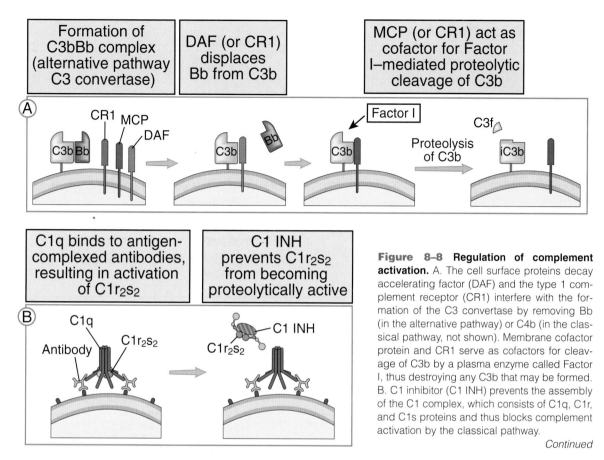

Ⓐ

| Formation of C3bBb complex (alternative pathway C3 convertase) | DAF (or CR1) displaces Bb from C3b | MCP (or CR1) act as cofactor for Factor I–mediated proteolytic cleavage of C3b |

Ⓑ

| C1q binds to antigen-complexed antibodies, resulting in activation of C1r₂s₂ | C1 INH prevents C1r₂s₂ from becoming proteolytically active |

Figure 8–8 Regulation of complement activation. A. The cell surface proteins decay accelerating factor (DAF) and the type 1 complement receptor (CR1) interfere with the formation of the C3 convertase by removing Bb (in the alternative pathway) or C4b (in the classical pathway, not shown). Membrane cofactor protein and CR1 serve as cofactors for cleavage of C3b by a plasma enzyme called Factor I, thus destroying any C3b that may be formed. B. C1 inhibitor (C1 INH) prevents the assembly of the C1 complex, which consists of C1q, C1r, and C1s proteins and thus blocks complement activation by the classical pathway.

Continued

are coated with large amounts of antibodies, as in some immunologic (hypersensitivity) diseases (see Chapter 11).

Inherited deficiencies of regulatory proteins cause excessive and pathologic complement activation. Deficiency of C1 INH is the cause of a disease called **hereditary angioneurotic edema,** in which excessive C1 activation and the production of vasoactive protein fragments lead to leakage of fluid (edema) in the larynx and many other tissues. A disease called **paroxysmal nocturnal hemoglobinuria** results from deficiency of an enzyme that synthesizes the glyco-lipid anchor for several membrane proteins, including the complement regulatory proteins DAF and MCP. Uncontrolled complement activation occurs on the erythrocytes of these patients and leads to lysis of the erythrocytes.

The effector mechanisms of humoral immunity that have been described so far may be active at any site in the body to which antibodies gain access. Antibodies also serve protective functions at two special anatomic sites, the mucosal organs and the fetus.

Functions of Antibodies at Special Anatomic Sites

As has been mentioned previously, antibodies are produced in peripheral lymphoid organs and readily enter the blood, from where they may go virtually anywhere. However, there are special mechanisms for transporting antibodies across epithelia and across the placenta, and antibodies play vital roles in defense in these locations.

Ⓒ Plasma proteins

Protein	Distribution	Function
C1 inhibitor (C1 INH)	Plasma; conc. 200 µg/mL	Inhibits C1r and C1s serine protease activity
Factor I	Plasma; conc. 35 µg/mL	Proteolytically cleaves C3b and C4b
Factor H	Plasma; conc. 480 mg/mL	Causes dissociation of alternative pathway C3 convertase subunits Cofactor for Factor I–mediated cleavage of C3b
C4 binding protein (C4BP)	Plasma; conc. 300 µg/mL	Causes dissociation of classical pathway C3 convertase subunits Cofactor for Factor I–mediated cleavage of C4b

Membrane proteins

Protein	Distribution	Function
Membrane cofactor protein (MCP, CD46)	Leukocytes, epithelial cells, endothelial cells	Cofactor for Factor I–mediated cleavage of C3b and C4b
Decay accelerating factor (DAF)	Blood cells, endothelial cells, epithelial cells	Causes dissociation of C3 convertase subunits
CD59	Blood cells, endothelial cells, epithelial cells	Blocks C9 binding and prevents formation of the MAC
Type 1 complement receptor (CR1, CD35)	Mononuclear phagocytes, neutrophils, B and T cells, erythrocytes, eosinophils, FDCs	Causes dissociation of C3 convertase subunits Cofactor for Factor I–mediated cleavage of C3b and C4b

Figure 8–8, cont'd   C. The major regulatory proteins of the complement system and their functions are listed.

Mucosal Immunity

IgA antibody is produced in mucosal lymphoid tissues, actively transported across epithelia, and binds to and neutralizes microbes that enter through mucosal organs (Fig. 8-9). Microbes are often inhaled or ingested, and antibodies that are secreted into the lumens of the respiratory or gastrointestinal tract bind to the microbes and prevent them from colonizing the host. This type of immunity is called mucosal immunity (or secretory immunity). The principal class of antibody produced in mucosal tissues is IgA. In fact, because of the vast surface area of the intestines, IgA accounts for 60% to 70% of the approximately 3 g of antibody produced daily by a healthy adult. The propensity of mucosal lymphoid tissues to produce IgA is at least in part because the principal cytokine that induces switching to this isotype, namely transforming growth factor-β, is produced at high levels in these tissues. Also, some of the IgA may be produced

Figure 8–9 Transport of IgA through epithelium. In the mucosa of the gastrointestinal and respiratory tracts, IgA is produced by plasma cells in the lamina propria and is actively transported through epithelial cells by an IgA-specific Fc receptor (called the poly-Ig receptor because it recognizes IgM as well). On the luminal surface, the IgA with a portion of the bound receptor is released. Here the antibody recognizes ingested or inhaled microbes and blocks their entry through the epithelium.

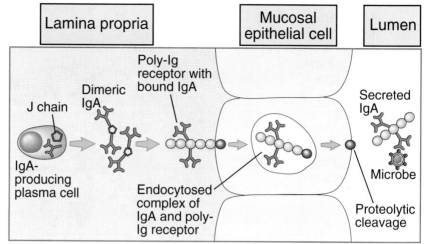

by a subset of B cells, called B-1 cells, that migrate to mucosal tissues and secrete IgA in response to non-protein antigens without T cell help.

The mucosal lymphoid tissues are located in the lamina propria, and IgA is produced in this region. This IgA has to be transported from the lamina propria into the lumen (which is the reverse of the usual transport of ingested molecules across the epithelium). Transport through the epithelium is carried out by a special Fc receptor, called the **poly-Ig receptor,** which is expressed on the basal surface of the epithelial cells. This receptor binds IgA, endocytoses it into vesicles, and transports it to the luminal surface. Here the receptor is cleaved by a protease, and the IgA is released into the lumen still carrying a portion of the bound poly-Ig receptor. The antibody can then recognize microbes in the lumen and block their binding to and entry through the epithelium. Mucosal immunity is the mechanism of protective immunity against poliovirus infection that is induced by oral immunization with the attenuated virus. Oral polio vaccine remains one of the most successful vaccines ever developed, and polio is likely to be the second disease to be eradicated worldwide by vaccination (smallpox being the first).

Neonatal Immunity

Maternal antibodies are actively transported across the placenta to the fetus and across the gut epithe-lium of neonates, protecting the newborn from infections. Newborn mammals have incompletely developed immune systems and are unable to mount effective immune responses against many microbes. During their early lives, they are protected from infections by antibodies acquired from their mothers. This is an excellent example of passive immunity. Neonates acquire maternal antibodies via two routes, both of which rely on a special Fc receptor called the **neonatal Fc receptor (FcRn).** During pregnancy, some classes of maternal IgG bind to the neonatal Fc receptor expressed in the placenta and the IgG is actively transported into the fetal circulation. After birth, neonates ingest maternal antibodies in milk. The neonate's intestinal epithelial cells also express the Fc receptor, which binds the ingested antibody and carries it across the epithelium. Thus, neonates acquire the IgG antibody profiles of their mothers and are protected from infectious microbes to which the mothers were exposed or vaccinated.

Evasion of Humoral Immunity by Microbes

Microbes have evolved numerous mechanisms to evade humoral immunity (Fig. 8-10). Many bacteria and viruses mutate their antigenic surface molecules and can no longer be recognized by antibodies produced in response to previous infections. Antigenic variation is commonly seen in viruses, such as

Mechanism of immune evasion	Examples	
Antigenic variation	Many viruses, e.g. influenza, HIV *Neisseria gonorrhoeae, E. coli, Salmonella typhimurium*	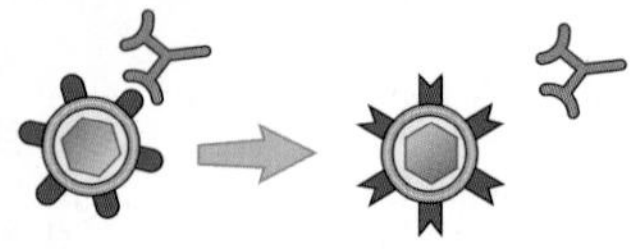
Inhibition of complement activation	Many bacteria	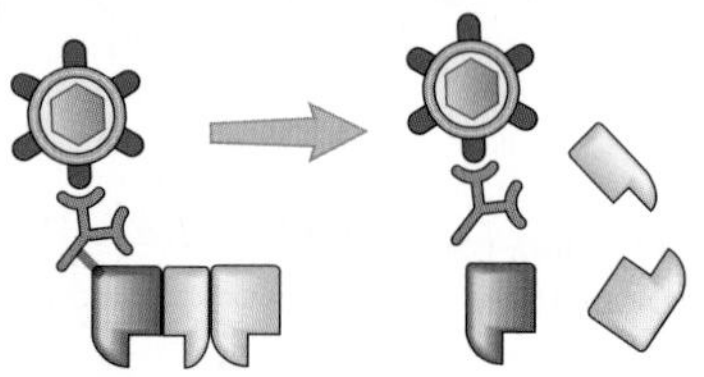
Resistance to phagocytosis	Pneumococcus	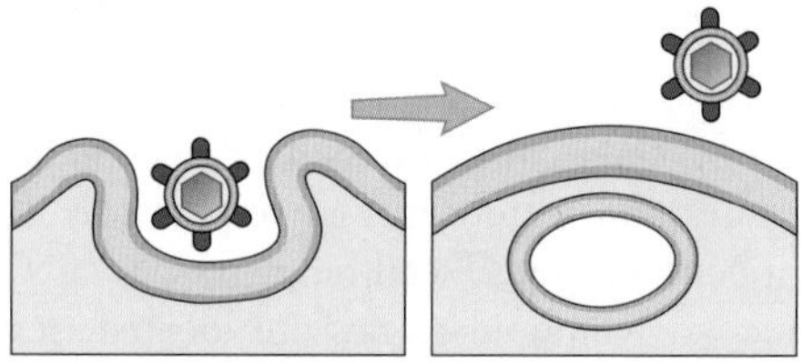

Figure 8–10   Evasion of humoral immunity by microbes. The principal mechanisms by which microbes evade humoral immunity are listed, with illustrative examples.

influenza, human immunodeficiency virus (HIV), and rhinovirus. There are so many variants of the major antigenic surface glycoprotein of HIV, called gp120, that antibodies against one HIV isolate may not protect against other HIV isolates. This is one reason why gp120 vaccines are of little or no effectiveness in protecting individuals from infection. Bacteria, such as *Escherichia coli*, vary the antigens contained in their pili and also evade antibody-mediated defense. The trypanosome parasite expresses new surface glycoproteins whenever it encounters antibodies against the original glycoprotein. As a result, infection with this protozoan parasite is characterized by waves of parasitemia, each wave consisting of an antigenically new parasite that is not recognized by antibodies produced against the parasites in the preceding wave. Other microbes inhibit complement activation or resist phagocytosis.

Vaccination

Vaccination is the process of stimulating protective adaptive immune responses against microbes by expo-

sure to nonpathogenic forms or components of the microbes. The development of vaccines against infections has been one of the great successes of immunology. The only human disease to be intentionally eradicated from the earth is smallpox, and this was achieved by a worldwide program of vaccination. Polio is likely to be the second such disease, and, as mentioned in Chapter 1, many other diseases have been largely controlled by vaccination (Fig. 1-2, Chapter 1). Several types of vaccines are in use and are being developed (Fig. 8-11). Some of the most effective vaccines are composed of attenuated microbes, which are treated to abolish their infectivity and pathogenicity while retaining their antigenicity. Immunization with these attenuated microbes stimulates the production of neutralizing antibodies against microbial antigens that protect vaccinated individuals from subsequent infections. For some infections, such as polio, the vaccines are given orally, to stimulate mucosal IgA responses that protect individuals from natural infection, which occurs by the oral route. Vaccines composed of microbial proteins

Type of vaccine	Examples	Form of protection
Live attenuated, or killed, bacteria	BCG, cholera	Antibody response
Live attenuated viruses	Polio, rabies	Antibody response; cell-mediated immune response
Subunit (antigen) vaccines	Tetanus toxoid, diphtheria toxoid	Antibody response
Conjugate vaccines	*Haemophilus influenzae*	Helper T cell–dependent antibody response
Synthetic vaccines	Hepatitis (recombinant proteins)	Antibody response
Viral vectors	Clinical trials of HIV antigens in canary pox vector	Cell-mediated and humoral immune responses
DNA vaccines	Clinical trials ongoing for several infections	Cell-mediated and humoral immune responses

Figure 8–11 Vaccination strategies. Examples of different types of vaccines and the nature of the protective immune responses induced by these vaccines are summarized.

and polysaccharides, called subunit vaccines, work in the same way. Some microbial polysaccharide antigens (which cannot stimulate T cell help) are chemically coupled to proteins, so that helper T cells are activated and high-affinity antibodies are produced against the polysaccharides. These are called conjugate vaccines, and they are excellent examples of the practical application of our knowledge of helper T cell–B cell interactions. Immunization with inactivated microbial toxins and with microbial proteins synthesized in the laboratory stimulate antibodies that bind to and neutralize the native toxins and the microbes, respectively.

One of the continuing challenges in vaccination is to develop vaccines that stimulate cell-mediated immunity against intracellular microbes. Injected or fed microbial antigens are extracellular antigens, and they induce mainly antibody responses. To elicit T cell–mediated immune responses, it may be necessary to deliver the antigens to the interior of cells, particularly professional antigen-presenting cells. Attenuated viruses can achieve this goal, but there are few

examples of viruses that have been successfully treated such that they remain able to infect cells and are both immunogenic and safe. Many newer approaches are being tried to stimulate cell-mediated immunity by vaccination. These approaches include incorporating microbial antigens into viral "vectors," which will infect host cells and produce the antigens inside the cells. A new technique is to immunize individuals with DNA encoding a microbial antigen in a bacterial plasmid. The plasmid is ingested by host antigen-presenting cells, and the antigen is produced inside the cells. Intracellular antigens induce cell-mediated immunity (see Chapters 5 and 6), which may be effective against infections by intracellular microbes. Many of these strategies are now undergoing clinical trials for different infections.

SUMMARY

▶ Humoral immunity is the type of adaptive immunity that is mediated by antibodies. Antibodies prevent infections by blocking the ability of microbes to invade host cells, and they eliminate microbes by activating several effector mechanisms.

▶ In antibody molecules, the antigen-binding (Fab) regions are spatially separate from the effector (Fc) regions. The ability of antibodies to neutralize microbes and toxins is entirely a function of the antigen-binding regions. Even Fc-dependent effector functions are activated after antibodies bind antigens.

▶ Antibodies are produced in lymphoid tissues and bone marrow, but they enter the circulation and are able to reach any site of infection. Heavy chain class switching and affinity maturation enhance the protective functions of antibodies.

▶ Antibodies neutralize the infectivity of microbes and the pathogenicity of microbial toxins by binding to and interfering with the ability of these microbes and toxins to attach to host cells.

▶ Antibodies coat (opsonize) microbes and promote their phagocytosis by binding to Fc receptors on phagocytes. The binding of antibody Fc regions to Fc receptors also stimulates the microbicidal activities of phagocytes.

▶ The complement system is a collection of circulating and cell surface proteins that play important roles in host defense. The complement system may be activated on microbial surfaces without antibodies (called the alternative pathway, a component of innate immunity) and after the binding of antibodies to antigens (the classical pathway, a component of adaptive humoral immunity). Complement proteins are sequentially cleaved, and active components, mainly C3b, become covalently attached to the surfaces where complement is activated. The late steps of complement activation lead to the formation of the cytolytic membrane attack complex. Different products of complement activation promote phagocytosis of microbes, induce cell lysis, and stimulate inflammation. Mammals express cell surface and circulating regulatory proteins that prevent inappropriate complement activation on host cells.

▶ IgA antibody is produced in the lamina propria of mucosal organs and is actively transported by a special Fc receptor through the epithelium into the lumen, where it blocks the ability of microbes to invade the epithelium.

▶ Neonates acquire IgG antibodies from their mothers through the placenta and from the milk through gut epithelium, using a neonatal Fc receptor to capture and transport the maternal antibodies.

▶ Microbes have developed strategies to resist or evade humoral immunity, such as varying their antigens and acquiring resistance to complement and phagocytosis.

▶ Most vaccines in current use work by stimulating the production of neutralizing antibodies. Many approaches are being tested to develop vaccines that can stimulate protective cell-mediated immune responses.

Review Questions

1 What regions of antibody molecules are involved in the functions of antibodies?

2 How do heavy chain class switching and affinity maturation improve the abilities of antibodies to combat infectious pathogens?

3 In what situations does the ability of antibodies to neutralize microbes protect the host from infections?

4 How do antibodies assist in the elimination of microbes by phagocytes?

5 How is the complement system activated, and why is it effective against microbes but does not react against host cells and tissues?

6 What are the functions of the complement system, and what components of complement mediate these functions?

7 How do antibodies prevent infections by ingested and inhaled microbes?

8 How do neonatal animals develop the capacity to protect themselves from infections even before their immune systems have reached maturity?

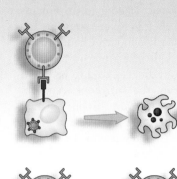

Immunologic Tolerance and Autoimmunity

Self-Nonself Discrimination in the Immune System and Its Failure

9

One of the remarkable characteristics of the normal immune system is that it is capable of reacting to an enormous variety of microbes, but it does not react against each individual's own (self) antigens. This unresponsiveness to self antigens, also called **immunologic tolerance,** is maintained despite the fact that the mechanisms by which lymphocyte receptors are expressed are not inherently biased to produce receptors for nonself antigens. In other words, lymphocytes with the ability to recognize self antigens are constantly being generated during the normal process of lymphocyte maturation. Furthermore, the immune system is readily accessible to many self antigens, so that unresponsiveness to these antigens cannot be maintained simply by concealing these antigens from lymphocytes. It follows that there must exist mechanisms that prevent immune responses to self antigens. These mechanisms are responsible for one of the cardinal features of the immune system, namely, its ability to discriminate between self and nonself (usually microbial) antigens. If these mechanisms fail, the immune system may attack the individual's own cells and tissues. Such reactions are called **autoimmunity,** and the diseases they cause are called autoimmune diseases.

In this chapter we will address the following questions.

- How does the immune system maintain its unresponsiveness to self antigens?

- What are the factors that may contribute to the development of autoimmunity?

This chapter begins with a discussion of the important principles and features of self-tolerance and autoimmunity. Following this the different mechanisms are discussed that maintain tolerance to self antigens, including how each mechanism may fail, resulting in autoimmunity.

Immunologic Tolerance: Significance and Mechanisms

Immunologic tolerance is a lack of response to antigens that is induced by exposure of lymphocytes to these antigens. When lymphocytes with receptors for a particular antigen are exposed to this antigen, any of three outcomes is possible (Fig. 9-1). The lymphocytes may be activated, leading to an immune response; antigens that elicit such a response are said to be immunogenic. The lymphocytes may be functionally inactivated or killed, resulting in tolerance; antigens that induce tolerance are said to be tolerogenic. In some situations, the antigen-specific lymphocytes may not react in any way; this phenomenon has been called ignorance, implying that the lymphocytes simply ignore the presence of the antigen. Normally, microbes are immunogenic, and self antigens are either tolerogenic or are ignored. The choice among lymphocyte activation, tolerance, and ignorance is determined by the nature of the antigen-specific lymphocytes and by the nature of the antigen and how it is displayed to the immune system. In fact, the same antigen may be administered in ways that induce an immune response or tolerance. This experimental observation has been exploited to analyze what factors determine whether activation or toler-

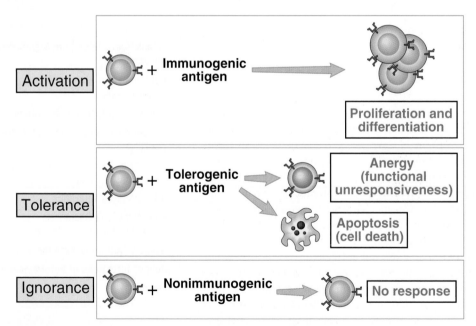

Figure 9–1   Consequences of the encounter of lymphocytes with antigens. Naive lymphocytes may be activated to proliferate and differentiate by immunogenic antigens. Tolerance is induced when tolerogenic antigens induce functional anergy (unresponsiveness) or apoptosis, leading to an inability of the cells to again respond to the same antigen even in an immunogenic form. Some antigens are ignored by lymphocytes, resulting in no response, but the lymphocytes are capable of responding to the same antigen in an immunogenic form.

ance develops as a consequence of encounter with an antigen.

The phenomenon of immunologic tolerance is important for several reasons. First, as we stated at the outset, self antigens normally induce tolerance. Second, if we learn how to induce tolerance in lymphocytes specific for a particular antigen, we may be able to use this knowledge to prevent or control unwanted immune reactions. Strategies for inducing tolerance are being tested to treat allergic and autoimmune diseases and to prevent the rejection of organ transplants. The same strategies may be valuable in gene therapy, to prevent immune responses against the products of newly expressed genes or vectors.

Immunologic tolerance to different self antigens may be induced when developing lymphocytes encounter these antigens in the generative lymphoid organs, called central tolerance, or when mature lymphocytes encounter self antigens in peripheral tissues, called peripheral tolerance (Fig. 9-2). Central tolerance is a mechanism of tolerance only to self antigens that are present in the generative lymphoid organs, namely, the bone marrow and thymus. Tolerance to self antigens that are not present in these organs must be induced and maintained by peripheral mechanisms. We do not know which, or how many, self antigens induce central or peripheral tolerance or are ignored by the immune system.

Autoimmunity: Principles and Pathogenesis

Autoimmunity is defined as an immune response against self (autologous) antigens and is an important cause of disease. It is estimated that at least 1% to 2% of individuals suffer from autoimmune diseases, although in many cases, diseases associated with uncontrolled immune responses are called autoimmune without any formal evidence that the responses are directed against self antigens.

The principal factors in the development of autoimmunity are the inheritance of susceptibility genes, which may contribute to failure of self-tolerance, and environmental triggers, such as infections, which may activate self-reactive lymphocytes (Fig. 9-3). Much has been learned from experimental animal models about how self-tolerance may fail and

how self-reactive lymphocytes may become pathogenic. Despite our growing knowledge of the immunologic abnormalities that may result in autoimmunity, we do not know the etiology of any human autoimmune disease. This lack of understanding is mainly because autoimmune diseases in humans are usually heterogeneous and multifactorial, the self antigens that are the inducers and targets of the autoimmune reactions are often unknown, and the diseases may present clinically long after the autoimmune reactions have been initiated. Autoimmunity may result in the production of antibodies against self antigens or the activation of T cells reactive with self antigens. How these antibodies and T cells damage tissues and cause disease is described in Chapter 11.

With this brief background, the discussion proceeds to the mechanisms of immunologic tolerance and how the failure of each mechanism may result in autoimmunity. Tolerance in CD4$^+$ helper T lymphocytes is described first, because more is known about this cell type than about any other. Recall that CD4$^+$ helper T cells control virtually all immune responses to protein antigens. Therefore, if helper T cells are made unresponsive to self protein antigens, this may be enough to prevent both cell-mediated and humoral immune responses against these antigens. Conversely, failure of tolerance in helper T cells may result in autoimmunity manifested by T cell–mediated attack against self antigens or by the production of autoantibodies against self proteins.

Central T Lymphocyte Tolerance

If immature T cells in the thymus recognize with high avidity self antigens present in the thymus, the lymphocytes die by apoptosis (Fig. 9-4). The lymphocytes that develop in the thymus consist of cells with receptors capable of recognizing many antigens, both self and foreign. If an immature lymphocyte strongly interacts with a self antigen, displayed as a peptide bound to a self major histocompatibility complex (MHC) molecule, that lymphocyte receives signals that trigger apoptosis, and the cell dies before it can complete its maturation. This process is also termed *negative selection* (see Chapter 4), and it is the princi-

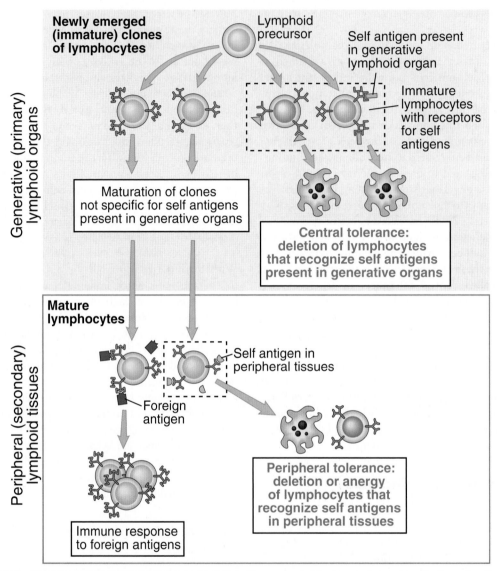

Figure 9–2 Central and peripheral tolerance to self antigens. Immature lymphocytes specific for self antigens may encounter these antigens in the generative lymphoid organs and are deleted (central tolerance). Mature self-reactive lymphocytes may be inactivated or deleted by encounter with self antigens in peripheral tissues (peripheral tolerance). B lymphocytes are shown here, but the same processes occur with T lymphocytes as well.

pal mechanism of central tolerance. Immature lymphocytes may interact strongly with an antigen if the antigen is present at high concentrations in the thymus and if the lymphocytes express receptors that recognize the antigen with high affinity. Antigens that induce negative selection tend to be present in higher concentrations in the thymus than antigens that induce positive selection and include proteins that are abundant throughout the body, such as plasma proteins and common cellular proteins. Surprisingly, many self proteins that have been thought to be expressed mainly or exclusively in peripheral

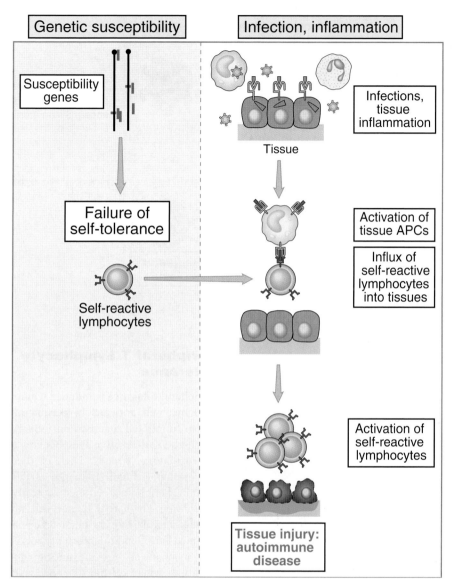

Figure 9–3 Postulated mechanisms of autoimmunity. In this proposed model of an organ-specific T cell–mediated auto-immune disease, various genetic loci may confer susceptibility to autoimmunity, probably by influencing the maintenance of self-tolerance. Environmental triggers, such as infections and other inflammatory stimuli, promote the influx of lymphocytes into tissues and the activation of self-reactive T cells, resulting in tissue injury.

tissues are actually expressed in some of the epithelial cells of the thymus. Therefore, negative selection of immature T cells may be important in protecting against responses to a wide variety of self protein antigens. Developing T cells that encounter these

proteins are deleted, thus preventing reactions against the peripheral self antigens. A transcription factor called AIRE (for autoimmune regulator) appears to be responsible for the thymic expression of such self protein antigens. Mutations in the *aire* gene are the

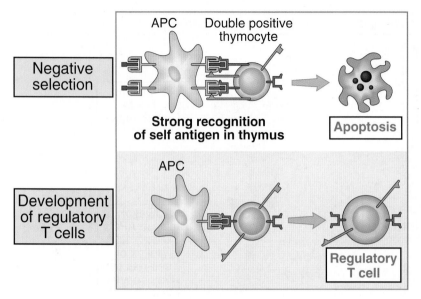

Figure 9–4 Central T cell tolerance. Strong recognition of self antigens by immature T cells in the thymus may lead to death of the cells (negative selection, or deletion). Self-antigen recognition in the thymus may also lead to the development of regulatory T cells that enter peripheral tissues.

cause of a rare autoimmune syndrome called APECED (autoimmune polyendocrinopathy with candidiasis and ectodermal dysplasia).

The lymphocytes that survive negative selection in the thymus go on to mature and are depleted of potentially dangerous autoreactive T cells. This process of central tolerance affects self-reactive CD4$^+$ T cells and CD8$^+$ T cells, which recognize self peptides displayed by class II MHC and class I MHC molecules, respectively. It is not known what signals induce apoptosis in immature lymphocytes that recognize antigens with high affinity in the thymus.

Some immature T cells that recognize self antigens in the thymus develop into regulatory T cells and enter peripheral tissues (see Fig. 9-4). The functions of regulatory T cells are described later in the chapter. What determines whether self antigens will induce negative selection or the development of regulatory T cells is not known.

Defective central tolerance is often postulated to be the reason why some autoimmune-prone inbred strains of mice contain abnormally large numbers of mature T cells specific for various self antigens. The mechanisms and consequences of failure of central tolerance in these mice are not well understood.

Peripheral T Lymphocyte Tolerance

Peripheral tolerance is induced when mature T cells recognize self antigens in peripheral tissues, leading to functional inactivation (anergy) or death, or when the self-reactive lymphocytes are suppressed by regulatory T cells. Each of these mechanisms of peripheral T cell tolerance is described in this section. Peripheral tolerance is clearly important for preventing T cell responses to self antigens that are present mainly in peripheral tissues and not in the thymus. Peripheral tolerance may also provide "back-up" mechanisms for preventing autoimmunity in situations where central tolerance is incomplete.

Anergy

Anergy is the functional inactivation of T lymphocytes that occurs when these cells recognize antigens without adequate levels of the costimulators (second signals) that are needed for full T cell activation (Fig. 9-5). In previous chapters we have pointed out that naive T lymphocytes need at least two signals for their proliferation and differentiation

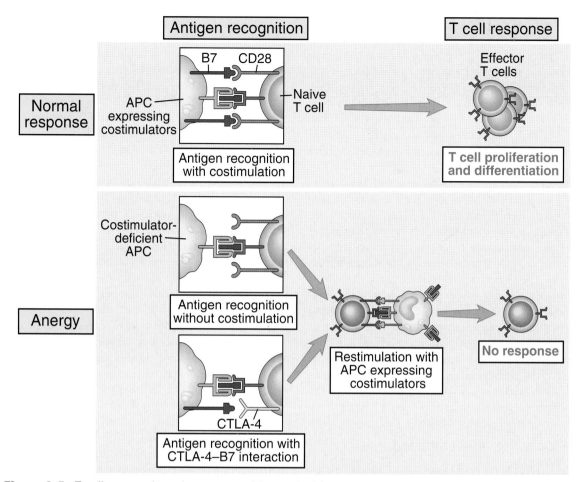

Figure 9–5 T cell anergy. An antigen presented by costimulator-expressing antigen-presenting cells (APCs) induces a normal T cell response. If the T cell recognizes antigen without costimulation, or in the presence of CTLA-4–B7 interactions, the T cell fails to respond and is rendered incapable of responding even if the antigen is subsequently presented by costimulator-expressing APCs.

into effector cells: signal 1 is always antigen, and signal 2 is provided by costimulators that are expressed on professional antigen-presenting cells (APCs) in response to microbes. It is believed that, normally, APCs in tissues and peripheral lymphoid organs are in a resting state, in which they express little or no costimulators such as B7 proteins (see Chapter 5). These APCs are constantly processing and displaying the self antigens that are present in the tissues. T lymphocytes with receptors for the self antigens are able to recognize the antigens and thus receive signals from their antigen receptors (signal 1), but the T cells do not receive the necessary second signals. Signal 1 without adequate signal 2 may induce long-lived T cell anergy. (Antigen recognition without costimulation may also induce no responses rather than anergy; see Fig. 5-6, Chapter 5.) In some cases, T cells that encounter self antigens may begin to express a molecule called CTLA-4 (CD152), which is a high-affinity receptor for B7 molecules that delivers inhibitory signals to the T cells. When a T cell sees a self antigen on an APC, CTLA-4 on the T cell may engage B7 molecules on the APC and inactivate the T cell. Recall that CD28 is the activating T cell receptor for B7 molecules and the major receptor for delivering second signals to T cells. It is not known how T cells choose to use one or the other receptor for B7, namely, CD28 to initiate responses or CTLA-4 to inhibit responses. One possibility is that resting APCs may express just enough B7 to engage the inhibitory receptor but not enough to activate the T cells.

Several experimental models support the importance of T cell anergy in the maintenance of self-tolerance. If high levels of B7 costimulators are artificially expressed in a tissue in a mouse, that animal develops autoimmune reactions against antigens in that tissue. Thus, artificially providing second signals "breaks" anergy and activates autoreactive T cells. If CTLA-4 molecules are blocked or deleted (by gene knockout) in a mouse, that mouse develops widespread autoimmunity against its own tissues. This result suggests that the inactivating receptor, CTLA-4, is constantly functioning to keep autoreactive T cells in check. There is great interest in determining if abnormalities in costimulators or CTLA-4 contribute to the development of autoimmune diseases in humans.

Deletion: Activation-Induced Cell Death

Repeated activation of mature T lymphocytes by self antigen, or recognition of self antigens without second signals, triggers pathways of apoptosis that result in elimination (deletion) of the self-reactive lymphocytes (Fig. 9-6). This process is called activation-induced cell death. There are two likely mechanisms of activation-induced death of lymphocytes. First, in CD4+ T cells, repeated activation leads to the coexpression of a death receptor called Fas (CD95) and its ligand, Fas ligand (FasL). FasL binds to Fas on the same or on a neighboring cell. This interaction generates signals through the Fas death receptor that culminate in the activation of caspases, cytosolic enzymes that induce apoptosis. Thus, the repeated activation of the T cell triggers an internal death program that prevents the T cell from continuing to respond. Self antigens may delete specific T cells because these antigens are present throughout

life and are capable of repeatedly stimulating lymphocytes. In contrast, most microbes are eliminated by immune responses, and microbial antigens are unlikely to be persistent enough to repeatedly stimulate specific lymphocytes. Interestingly, the T cell growth factor interleukin-2 (IL-2) potentiates Fas-mediated apoptosis. Thus, the same cytokine can function to initiate and terminate T cell responses. How the balance between these two opposing actions is determined is not known.

The second postulated mechanism of activation-induced cell death is that antigen recognition induces the production of pro-apoptotic proteins in T cells. In immune responses to microbes, the activity of these proteins is counteractive by anti-apoptotic proteins that are induced by costimulation and by other, largely undefined, second signals generated during innate immune responses. But self antigens do not stimulate production of anti-apoptotic proteins, resulting in death of the cells that recognize the self antigens. This pathway of activation-induced cell death does not involved death receptors such as Fas.

The best evidence supporting the role of Fas-mediated apoptosis in self-tolerance has come from genetic studies. Mice with mutations in the *fas* and *fasL* genes and children with mutations in *fas* all develop autoimmune diseases with lymphocyte accumulation. The human disease, called the autoimmune lymphoproliferative syndrome, is rare and the only known example of a defect in apoptosis causing a complex autoimmune phenotype.

Immune Suppression

On encounter with self antigens, some self-reactive T lymphocytes may develop into regulatory cells whose function is to prevent or suppress the activation of other, potentially harmful, self-reactive lymphocytes (Fig. 9-7). Regulatory T cells may develop in the thymus (see Fig. 9-5) or in peripheral lymphoid organs. We do not know what special features of antigen recognition lead to the development of regulatory cells and not effector cells, the usual consequence of lymphocyte activation. Most regulatory T cells are CD4+ and express high levels of CD25, the α chain of the IL-2 receptor, but the heterogeneity of this population is undefined. We also know little

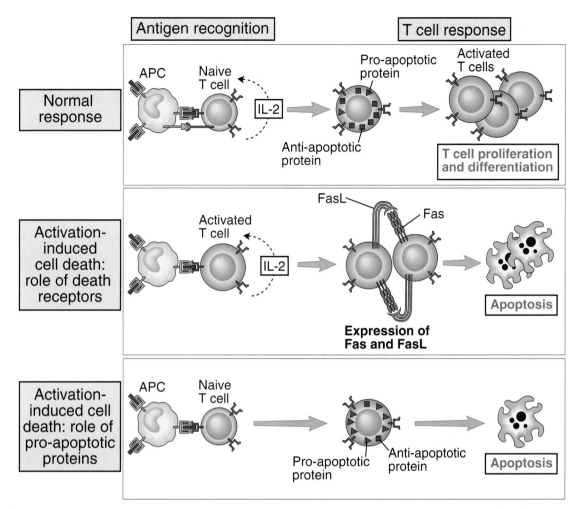

Figure 9–6   Activation-induced death of T lymphocytes. T cells respond to antigen presented by normal APCs by secreting IL-2, expressing anti-apoptotic proteins, and undergoing proliferation and differentiation. In one form of activation-induced cell death, restimulation of recently activated T cells by antigen leads to coexpression of Fas and Fas ligand (FasL), engagement of Fas, and apoptotic death of the T cells. Note that FasL on one T cell may engage Fas either on a neighboring cell (as shown) or on the same cell. Fas-independent activation–induced cell death may also occur when antigen recognition by T cells without costimulation or innate immunity leads to expression of intracellular pro-apoptotic proteins.

about the mechanisms by which regulatory T cells inhibit immune responses *in vivo*. Some regulatory cells produce cytokines, such as TGFβ and IL-10, which block the activation of lymphocytes and macrophages. Regulatory cells may also directly interact with and suppress other lymphocytes or APCs, by undefined mechanisms that do not involve cytokines.

The best evidence that active suppression plays a role in self-tolerance has come from complex animal models. It is thought that normal mice contain $CD25^+CD4^+$ T cells that have seen self antigens and become regulatory cells. In one experimental model, if T cells depleted of $CD25^+$ lymphocytes are transferred into a mouse that does not have any lymphocytes of its own, this mouse develops a disseminated autoimmune disease involving multiple organs. The interpretation of this experiment is that regulatory T cells, which are contained within the $CD25^+$ cell

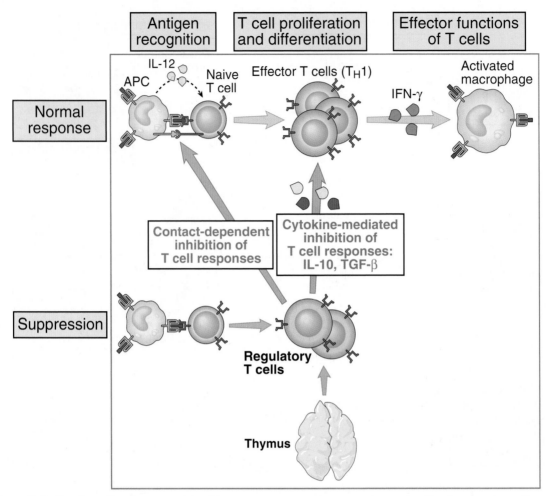

Figure 9–7   T cell–mediated suppression of immune responses. In a normal response, T cells recognize antigen and proliferate and differentiate into effector cells. A typical T_H1 response is shown, in which the APCs secrete IL-12, which stimulates differentiation of the naive T cells into T_H1 effectors that produce IFN-γ and activate macrophages in the effector phase of the response. Some T cells may differentiate into regulatory cells in the peripheral tissues or the thymus, and these regulatory cells inhibit the activation and differentiation of naive T cells, by contact-dependent mechanisms, or they may secrete cytokines that inhibit the effector phase of T cell responses.

population, normally control autoreactive lymphocytes and, in the absence of the regulators, the autoreactive lymphocytes are released from their control and attack self tissues. The role of regulatory cells in maintaining self-tolerance in humans is an issue that is being actively investigated.

Several important points emerge from this discussion of the mechanisms of T cell tolerance. First, self antigens differ from foreign microbial antigens in

several ways, which contribute to the choice between tolerance induced by the former and activation by the latter (Fig. 9-8). Self antigens are present in the thymus, where they induce central tolerance; in contrast, microbial antigens are actively transported to and concentrated in peripheral lymphoid organs. Self antigens are displayed by resting APCs in the absence of innate immunity and second signals, thus favoring the induction of T cell anergy or death. In contrast,

Feature of antigen	Tolerogenic self antigens	Immunogenic foreign antigens
	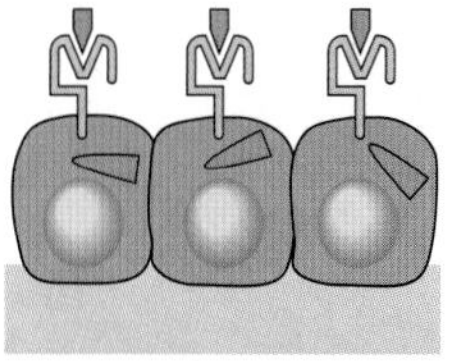 Tissue	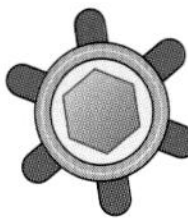 Microbe
Presence in generative organs	Yes (some self antigens): high concentrations induce negative selection and regulatory T cells (central tolerance)	No: microbial antigens are concentrated in peripheral lymphoid organs
Presentation with second signals (innate immunity)	No: deficiency of second signals may lead to T cell anergy or apoptosis	Yes: typically seen with microbes; second signals promote lymphocyte survival and activation
Persistence of antigen	Long-lived (throughout life); repeated T cell activation induces apoptosis	Usually short lived; immune response eliminates antigen

Figure 9–8 **Features of protein antigens that influence the choice between T cell tolerance and activation.** This table summarizes some of the characteristics of self and foreign (e.g., microbial) protein antigens that determine why the self antigens induce tolerance and microbial antigens stimulate T cell–mediated immune responses.

microbes elicit innate immune reactions, leading to the expression of costimulators and cytokines that function as second signals and promote T cell proliferation and differentiation into effector cells. Self antigens are present throughout life and may therefore cause repeated T cell activation and activation-induced cell death. Most microbes are rapidly eliminated by immune responses, before they are able to cause active death of specific lymphocytes. Second, it is apparent that much of our understanding of the mechanisms of T cell tolerance, and their roles in preventing autoimmunity, is based on studies with experimental animal models. Extending these studies to humans remains an important, and often daunting, challenge.

B Lymphocyte Tolerance

Self polysaccharides, lipids, and nucleic acids are T-independent antigens that are not recognized by T cells. These antigens must induce tolerance in B lymphocytes to prevent autoantibody production. B cell tolerance to self protein antigens has also been demonstrated experimentally. The principles of central and peripheral tolerance in the B lymphocyte compartment are similar to those of T cell tolerance.

Central B Cell Tolerance

When immature B lymphocytes interact strongly with self antigens in the bone marrow, the B cells are either killed (negative selection) or they change their receptor specificity (Fig. 9-9). The process of deletion is very similar to negative selection of immature T lymphocytes. As in the T cell compartment, negative selection of B cells eliminates lymphocytes with high-affinity receptors for abundant, and usually widely expressed, cell membrane or soluble self antigens. Immature B cells use a second mechanism to prevent autoimmunity. When these B cells recognize self antigens in the bone marrow, the cells may reactivate their immunoglobulin (Ig) gene recombination machinery and begin to express a new Ig light chain (see Chapter 4). This new light chain associates with

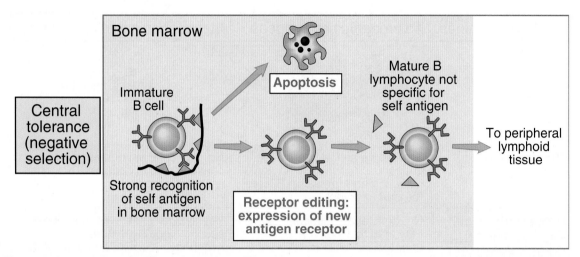

Figure 9–9   Negative selection and receptor editing in immature B lymphocytes. An immature B cell that strongly recognizes self antigens (in this case, a multivalent self antigen with several epitopes) in the bone marrow is either killed by apoptosis or changes its antigen receptor.

the previously expressed Ig heavy chain to produce a new antigen receptor that is no longer specific for the self antigen. This process of changing receptor specificity is called *receptor editing*. It is not known how many, or which, self antigens present in the bone marrow induce apoptosis or receptor editing and why any self-reactive B lymphocyte undergoes one or the other fate. It is possible that failure of central tolerance in developing B cells may result in autoimmunity, but there are no convincing examples illustrating this phenomenon.

Peripheral B Cell Tolerance

Mature B lymphocytes that encounter high concentrations of self antigens in peripheral lymphoid tissues become anergic and cannot again respond to that self antigen (Fig. 9-10). According to one hypothesis, if B cells recognize an antigen and do not receive T cell help (because helper T cells are absent or tolerant), the B cells become anergic. Presumably, T-independent antigens activate B lymphocytes without T cell help only when such antigens trigger strong signals in the B cells (see Chapter 7). Anergic B cells may leave lymphoid follicles and are subsequently excluded from the follicles. These excluded B cells may die because they do not receive necessary

survival stimuli. It is suspected that diseases associated with autoantibody production, such as systemic lupus erythematosus, are caused by defective tolerance in both B lymphocytes and helper T cells.

After discussing how immunologic tolerance to self antigens may be maintained, and why it may fail, it is important to point out that the development of autoimmunity is influenced by several factors in addition to primary lymphocyte defects. The most important of these factors are inherited genes and infections; how these may contribute to autoimmunity is described in the sections that follow.

Genetic Factors in Autoimmunity

Multiple genes predispose to autoimmune diseases, the most important of these being MHC genes. The genetic predisposition to autoimmunity was appreciated when it was noted that if one of two identical twins develops an autoimmune disease, the other twin is more likely to develop the same disease than an unrelated member of the general population. Furthermore, this increased incidence is greater among monozygotic (identical) twins than among dizygotic twins. Family studies and, more recently, genome

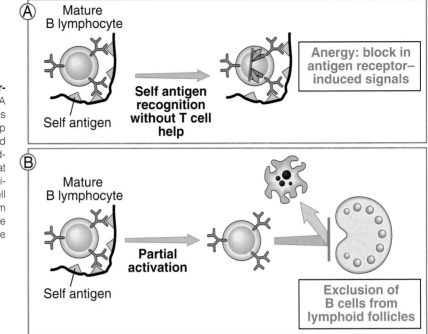

Figure 9–10   Peripheral tolerance in B lymphocytes. A. A mature B cell that recognizes a self antigen without T cell help is functionally inactivated and becomes incapable of responding to that antigen. B. B cells that are partially activated by recognition of self antigens without T cell help may be excluded from lymphoid follicles and may die by apoptosis because they are deprived of survival stimuli.

scanning techniques, as well as breeding studies in animals, have formally established that autoimmune diseases usually have a complex association with multiple gene loci.

Many autoimmune diseases in humans and inbred animals are linked to particular MHC alleles (Fig. 9-11). The association between HLA alleles and autoimmune diseases in humans was recognized many years ago and was one of the first lines of evidence that T cells played an important role in these disorders (since the function of MHC molecules is to present peptide antigens to T cells). The incidence of a particular autoimmune disease is often greater in individuals who inherit a particular HLA allele(s) than in the general population. This increased incidence is called the "relative risk" of an HLA-disease association. It is important to point out that an HLA allele may increase the risk of developing a particular autoimmune disease, but the HLA allele is not, by itself, the cause of the disease. In fact, the vast majority of individuals who inherit an HLA allele that is frequently disease associated never develop that disease. Particular MHC alleles may contribute to the development of autoimmunity because they are inefficient at displaying self antigens, leading to defective negative selection of T cells, or because peptide antigens presented by these MHC alleles may fail to stimulate regulatory T cells.

Numerous non-HLA genes are also associated with various autoimmune diseases (Fig. 9-12). Some of these associated genes are known, and their roles in the development of autoimmunity have been the focus of many hypotheses. Modern techniques for gene mapping and genomics have enormously expanded the number and diversity of genetic loci thought to be associated with various autoimmune diseases. At this time, many of the associations are with large chromosomal segments and the actual genes involved have not been identified.

Role of Infections in Autoimmunity

Infections may activate self-reactive lymphocytes and lead to the development of autoimmune diseases. Clinicians have recognized for many years that

Evidence	Examples		
	Disease	HLA allele	Relative risk
"Relative risk" of developing an autoimmune disease in individuals who inherit particular HLA allele(s) compared to individuals lacking these alleles	Ankylosing spondylitis	B27	90
	Rheumatoid arthritis	DR4	4
	Insulin-dependent diabetes mellitus	DR3/DR4	25
	Pemphigus vulgaris	DR4	14
Animal models: breeding studies establish association of disease with particular MHC alleles	Insulin-dependent diabetes mellitus (nonobese diabetic mouse strain)	I-A^{g7}	
Genome scanning methods reveal association of disease with MHC locus	Insulin-dependent diabetes mellitus	DR	

Figure 9–11   Association of autoimmune diseases with alleles of the MHC locus. Several lines of evidence support the association of certain MHC alleles with certain autoimmune diseases. Family and linkage studies show that individuals who inherit particular HLA alleles are more likely to develop some autoimmune diseases than individuals lacking these alleles ("relative risk"). Selected examples of HLA disease associations are listed. For instance, individuals who have the HLA-B27 allele are 90 to 100 times more likely to develop the disease ankylosing spondylitis than B27-negative individuals; other diseases show varying degrees of association with other HLA alleles. Breeding studies in animals have shown that the incidence of some autoimmune diseases correlates strongly with the inheritance of particular MHC alleles (e.g., insulin-dependent [type 1] diabetes mellitus with the mouse class II allele called I-A^{g7}). Genome scanning studies have also revealed the association of MHC with autoimmune diseases in humans and mice (e.g., HLA-DR and type 1 diabetes in humans).

Gene(s)	Disease association	Mechanism
Complement proteins (C2, C4)	Lupus-like disease	Defective clearance of immune complexes? Defects in B cell tolerance?
Fas, FasL	Lpr, gld mouse strains; human ALPS	Defective elimination of self-reactive T and B lymphocytes by AICD
AIRE	Autoimmune polyendocrinopathy with candidiasis and ectodermal dysplasia	Defective elimination of self-reactive T cells in the thymus

Figure 9–12   The roles of some non-MHC genes in autoimmunity. Shown here are examples of some genes other than MHC genes that may contribute to the development of autoimmune diseases. Lpr refers to the mouse mutation called "lymphoproliferation," and gld to "generalized lymphoproliferative disease." AICD, activation-induced cell death; ALPS, autoimmune lymphoproliferative syndrome.

the clinical manifestations of autoimmunity are often preceded by infectious prodromes. This association between infections and autoimmune tissue injury has been formally established in animal models. Infections may contribute to autoimmunity in several ways (Fig. 9-13). An infection of a tissue may induce a local innate immune response, and this may lead to increased expression of costimulators and cytokines by tissue APCs. As a result, these activated tissue APCs may be able to stimulate self-reactive T cells that encounter self antigens in the tissue. In other words, infection may "break" T cell anergy and promote the survival and activation of self reactive lymphocytes. Some infectious microbes may produce peptide antigens that are similar to, and cross-react with, self antigens. In these cases, immune responses to the microbial peptide may result in an immune attack against self antigens. Such cross-reactions between microbial and self antigens are termed *molecular mimicry*. Although the contribution of molecular mimicry to autoimmunity has fascinated immunologists, its actual significance in the development of

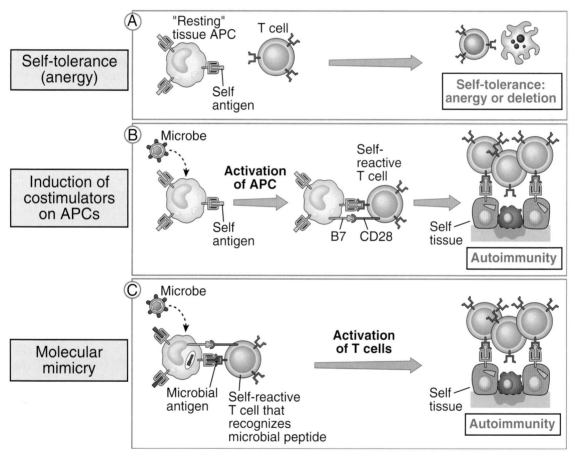

Figure 9–13 Mechanisms by which microbes may promote autoimmunity. A. Normally, encounter of mature T cells with self antigens presented by resting tissue APCs results in peripheral tolerance by anergy or deletion. B. Microbes may activate the APCs to express costimulators; and when these APCs present self antigens, the specific T cells are activated rather than rendered tolerant. C. Some microbial antigens may cross-react with self antigens (mimicry). Therefore, immune responses initiated by the microbes may become directed at self cells and tissues. This figure illustrates concepts as they apply to T cells; molecular mimicry may also apply to self-reactive B lymphocytes.

autoimmune diseases remains unknown. Infections may also injure tissues and release antigens that are normally sequestered from the immune system. For instance, some sequestered antigens (e.g., in the testis and eye) are normally not seen by the immune system and are ignored. Release of these antigens (e.g., by trauma or infection) may initiate an autoimmune reaction against the tissue.

SUMMARY

▶ Immunologic tolerance is specific unresponsiveness to an antigen induced by exposure of lymphocytes to that antigen. All individuals are tolerant of (unresponsive to) their own (self) antigens. Tolerance against antigens may be induced by administering that antigen in particular ways, and this strategy may be useful for treating immunologic disease and for preventing the rejection of transplants.

▶ Autoimmune diseases result from a failure of self-tolerance. Multiple factors contribute to autoimmunity, including immunologic abnormalities, susceptibility genes, and infections.

▶ Central tolerance is induced by the death of immature lymphocytes that encounter antigens in the generative lymphoid organs. Peripheral tolerance results from the recognition of antigens by mature lymphocytes in peripheral tissues.

▶ Central tolerance (negative selection) of T cells is the result of high-affinity recognition of antigens in the thymus, which tend to be widely disseminated self antigens. Central tolerance may eliminate the potentially most dangerous T cells, which express high-affinity receptors for disseminated self antigens.

▶ Peripheral tolerance in T cells is induced by multiple mechanisms. Anergy (functional inactivation) results from the recognition of antigens without costimulators (second signals) or when T cells use inhibitory receptors to recognize costimulators. Deletion (death by apoptosis) occurs when T cells repeatedly encounter self antigens. Some self-reactive T cells suppress potentially pathogenic T cells.

▶ In B lymphocytes, central tolerance is induced when immature cells recognize self antigens in the bone marrow and peripheral tolerance by anergy is induced when mature B cells recognize self antigens without T cell help.

▶ Many genes contribute to the development of autoimmunity. The strongest associations are between HLA genes and various T cell–mediated autoimmune diseases.

▶ Infections predispose to autoimmunity, by causing inflammation and inducing the aberrant expression of costimulators, or because of cross-reactions between microbial and self antigens.

⇄ Review Questions

1 What is immunologic tolerance? What are some of its important features, and why is it important?

2 How is central tolerance induced in T lymphocytes and B lymphocytes?

3 How is functional anergy induced in T cells? How may anergy be "broken" to give rise to autoimmune disorders?

4 What are some of the genes that contribute to autoimmunity? How may MHC genes play a role in the development of autoimmune diseases?

5 What are some possible mechanisms by which infections promote the development of autoimmunity?

Immune Responses Against Tumors and Transplants

Immunity to Noninfectious Transformed and Foreign Cells

10

Cancer and organ transplantation are two clinical situations in which the role of the immune system has received a great deal of attention. In cancer, it is widely believed that enhancing immunity against the tumors holds much promise for treatment. In organ transplantation, of course, the situation is precisely the reverse: immune responses against the transplants are a barrier to successful transplantation, and learning how to suppress these responses is a major goal of transplant immunologists. Because of the importance of the immune system in tumors and transplants, tumor immunology and transplantation immunology have become subspecialties in which researchers and clinicians come together to address both fundamental and clinical questions.

Immune responses against tumors and transplants share several characteristics. These are situations in which the immune system is not responding to microbes, as it usually does, but to noninfectious cells that are perceived as foreign. The antigens that mark tumors and transplants as foreign may be expressed in virtually any cell type that is the target of malignant transformation or is grafted from one individual to another. Therefore, there have to be special mechanisms for inducing immune responses against diverse cell types. Also, an important, and perhaps major, mechanism by which tumor cells and the cells of tissue transplants are destroyed involves cytolytic T lymphocytes (CTLs). For all these reasons, immunity to tumors and transplants are discussed in one chapter, focusing on the following questions:

- What are the antigens in tumors and tissue transplants that are recognized as foreign by the immune system?

- How does the immune system recognize and react to tumors and transplants?

- How can the immune responses to tumors and grafts be manipulated to enhance tumor rejection and inhibit graft rejection?

Tumor immunity is discussed first, and then transplantation, with an emphasis on the principles that are common to both.

Immune Responses Against Tumors

Since the 1950s it has been thought that a physiologic function of the adaptive immune system is to prevent the outgrowth of transformed cells or to destroy these cells before they become harmful tumors. This phenomenon is called **immune surveillance.** Several lines of evidence support the idea that immune surveillance against tumors is important for preventing tumor growth (Fig. 10-1). However, the fact that tumors develop in otherwise healthy immunocompetent individuals indicates that tumor immunity is often weak and is easily overwhelmed by rapidly growing tumors. Immunologists have been interested in defining the kinds of tumor antigens against which the immune system reacts and how antitumor immunity may be maximally enhanced.

Tumor Antigens

Malignant tumors express various types of molecules that may be recognized by the immune system as foreign antigens (Fig. 10-2) If the immune system of an individual is able to react against a tumor in that individual, it follows that the tumor must express antigens that are seen as nonself by that individual's immune system. In experimental tumors induced by chemical carcinogens or radiation, the tumor antigens may be mutants of normal cellular proteins. Virtually any protein may be mutagenized randomly in different tumors, and usually these proteins play no role in tumorigenesis. Such mutants of diverse cellular

Evidence	Conclusion
Histopathologic and clinical observations: lymphocytic infiltrates around some tumors and enlargement of draining lymph nodes correlate with better prognosis	Immune responses against tumors inhibit tumor growth
Experimental: transplants of a tumor are rejected by animals previously exposed to that tumor; immunity to tumor transplants can be transferred by lymphocytes from a tumor-bearing animal	Tumor rejection shows features of adaptive immunity (specificity, memory) and is mediated by lymphocytes
Clinical and experimental: Immunodeficient individuals have an increased incidence of some types of tumors	The immune system protects against the growth of tumors (the concept of "immune surveillance")

Figure 10–1   Evidence supporting the concept that the immune system reacts against tumors. Several lines of clinical and experimental evidence indicate that defense against tumors is mediated by reactions of the adaptive immune system.

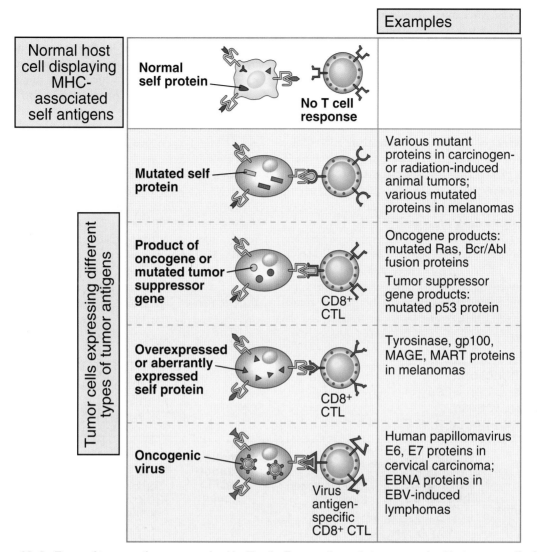

Figure 10–2   Types of tumor antigens recognized by T cells. Tumor antigens that are recognized by tumor-specific CD8+ T cells may be mutated forms of normal self proteins, products of oncogenes or tumor suppressor genes, overexpressed or aberrantly expressed self proteins, or products of oncogenic viruses. Tumor antigens may also be recognized by CD4+ T cells, but less is known about the role that CD4+ T cells play in tumor immunity. EBNA, Epstein-Barr virus nuclear antigen.

proteins are much less common in spontaneous human tumors than in experimentally induced tumors. Some tumor antigens are products of mutated or translocated oncogenes or tumor suppressor genes that are presumably involved in the process of malignant transformation. Surprisingly, in several human tumors, the antigens that elicit immune responses

appear to be entirely normal proteins that are either overexpressed or whose expression is normally limited to particular tissues or stages of development but is dysregulated in the tumors. One would expect that these normal self antigens would not elicit immune responses, but their aberrant expression may be enough to elicit such responses. For example, self proteins that are expressed only in embryonic tissues may not induce tolerance in adults. In tumors induced by oncogenic viruses, the tumor antigens are usually products of the viruses.

Immune Mechanisms of Tumor Rejection

The principal immune mechanism of tumor eradication is killing of tumor cells by cytolytic T lymphocytes (CTLs) specific for tumor antigens. The majority of tumor antigens that elicit immune responses in tumor-bearing individuals are endogenously synthesized cytosolic proteins that are displayed as class I MHC–associated peptides. Therefore, these antigens are recognized by class I MHC–restricted CD8$^+$ CTLs, whose function is to kill cells producing the antigens. The role of CTLs in tumor rejection has been established in animal models, in which transplants of tumors can be destroyed by transferring tumor-reactive CD8$^+$ T cells into the tumor-bearing animals.

CTL responses against tumors are often induced by recognition of tumor antigens on host antigen-presenting cells (APCs), which ingest tumor cells or their antigens and present the antigens to T cells (Fig. 10-3). Tumors may arise from virtually any nucleated cell type. These cells are able to display class I MHC–associated peptides (because all nucleated cells express class I MHC molecules), but often the tumor cells do not express costimulators or class II MHC molecules. We know, however, that the activation of naive CD8$^+$ T cells to proliferate and differentiate into active CTLs requires not only recognition of antigen (class I MHC-associated peptide) but also costimulation and/or help from class II MHC–restricted CD4$^+$ T cells (see Chapter 5). How then can tumors of different cell types stimulate CTL responses? The likely answer is that tumor cells are ingested by the host's professional APCs (e.g.,

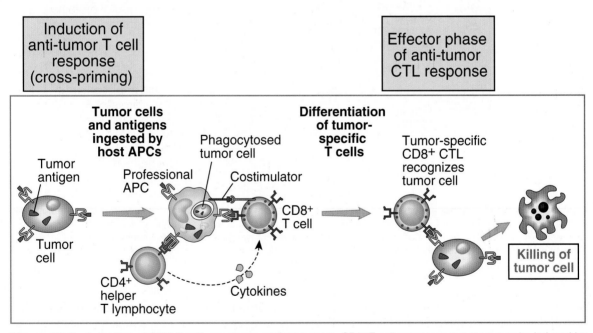

Figure 10–3   Induction of CD8$^+$ T cell responses against tumors. CD8$^+$ T cell responses to tumors may be induced by cross-priming (also called cross-presentation), in which the tumor cells and/or tumor antigens are taken up by professional APCs, processed, and presented to T cells. In some cases, B7 costimulators expressed by the APCs provide the second signals for the differentiation of the CD8$^+$ T cells. The APCs may also stimulate CD4$^+$ helper T cells, which provide the second signals for CTL development (see Chapter 5, Fig. 5-7). Differentiated CTLs kill tumor cells without a requirement for costimulation or T cell help.

dendritic cells), and the antigens of the tumor cells are processed and displayed by the host APC's class I and class II MHC molecules. Thus, tumor antigens may be recognized by CD8$^+$ T cells and by CD4$^+$ T cells much like any other protein antigens displayed by professional APCs. At the same time, the professional APCs express costimulators that provide "second signals" for the activation of the T cells. This process is called cross-presentation or cross-priming, because one cell type (the professional APC) presents antigens of another cell (the tumor cell) and activates (or primes) T lymphocytes specific for the second cell type. The concept of cross-presentation has been exploited to develop methods for vaccinating against tumors, as is discussed later in this chapter. Once naive CD8$^+$ T cells have differentiated into effector CTLs, they are able to kill tumor cells expressing the relevant antigens without a requirement for costimulation or T cell help. Thus, CTLs may be induced by cross-presentation of tumor antigens by host APCs but the CTLs are effective against the tumor itself.

Several other immune mechanisms may play a role in tumor rejection. Antitumor CD4$^+$ T cell responses and antibodies have been detected in patients, but there is little convincing evidence that these responses actually protect individuals against tumor growth. Experimental studies have shown that activated macrophages and natural killer (NK) cells are capable of killing tumor cells *in vitro*, but again the protective role of these effector mechanisms in tumor-bearing individuals is unclear.

Evasion of Immune Responses by Tumors

Immune responses often fail to check tumor growth, because these responses are ineffective or because tumors evolve to evade immune attack. The immune system faces a daunting challenge if it is to be effective against malignant tumors, because immune responses must kill all tumor cells and tumors grow rapidly. Often, the growth simply outstrips immune defenses. Immune responses against tumors may be weak because many tumor antigens are weakly immunogenic, perhaps because they differ only slightly from self antigens.

Growing tumors also develop mechanisms for evading immune responses (Fig. 10-4). Some tumors stop expressing the antigens that are the targets of immune attack. These tumors are called "antigen loss variants." If the lost antigen is not involved in maintaining the malignant properties of the tumor, the variant tumor cells continue to grow and spread. Other tumors stop expressing class I MHC molecules, and thus cannot display antigens to CD8$^+$ T cells. Because NK cells recognize cells lacking class I MHC molecules, they may provide a mechanism for killing class I MHC–negative tumors. Yet other tumors may produce molecules, such as transforming growth factor-β, that suppress immune responses.

Immunologic Approaches for Cancer Therapy

The main strategies for cancer immunotherapy aim to provide antitumor effectors (antibodies and T cells) to patients, actively immunize patients against their tumors, and stimulate the patients' own antitumor immune responses. At the present time, the treatment of disseminated cancers (which cannot be surgically resected) relies on chemotherapy and irradiation, both of which have devastating effects on normal nontumor tissues. Because the immune response is highly specific, it has long been hoped that tumor-specific immunity may be used to selectively eradicate tumors without injuring the patient. Immunotherapy remains a major goal of tumor immunologists, and many approaches to therapy have been tried in experimental animals and in humans.

One of the earliest strategies for tumor immunotherapy relied on various forms of passive immunization, in which immune effectors are injected into cancer patients. Monoclonal antibodies against various tumor antigens, often coupled to potent toxins, have been tried in many cancers. The antibodies bind to tumor antigens and either activate host effector mechanisms, such as phagocytes or the complement system, or deliver the toxins to the tumor cells. One such antibody, against the product of the *HER2/neu* oncogene that is overexpressed in some breast cancers, is now approved for use in patients with these tumors. Antibodies specific for CD20, which is expressed on B cells, are used to

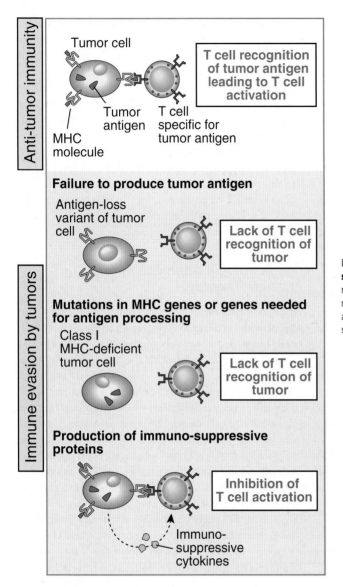

Figure 10–4 How tumors evade immune responses. Antitumor immunity develops when T cells recognize tumor antigens and are activated. Tumor cells may evade immune responses by losing expression of antigens or MHC molecules or by producing immuno-suppressive cytokines.

treat B cell tumors, usually in combination with chemotherapy. Because CD20 is not expressed by hematopoietic stem cells, normal B cells are replenished after the antibody treatment is stopped. T lymphocytes may be isolated from the blood or tumor infiltrates of a patient, expanded by culture with growth factors, and injected back into the same patient. The T cells presumably contain tumor-specific CTLs, which find the tumor and destroy it.

This approach, called "adoptive cellular immunotherapy," is being tried in several metastatic cancers, but results have been variable among different patients and tumors.

Many new strategies for cancer immunotherapy rely on boosting the host's own immune responses against tumors (Fig. 10-5). One way of stimulating immune responses against tumors is to vaccinate patients with their own tumor cells or antigens from

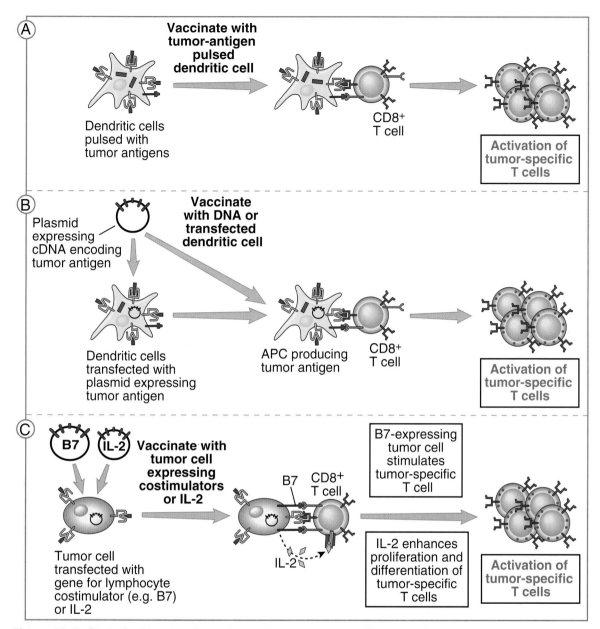

Figure 10–5 **Strategies for enhancing antitumor immune responses.** Tumor-specific immune responses may be stimulated by vaccinating with host dendritic cells that have been pulsed (incubated) with tumor antigens (A) or with plasmids containing complementary DNAs encoding tumor antigens that are injected directly into patients or used to transfect dendritic cells (B) or by vaccinating with tumor cells transfected with genes encoding B7 costimulators or the T cell growth factor interleukin-2 (C).

these cells. An important reason for defining tumor antigens is to produce and use these antigens to vaccinate individuals against their own tumors. Vaccines may be administered as recombinant proteins with adjuvants. More recently, there has been great interest in growing dendritic cells from individuals (by isolating precursors from the blood and expanding them by culture with growth factors), exposing the dendritic cells to tumor cells or tumor antigens, and using these "tumor-pulsed" dendritic cells as vaccines. It is hoped that the dendritic cells bearing tumor antigens will mimic the normal pathway of cross-presentation and will generate CTLs against the tumor cells. Another approach to vaccination uses a plasmid containing a complementary DNA (cDNA) encoding a tumor antigen. Injection of the plasmid results in the cDNA being expressed in host cells, including APCs, that take up the plasmid. The host cells produce the tumor antigen, thus inducing specific T cell responses.

Problems in identifying immunogenic tumor antigens and in developing effective vaccines have convinced some tumor immunologists that the best therapeutic strategy may be to let patients generate their own tumor-specific immune responses and to design therapies to optimize these responses. One approach for achieving this goal is to treat patients with cytokines that stimulate immune responses. The first cytokine to be used in this way was interleukin-2 (IL-2), but its applications are limited by serious toxic effects. Many other cytokines have been tried as systemic therapy or local administration at sites of

tumors. In a variation of this approach, a cytokine gene may be expressed in tumor cells and used to immunize the patient (see Fig. 10-5). In this way, it is hoped that T cell responses against tumor antigens become enhanced. The same principle underlies experimental studies in which the costimulator B7 is expressed in tumor cells, and the B7-expressing tumor cells are used as tumor vaccines. An interesting recent variation on the idea of boosting host immune responses against tumors is to eliminate normal inhibitory signals for lymphocytes. In some animal models, blocking the inhibitory T cell receptor CTLA-4 (which, as discussed in Chapter 9, shuts off T cell responses) has led to strong immune responses against transplanted tumors. Many of these new strategies for stimulating antitumor immunity are based on our improved understanding of lymphocyte activation and regulation and are thus rational (rather than empirical) strategies.

Immune Responses Against Transplants

From the advent of tissue transplantation, it was realized that individuals reject grafts from other individuals in a normal, outbred population. Rejection results from inflammatory reactions that damage the transplanted tissues. Studies in the 1940s and 1950s established that graft rejection is an immunologic phenomenon, because it shows specificity and memory and is mediated by lymphocytes (Fig. 10-6). Much of the knowledge about the immunology of

Evidence	Conclusion
Prior exposure to donor MHC molecules leads to accelerated graft rejection	Graft rejection shows memory and specificity, two cardinal features of adaptive immunity
The ability to reject a graft rapidly can be transferred to a naive individual by lymphocytes from a sensitized individual	Graft rejection is mediated by lymphocytes
Depletion or inactivation of T lymphocytes by drugs or antibodies results in reduced graft rejection	Graft rejection can be mediated by T lymphocytes

Figure 10–6 **Evidence indicating that the rejection of tissue transplants is an immune reaction.** Clinical and experimental evidence indicates that rejection of grafts is a reaction of the adaptive immune system.

transplantation came from studies with inbred animals, particularly mice, that were bred so that all members of an inbred strain are identical to each other and different from the members of other strains. Transplants exchanged between animals of the same and other inbred strains showed that grafts among members of an inbred strain are accepted and grafts among different strains are rejected. It was soon established that graft rejection is determined by inherited genes whose products are expressed in all tissues. The language of transplantation immunology evolved from these studies. The individual that provides the graft is called the donor, and the individual in whom the graft is placed is the recipient or host. Animals that are identical to one another (and grafts exchanged among these animals) are said to be syngeneic; animals (and grafts) of one species that differ from other animals of the same species are said to be allogeneic; and animals (and grafts) of different species are xenogeneic. Allogeneic and xenogeneic grafts, also called allografts and xenografts, are always rejected. The antigens that serve as the targets of rejection are called alloantigens and xenoantigens, and the antibodies and T cells that react against these antigens are said to be alloreactive and xenoreactive, respectively. In the clinical situation, transplants are usually exchanged among allogeneic individuals, who are members of an outbred species who differ from one another (except, of course, for identical twins). Most of our discussion focuses on immune responses to allografts.

Transplantation Antigens

The antigens of allografts that serve as the principal targets of rejection are proteins encoded in the major histocompatibility complex (MHC). As we mentioned in Chapter 3, the MHC was discovered (and named) on the basis of its role in the rejection of grafts exchanged between mice of different inbred strains. Homologous genes and molecules are present in all mammals; the human MHC is the human leukocyte antigen (HLA) complex. It took over 20 years after the discovery of the MHC to show that the physiologic function of MHC molecules is to display peptide antigens for recognition by T lymphocytes (see Chapter 3). Recall that every human being

expresses six class I MHC alleles (one allele of HLA-A, B, and C from each parent) and at least six class II MHC alleles (one allele of HLA-DR, DQ, and DP from each parent, and some combinations of these). MHC genes are highly polymorphic; it is estimated that there are at least 120 alleles of HLA-A genes and 250 alleles of HLA-B genes in the population. Therefore, every individual is likely to express some MHC proteins that appear foreign to another individual's immune system, except in the case of identical twins. All the MHC molecules may be targets of rejection, although HLA-C and HLA-DP have limited polymorphism and are probably of minor significance.

In each individual, all CD4$^+$ T cells and CD8$^+$ T cells are selected during their maturation to recognize peptides displayed by that individual's (self) MHC molecules. This selection is the basis of the "self MHC restriction" of T lymphocytes, a fundamental property of T cells. If all mature T cells are selected to recognize only peptides displayed by self MHC molecules, why should T cells from one individual recognize as foreign the MHC molecules of another (allogeneic) individual? In fact, recognition of the MHC antigens on another individual's cells is one of the strongest immune responses known. The reason why individuals react against MHC molecules of other individuals is now understood quite well. Recall that as a result of positive selection in the thymus, mature T cells strongly recognize self MHC molecules displaying foreign peptides. Allogeneic MHC molecules, containing peptides derived from the allogeneic cells, look like self MHC molecules + bound foreign peptides (Fig. 10-7). Therefore, recognition of allogeneic MHC molecules in allografts is an example of an immunologic cross-reaction. Many clones of T cells specific for different foreign peptides bound to the same self MHC molecule may cross-react with any one allogeneic MHC molecule, as long as the allogenic MHC molecule resembles complexes of self MHC plus foreign peptides. As a result, many self MHC–restricted T cells specific for different peptide antigens may recognize any one allogeneic MHC molecule. This is the main reason why recognition of allogeneic MHC molecules is a very strong T cell reaction.

Although MHC proteins are the major antigens that stimulate graft rejection, other polymorphic

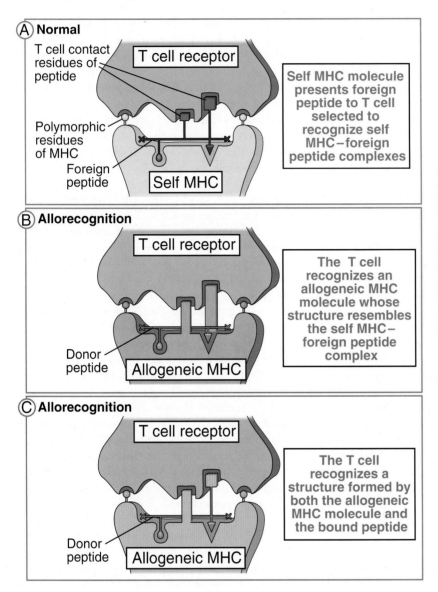

(A) Normal

T cell contact residues of peptide

T cell receptor

Self MHC molecule presents foreign peptide to T cell selected to recognize self MHC–foreign peptide complexes

Polymorphic residues of MHC

Foreign peptide

Self MHC

(B) Allorecognition

T cell receptor

The T cell recognizes an allogeneic MHC molecule whose structure resembles the self MHC–foreign peptide complex

Donor peptide

Allogeneic MHC

(C) Allorecognition

T cell receptor

The T cell recognizes a structure formed by both the allogeneic MHC molecule and the bound peptide

Donor peptide

Allogeneic MHC

Figure 10–7 Recognition of allogeneic MHC molecules by T lymphocytes. Recognition of allogeneic MHC molecules may be thought of as a cross reaction in which a T cell specific for a self MHC molecule–foreign peptide complex (A) also recognizes an allogeneic MHC molecule whose structure resembles that of a self MHC molecule–foreign peptide complex (B, C). Peptides derived from the graft (labeled "donor peptides") may not contribute to allorecognition (B), or they may form part of the complex that the T cell sees (C). As discussed later in the chapter, the type of T cell recognition depicted in B and C is called direct allorecognition.

proteins may also play a role in rejection. Non-MHC antigens that induce graft rejection are called minor histocompatibility antigens, and most of them are allelic forms of normal cellular proteins that happen to differ between donor and recipient. The rejection reactions that minor histocompatibility antigens elicit are usually not as strong as reactions against foreign MHC proteins. Two situations in which minor antigens are important targets of rejection are blood transfusion and bone marrow transplantation; these are discussed later in the chapter.

Induction of Immune Responses Against Transplants

The induction of T cell–mediated immune responses against tissue transplants has the same barrier as responses against tumors: because a graft may contain many cell types, often including epithelial and connective tissue cells, how can the immune system recognize and react against all these cells? The answer is that T cells in the graft recipient may recognize donor alloantigens in the graft in different ways, depending on what cells in the graft are displaying these alloantigens.

T cells may recognize allogeneic MHC molecules in the graft displayed by professional APCs, or graft alloantigens may be processed and presented by the host's professional APCs (Fig. 10-8). When T cells in the recipient recognize donor allogeneic MHC molecules on graft APCs, the T cells are activated; this process is called direct allorecognition (or direct presentation of alloantigens). Direct recognition can only occur if the graft contains donor-derived professional APCs, such as dendritic cells. Direct recognition stimulates the development of alloreactive T cells (e.g., CTLs) that recognize and attack the cells of the graft. However, if the graft does not contain professional APCs, how does it stimulate T cells? A plausible answer is that graft cells are ingested by professional APCs in the recipient and the donor alloantigens are processed and presented by the self MHC molecules on recipient APCs. This process is called indirect allorecognition (or indirect presentation) and is similar to the cross-presentation of tumor antigens discussed earlier. The professional APCs that present alloantigens by the direct or indirect pathway also provide costimulators and can stimulate helper T cells as well as alloreactive CTLs. However, if alloreactive CTLs are induced by the indirect pathway,

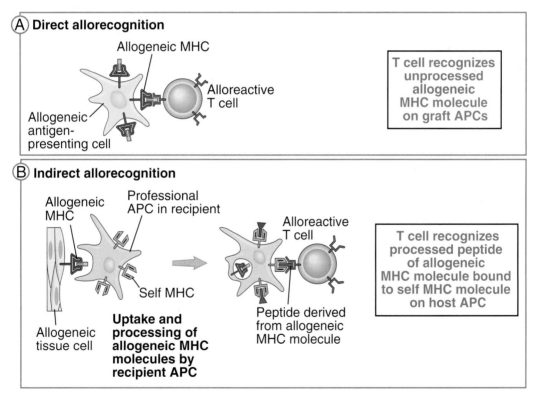

Figure 10–8 Direct and indirect recognition of alloantigens. A. Direct alloantigen recognition occurs when T cells bind directly to intact allogeneic MHC molecules on professional APCs in a graft, as illustrated in Figure 10-7. B. Indirect alloantigen recognition occurs when allogeneic MHC molecules from graft cells are taken up and processed by recipient APCs, and peptide fragments of the allogeneic MHC molecules are presented by recipient (self) MHC molecules. Recipient APCs may also process and present graft proteins other than allogeneic MHC molecules.

these CTLs should be specific for alloantigens displayed by self MHC molecules on host APCs. How can these CTLs recognize the allogeneic MHC molecules of the graft (where there is no self MHC)? This question remains unanswered. It is possible that when graft alloantigens are presented by the indirect pathway, the major responding T cell population consists of CD4$^+$ T cells. These T cells may enter the graft together with host APCs, recognize graft antigens displayed by the APCs, and secrete cytokines that injure the graft by a delayed-type hypersensitivity (DTH) reaction. We do not know the relative importance of the direct and indirect pathways of allorecognition in the rejection of allografts. It has been suggested that the direct pathway is most important for CTL-mediated acute rejection and that the indirect pathway plays a greater role in chronic rejection.

The **mixed lymphocyte reaction** (MLR) is an *in vitro* model of T cell recognition of alloantigens. In this model, T cells from one individual are cultured with leukocytes of another individual and the responses of the T cells are assayed. The magnitude of this response is proportional to the extent of the MHC differences between these individuals and is a rough predictor of the outcomes of grafts exchanged between these individuals.

Immune Mechanisms of Graft Rejection

Graft rejection is classified into hyperacute, acute, and chronic, based on clinical and pathologic features (Fig. 10-9). This historical classification was devised by clinicians, and it has stood the test of time remarkably well. It has also become apparent that each type of rejection is mediated by a particular type of immune response.

Hyperacute rejection occurs within minutes of transplantation and is characterized by thrombosis of graft vessels and ischemic necrosis of the graft. Hyperacute rejection is mediated by circulating antibodies, specific for antigens on graft endothelial cells, that are present before transplantation, perhaps because of prior transfusions and reactions against alloantigens in the transfused blood cells. These antibodies bind to antigens in the graft vascular endothelium, activate the complement and clotting systems, and lead to injury to the endothelium and clot formation. Hyperacute rejection is not a common problem in clinical transplantation, because every recipient is tested for antibodies against the cells of the potential donor. (The test is called a cross-match.) However, hyperacute rejection is the major barrier to xenotransplantation, as discussed later.

Acute rejection occurs within days or weeks after transplantation and is the principal cause of early graft failure. Acute rejection is mediated mainly by T cells, which react against alloantigens in the graft. These T cells may be CTLs that directly destroy graft cells, or the T cells may react against cells in graft vessels, leading to vascular damage. Antibodies also contribute to acute rejection, especially the vascular component of this reaction. Current immunosuppressive therapy is designed mainly to prevent and reduce acute T cell–mediated rejection, as is discussed later.

Chronic rejection is an indolent form of graft damage that occurs over months or years and leads to progressive loss of graft function. Chronic rejection may be manifested as fibrosis of the graft, or gradual narrowing of graft vessels, called graft arteriosclerosis. In both lesions, the culprits are believed to be T cells that react against graft alloantigens and secrete cytokines, which stimulate the proliferation and activities of fibroblasts and vascular smooth muscle cells in the graft. As treatment for acute rejection has improved, chronic rejection is becoming the principal cause of graft failure.

Figure 10–9   Mechanisms of graft rejection. A. In hyperacute rejection, preformed antibodies react with alloantigens on the vascular endothelium of the graft, activate complement, and trigger rapid intravascular thrombosis and necrosis of the vessel wall. B. In acute cellular rejection CD8$^+$ T lymphocytes reactive with alloantigens on graft endothelial cells and parenchymal cells cause damage to these cell types. Inflammation of the endothelium is sometimes called "endothelialitis." Alloreactive antibodies may also contribute to vascular injury. C. In chronic rejection with graft arteriosclerosis, T cells reactive with graft alloantigens may produce cytokines that induce proliferation of endothelial cells and intimal smooth muscle cells, leading to luminal occlusion. This type of rejection is probably a chronic DTH reaction to alloantigens in the vessel wall.

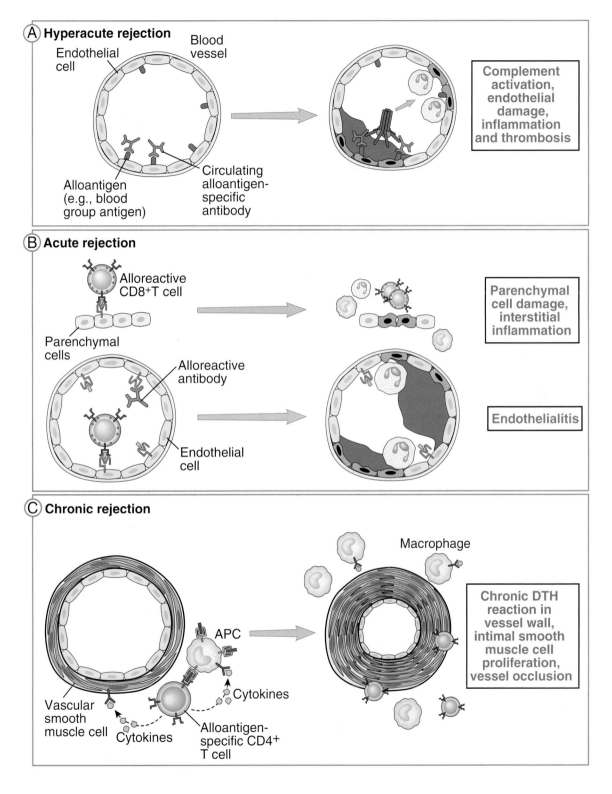

A Hyperacute rejection

Endothelial cell

Blood vessel

Alloantigen (e.g., blood group antigen)

Circulating alloantigen-specific antibody

Complement activation, endothelial damage, inflammation and thrombosis

B Acute rejection

Alloreactive CD8+T cell

Parenchymal cells

Parenchymal cell damage, interstitial inflammation

Alloreactive antibody

Endothelialitis

Endothelial cell

C Chronic rejection

Macrophage

APC

Cytokines

Chronic DTH reaction in vessel wall, intimal smooth muscle cell proliferation, vessel occlusion

Vascular smooth muscle cell

Cytokines

Alloantigen-specific CD4+ T cell

Prevention and Treatment of Graft Rejection

The mainstay of preventing and treating the rejec-tion of organ transplants is immunosuppression, designed mainly to inhibit T cell activation and effector functions (Fig. 10-10). The most useful immunosuppressive drug in clinical transplantation is cyclosporine, which functions by blocking the T cell phosphatase that is required to activate the transcrip-tion factor NFAT and thus inhibits transcription of cytokine genes in the T cells. The advent of cyclosporine as a clinically useful drug has opened up a new era in transplantation and allowed the transplantation of heart, liver, and lung. Many other immunosuppressive agents are used as adjuncts to or instead of cyclosporine (see Fig. 10-10). All these immunosuppressive drugs carry the problem of non-specific immunosuppression (i.e., the drugs inhibit responses to more than the graft). Therefore, patients treated with these drugs become susceptible to infec-tions, particularly infections by intracellular microbes, and have an increased incidence of cancers, especially tumors caused by oncogenic viruses.

The matching of donor and recipient HLA alleles by tissue typing had an important role in minimizing graft rejection in the days before cyclosporine became available for clinical use. However, now immuno-

Drug	Mechanism of action
Cyclosporine and FK506	Blocks T cell cytokine production by inhibiting activation of the NFAT transcription factor
Mycophenolate mofetil	Blocks lymphocyte proliferation by inhibiting guanine nucleotide synthesis in lymphocytes
Rapamycin	Blocks lymphocyte proliferation by inhibiting IL-2 signaling
Corticosteroids	Reduce inflammation by inhibiting macrophage cytokine secretion
Anti-CD3 monoclonal antibody	Depletes T cells by binding to CD3 and promoting phagocytosis or complement-mediated lysis (Used to treat acute rejection)
Anti-IL-2 receptor antibody	Inhibits T cell proliferation by blocking IL-2 binding. May also opsonize and help eliminate activated IL-2R–expressing T cells
CTLA4-Ig	Inhibits T cell activation by blocking B7 costimulator binding to T cell CD28; used to induce tolerance (experimental)
Anti-CD40 ligand	Inhibits macrophage and endothelial activation by blocking T cell CD40 ligand binding to macrophage CD40 (experimental)

Figure 10–10   Treatments for graft rejection. Agents that are commonly used to treat the rejection of organ grafts, and the mechanisms of action of these agents, are listed. FK506 is a drug that works like cyclosporine, but FK506 is not used as widely.

suppression is so effective that HLA matching is not considered necessary for many types of organ transplants, especially because recipients are often too sick to wait for the closest match.

The long-term goal of transplant immunologists is to induce immunologic tolerance specifically for the graft alloantigens. If this is achieved, it will allow graft acceptance without shutting off any other immune responses in the host. Attempts to induce graft-specific tolerance are ongoing in experimental models (e.g., by blocking costimulators at the time of transplantation and by stimulating alloreactive T cells to become regulatory cells).

A major problem in transplantation is the shortage of suitable donor organs. **Xenotransplantation** is a possible solution for this problem. Experimental studies with xenotransplants have shown that hyperacute rejection is a major problem with these grafts. The reason for the high incidence of hyperacute rejection of xenografts is that individuals often contain antibodies that react with cells from other species. These antibodies are called "natural anti-bodies" because their production does not require prior exposure to the xenoantigens. It is thought that these antibodies are produced against bacteria that normally inhabit the gut and the antibodies cross-react with cells of other species. Xenografts are also subject to acute rejection much like allografts. Attempts are ongoing to genetically modify xenogeneic tissues in ways that prevent their rejection by recipients of other species.

Transplantation of Blood Cells and Bone Marrow Cells

Transplantation of blood cells is called **transfusion** and is the oldest form of transplantation in clinical medicine. The major barrier to transfusion is the presence of foreign blood group antigens, the prototypes of which are the ABO antigens. These antigens are expressed on red blood cells, endothelial cells, and many other cell types. ABO molecules are glycosphingolipids containing a core glycan with sphingolipids attached. The names A and B refer to the terminal sugars (*N*-acetylgalactosamine and galactose, respectively); AB means that both are present; and O means that neither is present. Individuals expressing one blood group antigen are tolerant to that antigen but contain antibodies against the other. It is believed that these antibodies are produced against similar antigens expressed by intestinal microbes and cross-react with the ABO blood group antigens. The preformed antibodies react against transfused blood cells expressing the target antigens, and the result may be severe **transfusion reactions.** This problem is avoided by matching blood donors and recipients, a standard practice in medicine. Because the blood group antigens are sugars, they do not elicit T cell responses. Blood group antigens other than the ABO antigens are also involved in transfusion reactions, and these are usually less severe.

Bone marrow transplantation is being used increasingly to correct hematopoietic defects or to restore bone marrow cells that have been damaged by irradiation and chemotherapy for cancer. The transplantation of bone marrow cells poses many special problems. Before transplantation, some of the bone marrow of the recipient has to be destroyed to create "space" to receive the transplanted marrow cells. The immune system reacts very strongly against allogeneic bone marrow cells, so that successful transplantation requires careful HLA matching of donor and recipient. If mature allogeneic T cells are transplanted with the marrow cells, these mature T cells can attack the recipient's tissues, resulting in a serious clinical reaction called **graft-versus-host disease.** Even if the graft is successful, recipients are often severely immunodeficient while their immune systems are being reconstituted. Despite these problems, there is great interest in bone marrow transplantation as a therapy for a wide variety of diseases and as an approach for gene replacement.

SUMMARY

▶ A physiologic function of the immune system is to eradicate tumors and prevent the growth of tumors.

▶ Tumor antigens may be products of oncogenes or tumor suppressor genes, mutated cellular proteins, overexpressed or aberrantly expressed molecules, and products of oncogenic viruses.

▶ Tumor rejection is mediated mainly by CTLs recognizing peptides derived from tumor antigens. The induction of CTL responses against tumor antigens often involves ingestion of tumor cells or their antigens by professional APCs and presentation of the antigens to T cells.

▶ Tumors may evade immune responses by losing expression of their antigens, shutting off expression of MHC molecules or molecules involved in antigen processing, and secreting cytokines that suppress immune responses.

▶ Immunotherapy for cancer aims to enhance anti-tumor immunity by passively providing immune effectors to patients or by actively boosting the host's own effectors. Approaches for active boosting include vaccination with tumor antigens or with tumor cells engineered to express costimulators and cytokines.

▶ Tissue transplants are rejected by the immune system, and the major determinants of rejection are MHC molecules.

▶ The antigens of allografts that are recognized by T cells are allogeneic MHC molecules that resemble peptide-loaded self MHC molecules that the T cells are selected to recognize. Graft antigens are either directly presented to recipient T cells, or the graft antigens are picked up and presented by host APCs.

▶ Grafts may be rejected by different mechanisms. Hyperacute rejection is mediated by preformed antibodies that cause endothelial injury and thrombosis of blood vessels in the graft. Acute rejection is mediated by T cells, which injure graft cells or endothelium, and by antibodies that bind to the endothelium. Chronic rejection is caused by T cells that produce cytokines that stimulate growth of vascular endothelial and smooth muscle cells and tissue fibroblasts.

▶ Treatment for graft rejection is designed to suppress T cell responses and inflammation. The mainstay of treatment is the immunosuppressive drug cyclosporine; many other agents are in clinical use now.

▶ Bone marrow transplants elicit strong rejection reactions, carry the risk of graft-versus-host disease, and often lead to temporary immunodeficiency in recipients.

⇄ Review Questions

1 What are the types of tumor antigens that the immune system reacts against? What is the evidence that tumor rejection is an immunologic phenomenon?

2 How do CD8⁺ T cells recognize tumor antigens, and how are these cells activated to differentiate into effector CTLs?

3 What are some of the mechanisms by which tumors may evade the immune response?

4 What are some strategies for enhancing host immune responses to tumor antigens?

5 Why do normal T cells, which recognize foreign peptide antigens bound to self MHC molecules, react strongly against the allogeneic MHC molecules of a graft?

6 What are the principal mechanisms of rejection of allografts?

7 What is the mixed leukocyte reaction, and what is its importance?

8 What are some of the problems associated with the transplantation of bone marrow cells?

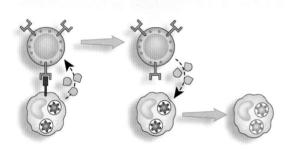

Hypersensitivity Diseases

Disorders Caused by Immune Responses

11

The concept that the immune system is required for defending the host against infections has been emphasized throughout this book. However, immune responses are themselves capable of causing tissue injury and disease. Disorders that are caused by immune responses are called **hypersensitivity diseases.** This term is derived from the idea that an immune response to an antigen may result in sensitivity to challenge with that antigen and, therefore, hypersensitivity is a reflection of excessive or aberrant immune responses. Hypersensitivity diseases may be caused by two types of abnormal immune responses. First, responses to foreign antigens may be dysregulated or uncontrolled, resulting in tissue injury. Second, the immune responses may be directed against self (autologous) antigens, as a result of the failure of self-tolerance (see Chapter 9). Responses against self antigens are termed *autoimmunity,* and hypersensitivity disorders caused by such responses are called *autoimmune diseases.*

This chapter describes the important features of hypersensitivity diseases, focusing on their pathogenesis. Details of the clinical and pathologic features of these diseases may be found in many other textbooks and are summarized only briefly in this chapter. The following questions are addressed:

- What factors contribute to the development of hypersensitivity diseases?
- What are the immunologic mechanisms that cause tissue injury and functional abnormalities in different types of hypersensitivity disorders?

- What are the major clinical and pathologic features of these diseases, and what principles underlie treatment of hypersensitivity diseases?

Types of Hypersensitivity Diseases

Hypersensitivity diseases are commonly classified on the basis of the principal immunologic mechanism that is responsible for tissue injury and disease (Fig. 11-1). We prefer the more informative descriptive designations rather than the numerical ones, and therefore these descriptors are used throughout this chapter. Immediate hypersensitivity (type I hypersensitivity) is a type of pathologic reaction that is caused by the release of mediators from mast cells. This reaction is most commonly triggered by the production of IgE antibody against environmental antigens and the binding of IgE to mast cells in various tissues. Antibodies other than IgE may cause diseases in two ways. Antibodies directed against cell or tissue antigens can damage these cells or tissues or impair their functions. These diseases are said to be antibody-mediated (type II hypersensitivity). Sometimes, antibodies against soluble antigens may form complexes with the antigens, and the immune complexes may deposit in blood vessels in various tissues and cause inflammation and tissue injury. Such diseases are called immune complex diseases (type III hypersensitivity). Finally, some diseases result from the reactions of T lymphocytes, often against self antigens in tissues. These T cell–mediated diseases are called type IV hypersensitivity.

In the remainder of this chapter, we describe the important features of each type of hypersensitivity disease.

Immediate Hypersensitivity

Immediate hypersensitivity is a rapid, IgE antibody– and mast cell–mediated vascular and smooth muscle reaction, often followed by inflammation, that occurs in some individuals on encounter with certain foreign antigens to which they have been exposed previously. Immediate hypersensitivity reactions are also called **allergy,** or **atopy,** and individuals

with a strong propensity to develop these reactions are said to be "atopic." Such reactions may affect various tissues and may be of varying severity in different individuals. Common types of immediate hypersensitivity reactions include hay fever, food allergies, bronchial asthma, and anaphylaxis. The clinical features of these reactions are discussed later in the chapter. Allergies are the most frequent disorders of the immune system, estimated to affect about 20% of the population.

The sequence of events in the development of immediate hypersensitivity reactions consists of the production of IgE antibodies in response to an antigen, binding of IgE to Fc receptors of mast cells, cross-linking of the bound IgE by reintroduced antigen, and release of mast cell mediators (Fig. 11-2). Some mast cell mediators cause a rapid increase in vascular permeability and smooth muscle contraction, resulting in many of the symptoms of these reactions. This vascular and smooth muscle reaction may occur within minutes of reintroduction of antigen into a previously sensitized individual. Other mast cell mediators are cytokines that recruit neutrophils and eosinophils to the site of the reaction over several hours. This inflammatory component of immediate hypersensitivity is called the **late phase reaction,** and it is mainly responsible for the tissue injury that results from repeated bouts of immediate hypersensitivity.

With this background, the discussion proceeds to the individual steps in immediate hypersensitivity reactions.

Production of IgE Antibody

In individuals who are prone to allergies, encounter with some antigens results in the activation of T_H2 cells and the production of IgE antibody (see Fig. 11-2). Normal individuals do not mount strong T_H2 responses to most foreign antigens. For unknown reasons, when some individuals encounter antigens such as proteins in pollen, certain foods, insect venoms, or animal dander, or if they are exposed to certain drugs such as penicillin, the dominant T cell response is the development of T_H2 cells. Any atopic individual may be allergic to one or more of these antigens. Immediate hypersensitivity develops as a consequence of the activation of T_H2 cells in response

Type of hypersensitivity	Pathologic immune mechanisms	Mechanisms of tissue injury and disease
Immediate hypersensitivity (Type I)	T_H2 cells, IgE antibody, mast cells, eosinophils 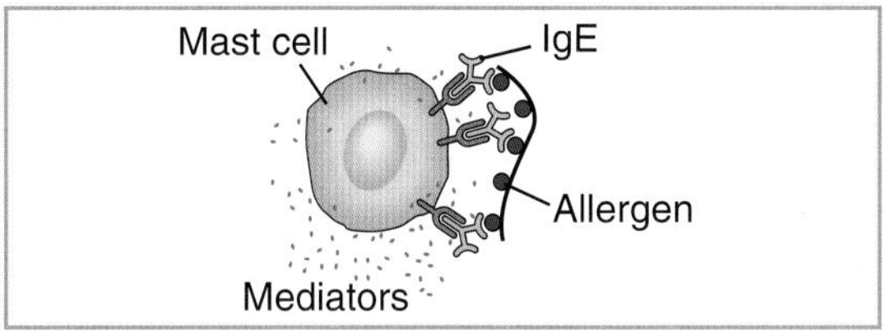	Mast cell–derived mediators (vasoactive amines, lipid mediators, cytokines) Cytokine-mediated inflammation (eosinophils, neutrophils)
Antibody-mediated diseases (Type II)	IgM, IgG antibodies against cell surface or extracellular matrix antigens 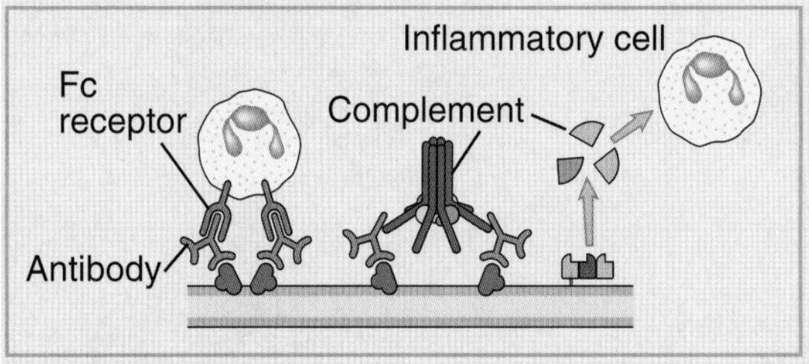	Complement- and Fc receptor–mediated recruitment and activation of leukocytes (neutrophils, macrophages) Opsonization and phagocytosis of cells Abnormalities in cellular function, e.g., hormone receptor signaling
Immune complex–mediated diseases (Type III)	Immune complexes of circulating antigens and IgM or IgG antibodies deposited in vascular basement membrane 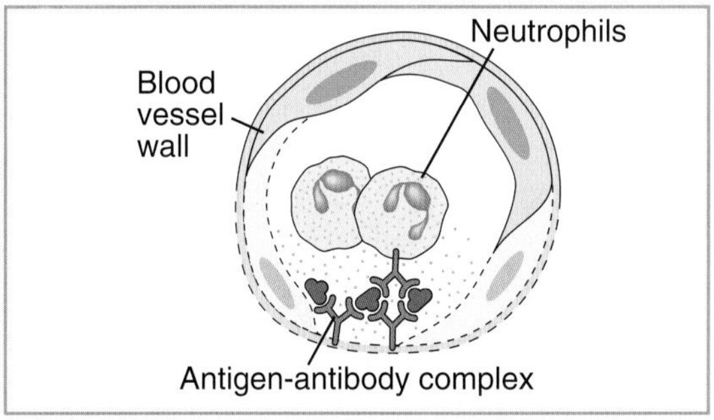	Complement and Fc receptor-mediated recruitment and activation of leukocytes
T cell–mediated diseases (Type IV)	1. CD4+ T cells (delayed-type hypersensitivity) 2. CD8+ CTLs (T cell–mediated cytolysis) 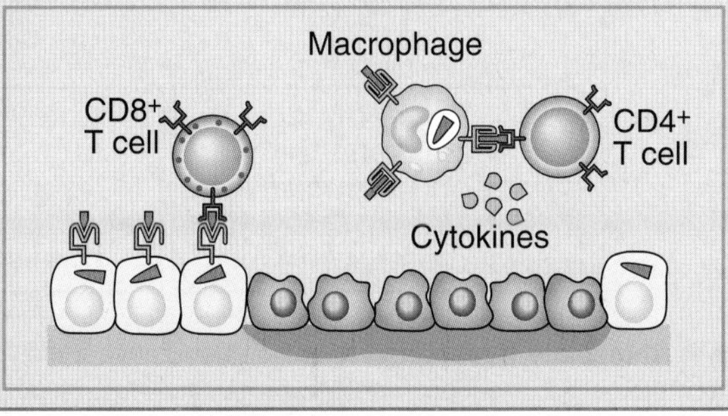	1. Macrophage activation, cytokine-mediated inflammation 2. Direct target cell lysis, cytokine-mediated inflammation

Figure 11–1 Types of hypersensitivity diseases. In the four major types of hypersensitivity reactions, different immune effector mechanisms cause tissue injury and disease.

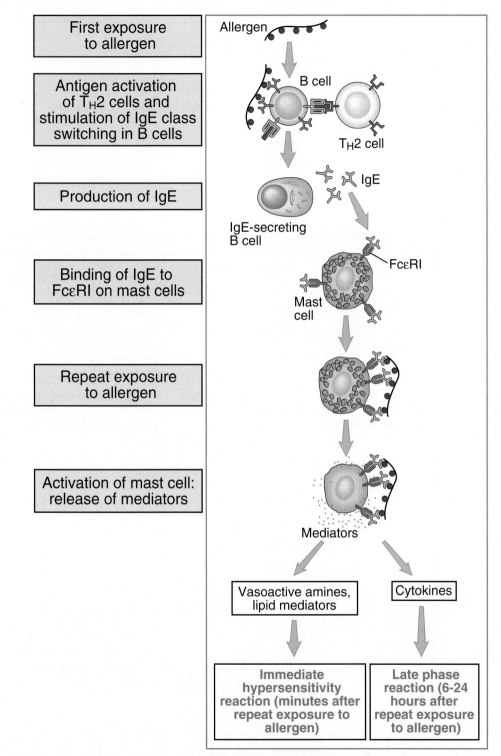

Figure 11-2 The sequence of events in immediate hypersensitivity. Immediate hypersensitivity diseases are initiated by the introduction of an allergen, which stimulates T_H2 reactions and IgE production. IgE binds to Fc receptors (FcεRI) on mast cells, and subsequent exposure to the allergen activates the mast cells to secrete the mediators that are responsible for the pathologic reactions of immediate hypersensitivity.

to protein antigens or chemicals that bind to proteins. Antigens that elicit immediate hypersensitivity (allergic) reactions are often called **allergens.**

Two of the cytokines secreted by T_H2 cells, interleukin (IL)-4 and IL-13, stimulate B lymphocytes specific for the foreign antigens to switch to IgE-producing cells. Therefore, atopic individuals produce large amounts of IgE antibody in response to antigens that do not elicit IgE responses in most people. We know that the propensity toward T_H2 development, IgE production, and immediate hypersensitivity has a strong genetic basis, with many different genes playing contributory roles.

Activation of Mast Cells and Secretion of Mediators

IgE antibody produced in response to an allergen binds to high-affinity Fc receptors specific for the ε heavy chain expressed on mast cells (Fig. 11-3).

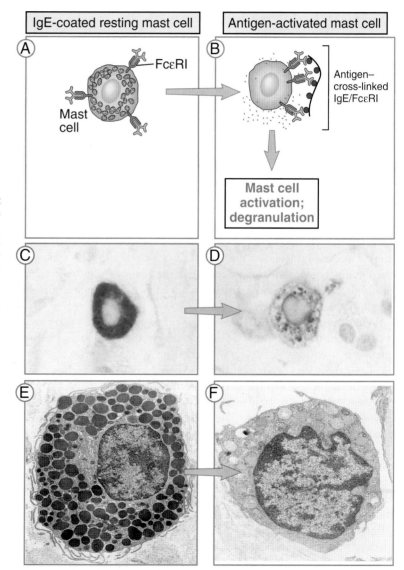

Figure 11–3 The activation of mast cells. Mast cells are sensitized by the binding of IgE to FcεRI receptors (A), and binding of the allergen to the IgE cross-links the Fcε receptors and activates the mast cells (B). Mast cell activation leads to degranulation, as seen in the light micrographs in which the granules are stained with a red dye (C, D) and in the electron micrographs of a resting and an activated mast cell (E, F). (Courtesy of Dr. Daniel Friend, Department of Pathology, Harvard Medical School, Boston, MA.)

Thus, in an atopic individual, mast cells are coated with IgE antibody specific for the antigen(s) to which the individual is allergic. This process of coating mast cells with IgE is called "sensitization," because coating with IgE specific for an antigen makes the mast cells sensitive to activation by subsequent encounter with that antigen. In normal individuals, by contrast, mast cells may carry IgE molecules of many different specificities, because many antigens may elicit small IgE responses, not enough to cause immediate hypersensitivity reactions. Mast cells are present in all connective tissues, and which of the body's mast cells are activated by cross-linking of allergen-specific IgE often depends on the route of entry of the allergen. For instance, inhaled allergens activate mast cells in the submucosal tissues of the bronchus, whereas ingested allergens activate mast cells in the wall of the intestine.

IgE binds to a high-affinity Fcε receptor, called FcεRI, that is expressed on the surface of mast cells. This receptor consists of three chains, one of which binds the Fc portion of the ε heavy chain very strongly, with a K_d of approximately 10^{-11} M. (The concentration of IgE in the plasma is approximately 10^{-9} M, so that even in normal individuals mast cells are always coated with IgE bound to FcεRI.) The other two chains of the receptor are signaling proteins. The same FcεRI is also present on basophils, the circulating counterpart of mast cells, but the role of basophils in immediate hypersensitivity is not as well established as the role of mast cells.

When mast cells sensitized by IgE are exposed to the allergen, the cells are activated to secrete their mediators (see Fig. 11-3). Thus, immediate hypersensitivity reactions occur after initial exposure to an allergen elicits specific IgE production and repeat exposure activates sensitized mast cells. Mast cell activation results from binding of the allergen to two or more IgE antibodies on the mast cell. When this happens, the IgE and the FcεRI molecules that are carrying the IgE are cross-linked, triggering biochemical signals from the signal-transducing chains of FcεRI. The signals lead to three types of responses in the mast cell: rapid release of granule contents (degranulation), synthesis and secretion of lipid mediators, and synthesis and secretion of cytokines.

The most important mediators produced by mast cells are vasoactive amines and proteases that are released from granules, products of arachidonic acid metabolism, and cytokines (Fig. 11-4). These mediators have different actions. The major amine, histamine, causes the dilatation of small blood vessels, increases vascular permeability, and stimulates the transient contraction of smooth muscles. Proteases may cause damage to local tissues. Arachidonic acid metabolites include prostaglandins, which cause vascular dilatation, and leukotrienes, which stimulate prolonged smooth muscle contraction. Cytokines induce local inflammation (the late phase reaction, described below). Thus, mast cell mediators are responsible for acute vascular and smooth muscle reactions and inflammation, the hallmarks of immediate hypersensitivity.

Cytokines produced by mast cells stimulate the recruitment of leukocytes, which cause the late phase reaction. The principal leukocytes involved in this reaction are eosinophils, neutrophils, and T_H2 cells. Mast cell–derived tumor necrosis factor (TNF) and IL-4 promote neutrophil- and eosinophil-rich inflammation. Chemokines produced by mast cells and by epithelial cells in the tissues also contribute to leukocyte recruitment. Eosinophils and neutrophils liberate proteases, which cause tissue damage, and T_H2 cells may exacerbate the reaction by producing more cytokines. Eosinophils are prominent components of many allergic reactions and are an important cause of tissue injury in these reactions. These cells are activated by the cytokine IL-5, which is produced by T_H2 cells and mast cells.

Clinical Syndromes and Therapy

Immediate hypersensitivity reactions have diverse clinical and pathologic features, all of which are attributable to mediators produced by mast cells in different amounts and in different tissues (Fig. 11-5). Some mild reactions, such as allergic rhinitis and sinusitis, which are commonly seen in **hay fever,** are reactions to inhaled allergens, such as the ragweed protein of pollen. Mast cells in the nasal mucosa produce histamine, which causes increased secretion of mucus. Late phase reactions may lead to more

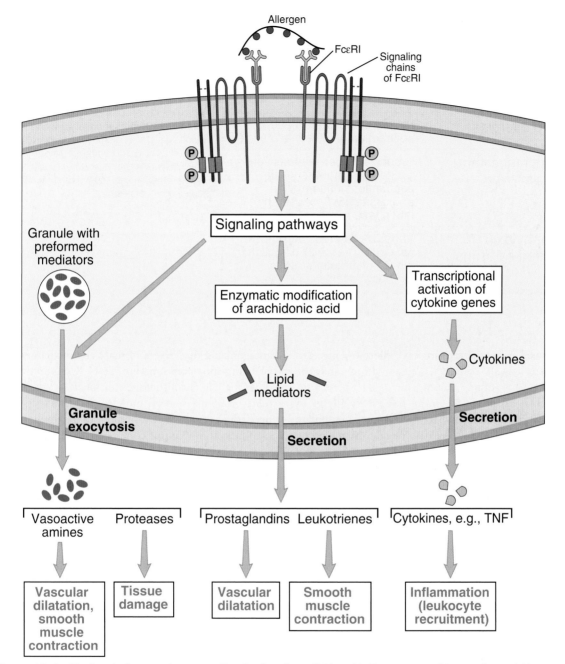

Figure 11–4   Biochemical events in mast cell activation. Cross-linking of IgE on a mast cell by an allergen initiates multiple signaling pathways from the signaling chains of the IgE Fc receptor (FcεRI), including the phosphorylation of ITAMs. These signaling pathways stimulate the release of mast cell granule contents (amines, proteases), the synthesis of arachidonic acid metabolites (prostaglandins, leukotrienes), and the synthesis of various cytokines. These mast cell mediators stimulate the various reactions of immediate hypersensitivity.

Clinical syndrome	Clinical and pathologic manifestations
Allergic rhinitis, sinusitis (hay fever)	Increased mucus secretion; inflammation of upper airways, sinuses
Food allergies	Increased peristalsis due to contraction of intestinal muscles
Bronchial asthma	Bronchial hyper-responsiveness caused by smooth muscle contraction; inflammation and tissue injury caused by late phase reaction
Anaphylaxis (may be caused by drugs, bee sting, food)	Fall in blood pressure (shock) caused by vascular dilatation; airway obstruction due to laryngeal edema

Figure 11–5 Clinical manifestations of immediate hypersensitivity reactions. The manifestations of some common immediate hypersensitivity reactions are listed. Immediate hypersensitivity may be manifested in many other ways, such as urticaria and eczema in the skin.

prolonged inflammation. In **food allergies,** ingested allergens trigger mast cell degranulation, and the released histamine causes increased peristalsis. **Bronchial asthma** is a form of respiratory allergy in which inhaled allergens (often undefined) stimulate bronchial mast cells to release mediators, including leukotrienes, which cause repeated bouts of bronchial constriction and airway obstruction. In chronic asthma, there are large numbers of eosinophils in the bronchial mucosa and excessive secretion of mucus in the airways, and the bronchial smooth muscle becomes hyper-reactive to various stimuli. Some cases of asthma are not associated with IgE production, although all are caused by mast cell activation. In some individuals, asthma may be triggered by cold or exercise; how these cause mast cell activation is unknown. The most severe form of immediate hypersensitivity is **anaphylaxis,** a systemic reaction characterized by edema in many tissues, including the larynx, accompanied by a fall in blood pressure. This reaction is caused by widespread mast cell degranulation in response to a systemic antigen, and it is life threatening because of the sudden fall in blood pressure and airway obstruction.

The therapy for immediate hypersensitivity reactions is aimed at inhibiting mast cell degranulation, antagonizing the effects of mast cell mediators, and **reducing inflammation** (Fig. 11-6). Commonly used drugs include antihistamines for hay fever, drugs that relax bronchial smooth muscles in asthma, and epinephrine in anaphylaxis. In diseases in which inflammation is an important component of the pathology, such as asthma, corticosteroids are used to inhibit inflammation. Many patients benefit from repeated administration of small doses of allergens, called **desensitization.** This treatment may work by changing the T cell response away from T_H2 dominance or by inducing tolerance (anergy) in allergen-specific T cells.

Before concluding the discussion of immediate hypersensitivity, it is important to address the question of why evolution has preserved an IgE antibody– and mast cell–mediated immune response whose major effects are pathologic. There is no good answer to this puzzle. It is known that IgE antibody and eosinophils are important mechanisms of defense against helminthic infections, and mast cells play a role in innate immunity against some bacteria. But it is not understood why common environmental antigens elicit reactions of T_H2 cells and mast cells that are capable of causing considerable damage.

Syndrome	Therapy	Mechanism of action
Anaphylaxis	Epinephrine	Causes vascular smooth muscle contraction; increases cardiac output (to counter shock); inhibits further mast cell degranulation
Bronchial asthma	Corticosteroids Phosphodiesterase inhibitors	Reduce inflammation Relax bronchial smooth muscles
Most allergic diseases	"Desensitization" (repeated administration of low doses of allergens)	Unknown; may inhibit IgE production and increase production of other Ig isotypes; may induce T cell tolerance
	Anti-IgE antibody (in clinical trials)	Neutralize and eliminate IgE
	Antihistamines	Block actions of histamine on vessels and smooth muscles
	Cromolyn	Inhibits mast cell degranulation

Figure 11–6 **Treatment of immediate hypersensitivity reactions.** Various drugs are used to treat immediate hypersensitivity reactions. The principal mechanisms of action of these drugs are summarized.

Diseases Caused by Antibodies and Antigen-Antibody Complexes

Antibodies, other than IgE, may cause disease by binding to their target antigens in cells and tissues or by forming immune complexes that deposit in blood vessels (Fig. 11-7). Antibody-mediated hypersensitivity diseases were recognized many years ago and are common forms of chronic immunologic diseases in humans. Antibodies against cells or extracellular matrix components may deposit in any tissue that expresses the relevant target antigen. Diseases caused by such antibodies are usually specific for a particular tissue. Immune complexes tend to deposit in blood vessels at sites of turbulence (branches of vessels) or high pressure (kidney glomeruli and synovium). Therefore, immune complex diseases tend to be systemic and often manifest as widespread vasculitis, arthritis, and nephritis.

Etiology of Antibody-Mediated Diseases

The antibodies that cause disease are most often autoantibodies against self antigens and less commonly are specific for foreign (e.g., microbial) antigens. The production of autoantibodies results from a failure of self-tolerance. In Chapter 9 the mechanisms by which self-tolerance may fail were discussed, but, as pointed out, it is still not understood why this happens in any human autoimmune disease. Autoantibodies may bind to self antigens in tissues, or they may form immune complexes with circulating self antigens.

There are few examples of diseases caused by antibodies that are produced against microbial antigens. Two of the best described are rare, late sequelae of streptococcal infections. After such infections, some individuals produce antistreptococcal antibodies that cross-react with an antigen in heart muscle. Deposition of these antibodies in the heart triggers an inflammatory disease called rheumatic fever. Other individuals make antistreptococcal antibodies that deposit in kidney glomeruli, causing poststreptococcal glomerulonephritis. Some immune complex diseases are caused by antibodies against microbial antigens forming complexes with the antigens.

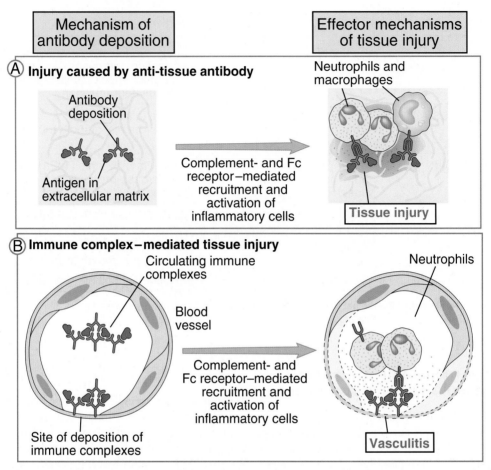

Figure 11–7   Types of antibody-mediated diseases. Antibodies (other than IgE) may cause tissue injury and disease by binding directly to their target antigens in cells and extracellular matrix (A, type II hypersensitivity) or by forming immune complexes that deposit mainly in blood vessels (B, type III hypersensitivity).

Mechanisms of Tissue Injury and Disease

Antibodies specific for cell and tissue antigens may deposit in tissues and cause injury by inducing local inflammation, or they may interfere with normal cellular functions (Fig. 11-8). Antibodies against tissue antigens and immune complexes deposited in vessels induce inflammation by attracting and activating leukocytes. IgG antibodies of the IgG1 and IgG3 subclasses bind to neutrophil and macrophage Fc receptors and activate these leukocytes, resulting in inflammation. The same antibodies, as well as IgM, activate the complement system by the classical pathway, resulting in the production of complement by-products that recruit leukocytes and induce inflammation. When leukocytes are activated at sites of antibody deposition, these cells produce substances such as reactive oxygen intermediates and lysosomal enzymes that damage the adjacent tissues. If antibodies bind to cells, such as erythrocytes and platelets, the cells are opsonized and may be ingested and destroyed by host phagocytes. Some antibodies may cause disease without directly inducing tissue injury. For instance, antibodies against hormone receptors may inhibit receptor function; in some cases of

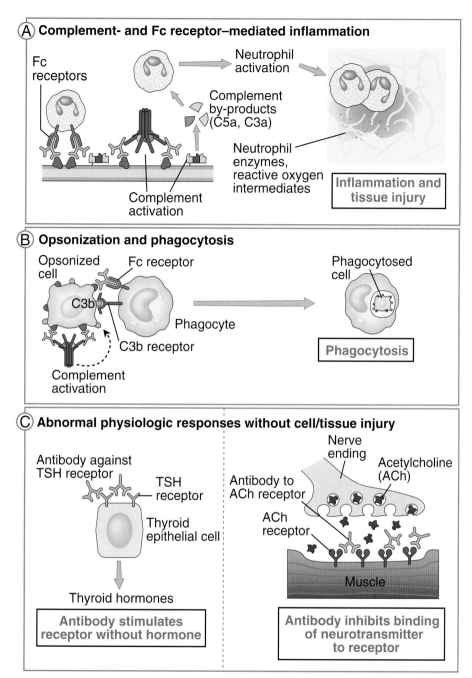

Figure 11–8   Effector mechanisms of antibody-mediated diseases. Antibodies may cause disease by inducing inflammation at the site of deposition (A), by opsonizing cells for phagocytosis (B), and by interfering with normal cellular functions, such as hormone receptor signaling (C). All three mechanisms are seen with antibodies that bind directly to their target antigens, but immune complexes cause disease mainly by inducing inflammation (A). TSH, thyroid-stimulating hormone; ACh, acetylcholine.

myasthenia gravis, antibodies against the acetylcholine receptor inhibit neuromuscular transmission and cause paralysis. Other antibodies may activate receptors without their physiologic hormone; in a form of hyperthyroidism called Graves' disease, antibodies against the receptor for thyroid-stimulating hormone stimulate thyroid cells even in the absence of the hormone.

Clinical Syndromes and Therapy

Many chronic hypersensitivity disorders in humans are known to be caused by, or are associated with, anti-tissue antibodies (Fig. 11-9) and immune complexes (Fig. 11-10). Therapy for these diseases is intended mainly to limit inflammation and its injurious consequences, with drugs such as corticosteroids. In severe cases, plasmapheresis is used to reduce levels of circulating antibodies or immune complexes. There is great interest in trying novel approaches for inhibiting the production of autoantibodies (e.g., by treating patients with antagonists that block CD40 ligand and thus inhibit helper T cell–dependent B cell activation). There is also great interest in inducing tolerance in cases in which the autoantigens are known. These newer therapies are at the stage of preclinical testing and early clinical trials.

Diseases Caused by T Lymphocytes

The role of T lymphocytes in human immunologic diseases has been increasingly recognized as methods for identifying and isolating these cells from lesions have improved and animal models of human diseases have been developed in which a pathogenic role of T cells can be established by experiments. In fact, much of the recent interest in the pathogenesis and treatment of human autoimmune diseases is focused on disorders in which tissue injury is caused mainly by T lymphocytes.

Etiology of T Cell–Mediated Diseases

Most T cell–mediated hypersensitivity diseases are believed to be caused by autoimmunity. The auto-immune reactions are usually directed against cellular antigens with restricted tissue distribution. Therefore, T cell–mediated autoimmune diseases tend to be limited to a few organs and are usually not systemic. Tissue injury may also accompany entirely normal T cell responses to microbes. For instance, in tuberculosis, there is a T cell–mediated immune response against M. *tuberculosis*, and the response becomes chronic because the infection is difficult to eradicate. The resultant granulomatous inflammation is the principal cause of injury to normal tissues at the site of infection and subsequent functional impairment. In hepatitis virus infection, the virus itself may not be highly cytopathic, but the cytolytic T lymphocyte (CTL) response to infected hepatocytes may cause liver injury.

Mechanisms of Tissue Injury

In different T cell–mediated diseases, tissue injury is caused by a delayed-type hypersensitivity response mediated by CD4⁺ T cells or by lysis of host cells by CD8⁺ CTLs (Fig. 11-11). The mechanisms of tissue injury are the same as the mechanisms used by T cells to eliminate cell-associated microbes. CD4⁺ T cells may react against cell or tissue antigens and secrete cytokines that induce local inflammation and activate macrophages. The actual tissue injury is caused by the macrophages and other inflammatory cells. CD8⁺ T cells specific for antigens on autologous cells may directly kill these cells. In many T cell–mediated autoimmune diseases, both CD4⁺ T cells and CD8⁺ T cells specific for self antigens are present, and both contribute to tissue injury.

Clinical Syndromes and Therapy

Many organ-specific autoimmune diseases in humans are believed to be caused by T cells, based on the identification of these cells in lesions and similarities with animal models in which the diseases are known to be T cell mediated (Fig. 11-12).

The therapy for T cell–mediated hypersensitivity disorders is designed to reduce inflammation, using corticosteroids and antagonists against cytokines such as TNF, and to inhibit T cell responses with immuno-

Disease	Target antigen	Mechanisms of disease	Clinicopathologic manifestations
Autoimmune hemolytic anemia	Erythrocyte membrane proteins (Rh blood group antigens, I antigen)	Opsonization and phagocytosis of erythrocytes	Hemolysis, anemia
Autoimmune (idiopathic) thrombocytopenic purpura	Platelet membrane proteins (gpIIb:IIIa integrin)	Opsonization and phagocytosis of platelets	Bleeding
Pemphigus vulgaris	Proteins in intercellular junctions of epidermal cells (epidermal cadherin)	Antibody-mediated activation of proteases, disruption of intercellular adhesions	Skin vesicles (bullae)
Goodpasture's syndrome	Noncollagenous protein in basement membranes of kidney glomeruli and lung alveoli	Complement- and Fc receptor–mediated inflammation	Nephritis, lung hemorrhages
Acute rheumatic fever	Streptococcal cell wall antigen; antibody cross-reacts with myocardial antigen	Inflammation, macrophage activation	Myocarditis, arthritis
Myasthenia gravis	Acetylcholine receptor	Antibody inhibits acetycholine binding, down-modulates receptors	Muscle weakness, paralysis
Graves' disease (hyperthyroidism)	Thyroid-stimulating hormone (TSH) receptor	Antibody-mediated stimulation of TSH receptors	Hyperthyroidism
Pernicious anemia	Intrinsic factor of gastric parietal cells	Neutralization of intrinsic factor, decreased absorption of vitamin B_{12}	Abnormal erythropoiesis, anemia

Figure 11–9   Human antibody-mediated diseases. Examples of human diseases that are caused by antibodies are listed. In most of these diseases, the role of antibodies is inferred from the detection of antibodies in the blood or the lesions, and in some cases by similarities with experimental models in which the involvement of antibodies can be formally established by transfer studies.

suppressive drugs such as cyclosporine. Antagonists of TNF have proved to be beneficial in patients with rheumatoid arthritis and inflammatory bowel disease. Many newer agents are being developed to inhibit T cell responses. These include antagonists against receptors for cytokines such as IL-2, and agents that block costimulators such as B7. There is also great hope for inducing tolerance in pathogenic T cells, but no successful clinical trials have been reported yet.

Disease	Antibody specificity	Mechanisms of disease	Clinicopathologic manifestations
Systemic lupus erythematosus	DNA, nucleoproteins, others	Complement- and Fc receptor–mediated inflammation	Nephritis, arthritis, vasculitis
Polyarteritis nodosa	Hepatitis B virus surface antigen	Complement- and Fc receptor–mediated inflammation	Vasculitis
Post-streptococcal glomerulonephritis	Streptococcal cell wall antigen(s)	Complement- and Fc receptor–mediated inflammation	Nephritis

Figure 11–10   Human immune complex diseases. Examples of human diseases that are caused by the deposition of immune complexes are listed. In these diseases, immune complexes are detected in the blood or in the tissues that are the sites of injury.

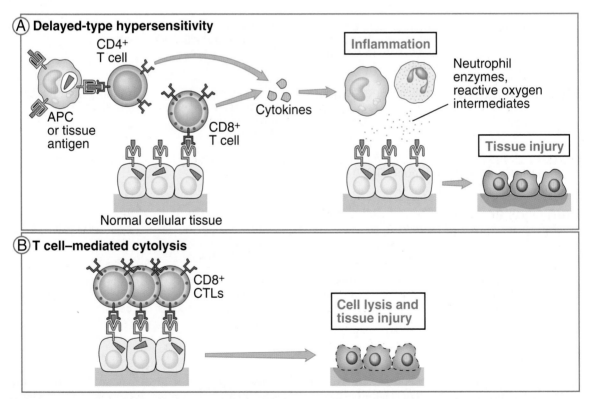

Figure 11–11   Mechanisms of T cell–mediated tissue injury. T cells may cause tissue injury and disease by two mechanisms: delayed hypersensitivity reactions (A), which may be triggered by CD4+ and CD8+ T cells and in which tissue injury is caused by activated macrophages and inflammatory cells, and direct killing of target cells (B), which is mediated by CD8+ CTLs.

Disease	Specificity of pathogenic T cells	Human disease	Animal models
Insulin-dependent (type I) diabetes mellitus	Islet cell antigens (insulin, glutamic acid decarboxylase, others)	Specificity of T cells not established	NOD mouse, BB rat, transgenic mouse models
Rheumatoid arthritis	Unknown antigen in joint synovium	Specificity of T cells and role of antibody not established	Collagen-induced arthritis, others
Experimental allergic encephalomyelitis	Myelin basic protein, proteolipid protein	Postulated: multiple sclerosis	Induced by immunization by CNS myelin antigens; transgenic mouse models
Inflammatory bowel disease	Unknown, ? role of intestinal microbes	Specificity of T cells not established	Induced by IL-2 or IL-10 gene knockout or lack of regulatory T cells

Figure 11–12 T cell–mediated diseases. Examples of T cell–mediated diseases in humans, and their corresponding animal models, are listed. In most of the human diseases the role of T cells is inferred from the detection and isolation of T cells reactive with self tissue antigens from the blood or lesions and from the similarity with experimental models in which the involvement of T cells has been established by transfer studies. In some autoimmune diseases, such as myasthenia gravis and thyroiditis, the lesions are caused by autoantibodies but the lesions may be transferred in experimental models by CD4$^+$ T cells. It is believed that in these disorders the T cells function as helper cells to stimulate the production of autoantibodies. The specificity of pathogenic T cells has been defined mainly in animal models.

SUMMARY

▶ Diseases caused by immune responses, called hypersensitivity diseases, may arise from uncontrolled or abnormal responses to foreign antigens or autoimmune responses against self antigens.

▶ Hypersensitivity diseases are classified according to the mechanism of tissue injury.

▶ Immediate hypersensitivity (type I, commonly called allergy) is caused by the production of IgE antibody against environmental antigens or drugs (allergens), sensitization of mast cells by the IgE, and degranulation of these mast cells on subsequent encounter with the allergen.

▶ The clinical and pathologic manifestations of immediate hypersensitivity are due to the actions of mediators secreted by the mast cells. These include amines, which dilate vessels and contract smooth muscles, arachidonic acid metabolites, which also contract muscles, and cytokines, which induce inflammation, the hallmark of the late phase reaction. Treatment of allergies is designed to inhibit the production of and antagonize the actions of mediators and to counteract their effects on end organs.

▶ Antibodies against cell and tissue antigens may cause tissue injury and disease (type II hypersensitivity). IgM and IgG antibodies promote the phagocytosis of cells to which they bind, induce inflammation by complement- and Fc receptor–mediated leukocyte recruitment, and may interfere with the functions of cells by binding to essential molecules and receptors.

▶ Antibodies may bind to circulating antigens to form immune complexes, which deposit in vessels and cause tissue injury (type III hypersensitivity). Injury is mainly due to leukocyte recruitment and inflammation.

▶ T cell–mediated diseases (type IV hypersensitivity) are caused by CD4$^+$ T cell–mediated delayed-type hypersensitivity reactions or by killing of host cells by CD8$^+$ CTLs.

Review Questions

1 What types of antigens may induce immune responses that cause hypersensitivity diseases?

2 What is the sequence of events in a typical immediate hypersensitivity reaction? What is the late phase reaction, and what is it caused by?

3 What are some examples of immediate hypersensitivity disorders, what is their pathogenesis, and how are they treated?

4 How do antibodies cause tissue injury and disease? What are some of the differences in the manifestations of diseases caused by antibodies against extracellular matrix proteins and by immune complexes that deposit in tissues?

5 What are some examples of diseases caused by antibodies or immune complexes, what is their pathogenesis, and what are their principal clinical and pathologic manifestations?

Congenital and Acquired Immunodeficiencies

12

Diseases Caused by Defective Immune Responses

Defects in the development and functions of the immune system result in increased susceptibility to infections and in an increased incidence of certain cancers. These consequences of defective immunity are predictable because, as emphasized throughout this book, the normal function of the immune system is to defend individuals against infections and some cancers. Disorders caused by defective immunity are called **immunodeficiency diseases.** Some of these diseases may result from genetic abnormalities in one or more components of the immune system; these are called **congenital** (or **primary**) **immunodeficiencies.** Other defects in the immune system may result from infections, nutritional abnormalities, or treatments that cause loss or inadequate function of various components of the immune system; these are called **acquired** (or **secondary**) **immunodeficiencies.** In this chapter we will describe the causes and pathogenesis of congenital and acquired immunodeficiencies. Among the acquired diseases, this chapter emphasizes the acquired immunodeficiency syndrome (AIDS), the disease that results from infection by the human immunodeficiency virus (HIV) and that is one of the most devastating health problems worldwide. The following questions will be addressed:

- What are the pathogenetic mechanisms of the common immunodeficiency diseases? (Information about the clinical features of these disorders may be found in textbooks of pediatrics and medicine.)

- How does HIV cause the clinical and pathologic abnormalities of AIDS?

- What approaches are being used to treat immunodeficiency diseases?

Congenital (Primary) Immunodeficiencies

Congenital immunodeficiencies are caused by genetic defects that lead to blocks in the maturation or functions of different components of the immune system. It is estimated that as many as 1 in 500 individuals in the United States and Europe suffer from congenital immune deficiencies of varying severity.

All congenital immunodeficiencies share several features, their hallmark being infectious complications (Fig. 12-1). However, different congenital immunodeficiency diseases may differ considerably in clinical and pathologic manifestations. Some of these disorders result in greatly increased susceptibility to infections that may be manifested early after birth and may be fatal unless the immunologic defects are corrected. Other congenital immunodeficiencies lead to mild infections and may be detected in adult life. In the following discussion, the pathogenesis of selected immunodeficiencies is summarized, several of which were mentioned in earlier chapters to illustrate the physiologic importance of various components of the immune system.

Defects in Lymphocyte Maturation

Many congenital immunodeficiencies are the result of genetic abnormalities that cause blocks in the maturation of B lymphocytes, T lymphocytes, or both (Figs. 12-2 and 12-3). Disorders manifesting as defects in both the B cell and T cell arms of the adaptive

Type of immunodeficiency	Histopathology and laboratory abnormalities	Common infectious consequences
B cell deficiencies	Absent or reduced follicles and germinal centers in lymphoid organs Reduced serum Ig levels	Pyogenic bacterial infections
T cell deficiencies	May be reduced T cell zones in lymphoid organs Reduced DTH reactions to common antigens Defective T cell proliferative responses to mitogens *in vitro*	Viral and other intracellular microbial infections (e.g., *Pneumocystis carinii*, atypical mycobacteria, fungi) Virus-associated malignancies (e.g., EBV-associated lymphomas)
Innate immune deficiencies	Variable, depending on which component of innate immunity is defective	Variable; pyogenic bacterial infections

Figure 12–1 **Features of immunodeficiency diseases.** The important diagnostic features and clinical manifestations of immune deficiencies affecting different components of the immune system are summarized. Within each group, different diseases, and even different patients with the same disease, may show considerable variation.

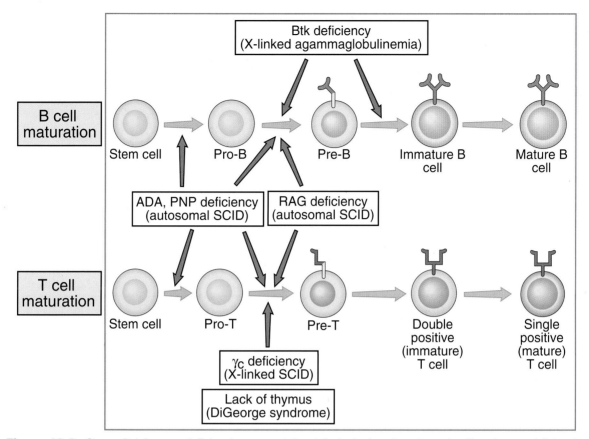

Figure 12–2 Congenital immunodeficiencies caused by defects in lymphocyte maturation. Immunodeficiencies caused by genetic defects in lymphocyte maturation are shown. Lymphocyte maturation pathways are described in more detail in Chapter 4. ADA, adenosine deaminase; PNP, purine nucleoside phosphorylase; RAG, recombination activating gene.

immune system are classified as **severe combined immunodeficiency (SCID)**.

Several different genetic abnormalities cause severe combined immunodeficiencies. About half of these cases are X-linked, affecting only male children. About 50% of cases of **X-linked SCID** are caused by mutations in a signaling subunit of a receptor for cytokines. This subunit is called the common γ chain (γc), because it is a component of the receptors for numerous cytokines, including interleukin (IL)-2, IL-4, IL-7, IL-9, and IL-15. (Because the γc chain was first identified as one of the three chains of the IL-2 receptor, it is often called the IL-2Rγ chain.) When the γc chain is not functional, immature lymphocytes at the pro-T cell and pro-B cell stages cannot proliferate in response to the major growth factor for these

cells, namely, IL-7. Defective responses to IL-7 result in reduced survival and maturation of lymphocyte precursors. In humans, the defect affects mainly T cell maturation. The consequence of this block is a profound decrease in the numbers of mature T cells, deficient cell-mediated immunity, and defective humoral immunity because of absent T cell help (even though B cells may mature almost normally).

About half the cases of **autosomal SCID** are caused by mutations in an enzyme called adenosine deaminase (ADA), which is involved in the breakdown of purines. Deficiency of ADA leads to the accumulation of toxic purine metabolites in cells that are actively synthesizing DNA, namely, proliferating cells. Lymphocytes, which actively proliferate during their maturation, are injured by these accumulating

Severe combined immunodeficiency (SCID)

Disease	Functional deficiencies	Mechanism of defect
X-linked SCID	Markedly decreased T cells; normal or increased B cells; reduced serum Ig	Cytokine receptor common γ chain gene mutations, defective T cell maturation due to lack of IL-7 signals
Autosomal recessive SCID due to ADA, PNP deficiency	Progressive decrease in T and B cells (mostly T); reduced serum Ig in ADA deficiency, normal B cells and serum Ig in PNP deficiency	ADA or PNP deficiency leads to accumulation of toxic metabolites in lymphocytes
Autosomal recessive SCID due to other causes	Decreased T and B cells; reduced serum Ig	Defective maturation of T and B cells; genetic basis unknown in most cases; may be mutations in *RAG* genes

B cell immunodeficiencies

Disease	Functional deficiencies	Mechanism of defect
X-linked agammaglobulinemia	Decrease in all serum Ig isotypes; reduced B cell numbers	Block in maturation beyond pre-B cells, because of mutation in B cell tyrosine kinase
Ig heavy chain deletions	IgG1, IgG2, or IgG4 absent; sometimes associated with absent IgA or IgE	Chromosomal deletion at 14q32 (Ig heavy chain locus)

T cell immunodeficiencies

Disease	Functional deficiencies	Mechanism of defect
DiGeorge syndrome	Decreased T cells; normal B cells; normal or decreased serum Ig	Anomalous development of 3rd and 4th branchial pouches, leading to thymic hypoplasia

Figure 12–3   Features of congenital immunodeficiencies caused by defects in lymphocyte maturation. The congenital immunodeficiencies in which the genetic blocks are known, and their principal features, are summarized.

toxic metabolites. ADA deficiency results in a block in T cell maturation more than in B cell maturation; defective humoral immunity is largely a consequence of the lack of T cell helper function. Another important cause of autosomal SCID is mutations in an enzyme that is involved in signaling by the γc

cytokine receptor chain. These mutations result in the same abnormalities as X-linked SCID due to γc mutations, described previously. Rare cases of autosomal SCID are caused by mutations in *RAG1* or *RAG2* genes, which encode the lymphocyte specific components of the VDJ recombinase that are required for immunoglobulin and T cell receptor gene recombinations and lymphocyte maturation (see Chapter 4). The cause of about 50% of both X-linked and autosomal cases of SCID is not known.

The most common clinical syndrome caused by a block in B cell maturation is **X-linked agammaglobulinemia.** In this disorder, B cells in the bone marrow fail to mature beyond the pre-B cell stage, resulting in a severe decrease or absence of mature B lymphocytes and serum immunoglobulins. The disease is caused by mutations in the gene encoding a kinase called the B cell tyrosine kinase (Btk), resulting in defective production or function of the enzyme. The exact role of Btk in B cell maturation is not known. The enzyme is activated by the pre-B cell receptor expressed in pre-B cells, and it is believed to participate in delivering biochemical signals that promote maturation of these cells. The gene for this enzyme is located on the X chromosome. Therefore, women who carry a mutant allele of the *Btk* gene on one of their X chromosomes are carriers of the disease, and male offspring who inherit the abnormal X chromosome are affected. Paradoxically, about a fourth of patients with X-linked agammaglobulinemia develop autoimmune diseases, notably arthritis. Why an immune deficiency should lead to a reaction typical of excessive or uncontrolled immune responses is not known.

Selective defects in T cell maturation are quite rare. The most frequent of these is the **DiGeorge syndrome,** which results from incomplete development of the thymus (and the parathyroid glands) and a failure of T cell maturation. Patients with this disease tend to improve with age, probably because the small amount of thymic tissue that does develop is able to support some T cell maturation.

SCID is fatal in early life unless the patient's immune system is reconstituted. The most widely used treatment is bone marrow transplantation, with careful matching of donor and recipient to avoid potentially serious graft-versus-host disease. For selective B cell defects, patients may be given antibodies isolated from healthy donors to provide passive immunity. Immunoglobulin replacement therapy has had enormous benefit in X-linked agammaglobulinemia. The ideal treatment for all congenital immunodeficiencies is replacement gene therapy. This treatment, however, remains a distant goal for most diseases. The most impressive results of successful gene therapy have been reported in patients with X-linked SCID, but so far very few patients have been treated, and the long-term effectiveness of the therapy is unknown. In all patients with these diseases, infections are treated with antibiotics as needed.

Defects in Lymphocyte Activation and Function

As understanding of the molecules involved in lymphocyte activation and function has improved, mutations and other abnormalities in these molecules that result in immunodeficiency disorders have also begun to be recognized. Many such disorders are now known (Fig. 12-4). The following section describes some of the diseases in which lymphocytes mature normally but the activation and effector functions of the cells are defective.

The **X-linked hyper-IgM syndrome** is characterized by defective B cell heavy chain class (isotype) switching, resulting in IgM being the major serum antibody, and severe deficiency of cell-mediated immunity against intracellular microbes. The disease is caused by mutations in CD40 ligand (CD40L), the helper T cell protein that binds to CD40 on B cells and macrophages and thus mediates T cell–dependent activation of B cells and macrophages. Failure to express functional CD40 ligand leads to defective T cell–dependent B cell responses, such as class switching in humoral immunity, and defective T cell–dependent macrophage activation in cell-mediated immunity.

Genetic deficiencies in the production of selected Ig isotypes are quite common; IgA deficiency is believed to affect as many as 1 in 700 individuals, but in most of these persons it causes no clinical problems. The defect causing these deficiencies is not known in the majority of cases; rarely, the deficiencies may be caused by mutations of Ig heavy chain constant region genes. **Common variable immunodeficiency** is a heterogeneous group of disorders that comprise the most common form of primary immunodeficiency. These disorders are characterized by poor antibody responses to infections and reduced serum levels of IgM, IgA, and often IgM. The underlying causes of common variable disease are poorly understood but include

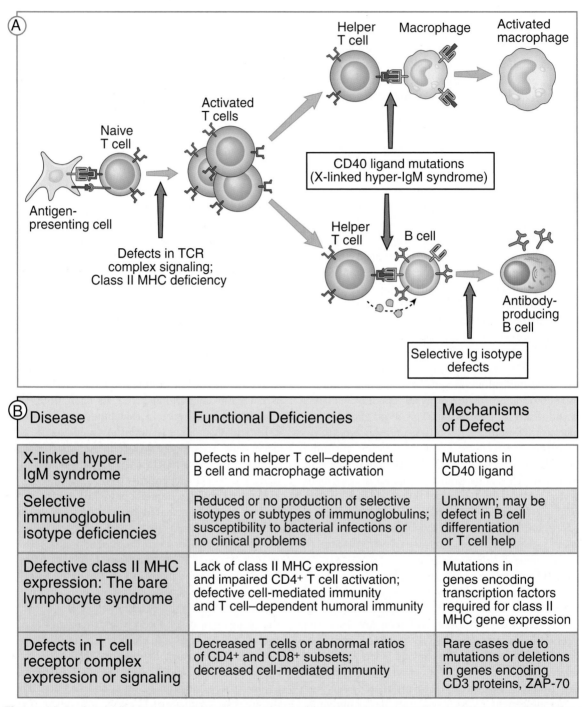

Figure 12–4 Congenital immunodeficiencies associated with defects in lymphocyte activation and effector functions. Congenital immunodeficiencies may be caused by genetic defects in the expression of molecules required for antigen presentation to T cells, T or B lymphocyte antigen receptor signaling, helper T cell activation of B cells and macrophages, and differentiation of antibody-producing B cells. Examples showing the sites where immune responses may be blocked are illustrated in A, and the features of some of these disorders are summarized in B.

defects in B call maturation and activation as well as defects in helper T cell function. Patients suffer from recurrent infections, autoimmune disease, and lymphomas.

Defective activation of T lymphocytes may result from deficient expression of major histocompatibility complex (MHC) molecules. The **bare lymphocyte syndrome** is a disease caused by a failure to express class II MHC molecules, as a result of mutations in the transcription factors that normally induce class II MHC expression. Recall that class II MHC molecules display peptide antigens for recognition by CD4$^+$ T cells and that this recognition is critical for maturation and activation of the T cells. The disease is manifested by a profound decrease in CD4$^+$ T cells, because of defective maturation of these cells in the thymus and defective activation in peripheral lymphoid organs. Occasional patients have been described in whom immunodeficiency is caused by mutations in T cell signal transducing molecules, cytokines, and various receptors.

Defects in Innate Immunity

Abnormalities in two components of innate immunity, phagocytes and the complement system, are important causes of immunodeficiency (Fig. 12-5). **Chronic granulomatous disease** is caused by mutations in the enzyme phagocyte oxidase, which catalyzes the production of microbicidal reactive oxygen intermediates in lysosomes (see Chapter 2). As a result, neutrophils and macrophages that phagocytose microbes are unable to kill the microbes. The immune system tries to compensate for this defective microbial killing by calling in more and more macrophages, and by activating T cells, which stimulate recruitment and activation of even more phagocytes. Therefore, collections of phagocytes accumulate around infections by intracellular microbes but the microbes cannot be destroyed effectively. These collections resemble granulomas, giving rise to the name of this disease. **Leukocyte adhesion deficiency** is caused by mutations in genes encoding integrins or in enzymes required for the expression of ligands for selectins. Integrins and selectin ligands are involved in the adhesion of leukocytes to other cells. As a result of these mutations, blood leukocytes do not bind firmly

to vascular endothelium and are not recruited normally to sites of infection.

Deficiencies of almost every complement protein, and many complement regulatory proteins, have been described, and some of these were mentioned in Chapter 8. C3 deficiency results in severe infections and is usually fatal. Deficiencies of C2 and C4, two components of the classical pathway of complement activation, result not in immunodeficiency but in immune complex–mediated diseases resembling lupus. A likely explanation for this association between complement deficiencies and lupus-like disease is that the classical complement pathway is involved in eliminating immune complexes that are constantly being formed during humoral immune responses. Failure to clear these immune complexes results in their deposition in tissues and immune complex disease. The observation that C2 and C4 deficiencies do not make individuals susceptible to infection suggests that the alternative pathway may be adequate for host defense. Deficiencies of complement regulatory proteins lead to excessive complement activation and not to immunodeficiencies (see Chapter 8).

The **Chédiak-Higashi syndrome** is an immunodeficiency disease in which the lysosomal granules of leukocytes do not function normally. The immune defect is thought to affect phagocytes and natural killer (NK) cells and is manifested by increased susceptibility to bacterial infections.

Lymphocyte Abnormalities Associated with Other Diseases

Some systemic diseases that involve multiple organ systems, and whose major manifestations are not immunologic, may have a component of immunodeficiency. The **Wiskott-Aldrich syndrome** is characterized by eczema, reduced blood platelets, and immunodeficiency. It is an X-linked disease, caused by a mutation in a gene that encodes a protein that binds to various adapter molecules and cytoskeletal components in hematopoietic cells. It is believed that because of the absence of this protein, platelets and leukocytes are small, do not develop normally, and fail to migrate normally. **Ataxia-telangiectasia** is a disease characterized by gait abnormalities (ataxia),

Disease	Functional Deficiencies	Mechanisms of Defect
Chronic granulomatous disease	Defective production of reactive oxygen intermediates by phagocytes	Mutations in genes encoding components of the phagocyte oxidase enzyme, most often cytochrome b558
Leukocyte adhesion deficiency-1	Absent or deficient expression of β2 integrins causing defective leukocyte adhesion-dependent functions	Mutations in gene encoding the β chain (CD18) of β2 integrins
Leukocyte adhesion deficiency-2	Absent or deficient expression of leukocyte ligands for endothelial E- and P-selectins, causing failure of leukocyte migration into tissues	Mutations in gene encoding a protein required for synthesis of the sialyl-Lewis X component of E- and P-selectin ligands
Complement C3 deficiency	Defect in complement cascade activation	Mutations in the C3 gene
Complement C2, C4 deficiency	Deficient activation of classical pathway of complement leading to failure to clear immune complexes and development of lupus-like disease	Mutations in C2 or C4 genes
Chédiak-Higashi syndrome	Defective lysosomal function in neutrophils, macrophages and dendritic cells, and defective granule function in natural killer cells	Mutation in a gene encoding a lysosomal trafficking regulatory protein

Figure 12–5 Congenital immunodeficiencies caused by defects in innate immunity. Immunodeficiency diseases caused by defects in various components of the innate immune system are listed.

vascular malformations (telangiectasia), and immunodeficiency. The disease is caused by mutations in a gene whose product may be involved in DNA repair. Defects in this protein may lead to abnormal DNA repair (e.g., during recombination of antigen receptor gene segments), resulting in defective lymphocyte maturation.

Acquired (Secondary) Immunodeficiencies

Deficiencies of the immune system often develop because of abnormalities that are not genetic but are acquired during life (Fig. 12-6). The most important of these abnormalities is HIV infection, and this is described later in the chapter. Protein-calorie malnutrition results in deficiencies of virtually all components of the immune system and is a common cause of immunodeficiency in underdeveloped countries. Cancer treatment with chemotherapeutic drugs and irradiation may damage proliferating cells, including bone marrow precursors and mature lymphocytes, resulting in immunodeficiency. Other treatments (e.g., to prevent graft rejection) are designed to suppress immune responses. Therefore, immunodeficiency is a frequent complication of such therapies.

Cause	Mechanism
Human immunodeficiency virus infection	Depletion of CD4+ helper T cells
Protein-calorie malnutrition	Metabolic derangements inhibit lymphocyte maturation and function
Irradiation and chemotherapy treatments for cancer	Decreased bone marrow precursors for all leukocytes
Cancer metastases to bone marrow	Reduced site of leukocyte development
Removal of spleen	Decreased phagocytosis of microbes

Figure 12–6 Acquired (secondary) immunodeficiency diseases. The most common causes of acquired immunodeficiencies, and how they lead to defects in immune responses, are listed.

Acquired Immunodeficiency Syndrome (AIDS)

It is a remarkable and tragic fact that although AIDS was recognized as a distinct disease entity as recently as the 1980s, in this brief period it has become one of the most devastating afflictions in the history of mankind. AIDS is caused by infection with the human immunodeficiency virus (HIV). It is estimated that there are more than 42 million HIV-infected individuals in the world, more than 21 million deaths attributable to this disease, and more than 3 million deaths annually. The infection continues to spread, especially in Africa and Asia; and in some countries in Africa, more than 30% of the population has been infected with HIV. The following section describes the important features of HIV, how it infects humans, and the disease it causes. The section concludes with a brief discussion of the current status of therapy and vaccine development.

The Human Immunodeficiency Virus (HIV)

HIV is a retrovirus that infects cells of the immune system, mainly CD4+ T lymphocytes, and causes progressive destruction of these cells. An infectious HIV particle consists of two RNA strands within a protein core, surrounded by a lipid envelope derived from infected host cells but containing viral proteins (Fig. 12-7). The viral RNA encodes structural proteins, various enzymes, and proteins that regulate transcription of viral genes and the viral life cycle.

The life cycle of HIV consists of the following sequential steps: infection of cells, production of viral DNA and its integration into the host genome, expression of viral genes, and production of viral particles (Fig. 12-8). HIV infects cells by virtue of its major envelope glycoprotein, called gp120 (for 120 kD glycoprotein), binding to CD4 and particular chemokine receptors (CXCR4 and CCR5) on human cells. Therefore, the virus can efficiently infect only cells expressing CD4 and these chemokine receptors. The major cell type that may be infected by HIV is the CD4+ T lymphocyte, but macrophages and dendritic cells are also infected by the virus. Different cell populations may use different chemokine receptors to bind slightly different strains of the virus. After binding to cellular receptors, the viral membrane fuses with the host cell membrane and the virus enters the cell's cytoplasm. Here the virus is uncoated by viral protease and its RNA is released. A DNA copy of the viral RNA is synthesized by the virus's reverse transcriptase enzyme (a process that is characteristic of all retroviruses), and the DNA integrates into the host cell's DNA by the action of the integrase enzyme. The integrated viral DNA is called a provirus. If the infected T cell, macrophage, or dendritic cell is

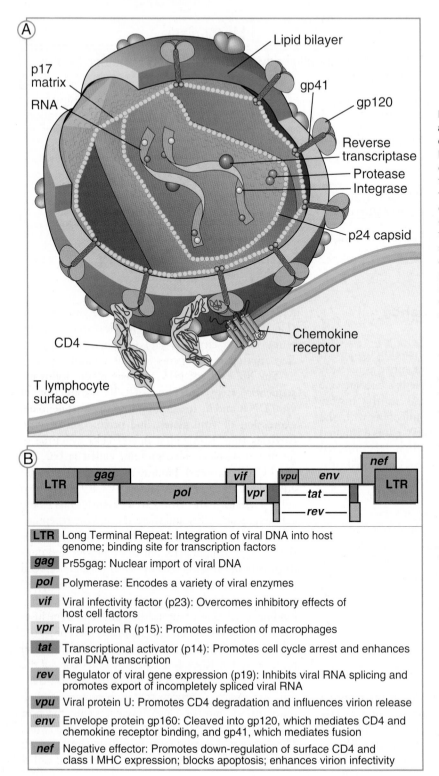

Figure 12–7 The structure and genes of the human immunodeficiency virus (HIV). A. An HIV-1 virion is shown next to a T cell surface. HIV-1 consists of two identical strands of RNA (the viral genome) and associated enzymes, including reverse transcriptase, integrase, and protease, packaged in a cone-shaped core composed of the p24 capsid protein with a surrounding p17 protein matrix, all surrounded by a phospholipid membrane envelope derived from the host cell. Virally encoded membrane proteins (gp41 and gp120) are bound to the envelope. CD4 and chemokine receptors on the host cell surface function as the receptors for HIV-1. (Adapted from the front cover of "The New Face of AIDS." Science 272:1841-2102, 1996. © Terese Winslow.) B. The HIV-1 genome consists of genes whose positions are indicated as differently colored blocks. Some genes contain sequences that overlap with sequences of other genes, as shown by overlapping blocks, but are read differently by host cell RNA polymerase. Similarly shaded blocks separated by lines (*tat, rev*) indicate genes whose coding sequences are separated in the genome and require RNA splicing to produce functional messenger RNA. The major functions of the proteins encoded by different viral genes are listed. LTR, long terminal repeat. (Adapted from Greene WC. AIDS and the Immune System. © 1993 by Scientific American, Inc. All rights reserved.)

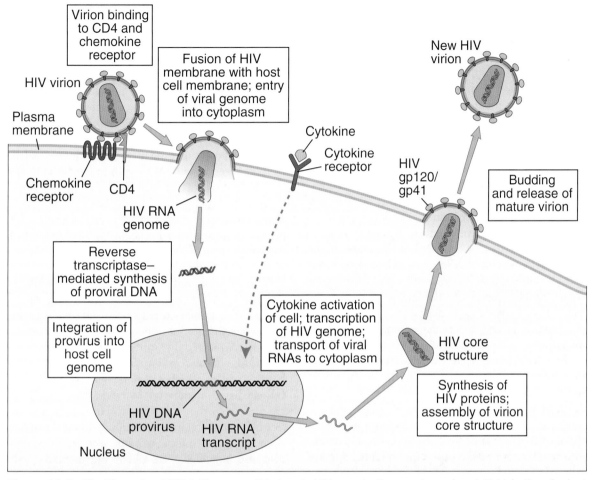

Figure 12–8   The life cycle of HIV-1. The sequential steps in HIV reproduction are shown, from initial infection of a host cell to release of a new virus particle (virion). For the sake of clarity, the production and release of only one new virion is shown. An infected cell actually produces many virions, each capable of infecting nearby cells, leading to spread of the infection.

activated by some extrinsic stimulus, such as another infectious microbe, the cell responds by turning on the transcription of many of its own genes and often by producing cytokines. An unfortunate consequence of this normal response is that the cytokines, and the process of cellular activation itself, may also activate the provirus, leading to production of viral RNAs and then proteins. The virus is now able to form a core structure, which migrates to the cell membrane, acquires a lipid envelope from the host, and is shed as an infectious viral particle, ready to infect another cell. It is possible that the integrated

HIV provirus remains latent within infected cells for months or years, hidden from the patient's immune system (and even from antiviral therapies, discussed later).

Most cases of AIDS are caused by HIV-1. A related virus, HIV-2, causes some cases of the disease.

Pathogenesis of AIDS

HIV establishes a latent infection in cells of the immune system and may be reactivated to produce infectious virus. This viral production leads to

death of infected cells, as well as to death of uninfected lymphocytes, subsequent immune deficiencies, and clinical AIDS (Fig. 12-9). HIV infection is acquired by sexual intercourse, contaminated needles used by intravenous drug users, transplacental transfer, or transfusion of infected blood or blood products. After infection there may be a brief, acute viremia, when the virus is detected in the blood, and the host may respond as in any mild viral infection. The virus infects CD4+ T cells, dendritic cells, and macrophages in the blood, sites of entry through epithelia, and, most of all, lymphoid organs such as lymph nodes. Dendritic cells may capture the virus as it enters through epithelia and transport it to peripheral lymphoid organs, where it infects T cells. The integrated provirus may be activated in infected cells, as described previously, leading to production of viral particles and spread of the infection. During the course of HIV infection, the major source of infectious viral particles is activated CD4+ T cells; dendritic cells and macrophages are reservoirs of infection.

The depletion of CD4+ T cells after HIV infection is due to a cytopathic effect of the virus, resulting from production of viral particles, as well as death of uninfected cells. Active viral gene expression and protein production may interfere with the synthetic machinery of the T cells. Therefore, infected T cells in which the virus is replicating are killed during this process. The loss of T cells during the progression to AIDS is much greater than the numbers of infected cells. The mechanism of this T cell loss remains poorly defined. One possibility is that T cells are chronically activated, perhaps by infections that are common in these patients, and the chronic stimulation culminates in apoptosis, by the pathway called activation-induced cell death.

Other infected cells, such as dendritic cells and macrophages, may also die, resulting in destruction of the architecture of lymphoid organs. Many studies have suggested that immune deficiency results from various functional abnormalities in T lymphocytes and other immune cells, in addition to destruction of these cells. However, the significance of these functional defects has not been established, and loss of T cells remains the most reliable indicator of disease progression.

Clinical Features of HIV Infection and AIDS

The clinical course of HIV infection is characterized by several phases, culminating in immune deficiency (Fig. 12-10). Early after HIV infection, patients may experience a mild acute illness with fever and malaise, correlating with the initial viremia. This illness subsides within a few days, and the disease enters a period of clinical latency. During this latency, there is usually a progressive loss of CD4+ T cells in lymphoid tissues and destruction of the architecture of the lymphoid tissues. Eventually, the blood CD4+ T cell count begins to decline, and when the count falls below 200 per mm^3 (the normal being about 1500 cells per mm^3), patients become susceptible to infections and are said to be suffering from AIDS.

The clinical and pathologic manifestations of full-blown AIDS are primarily the result of increased susceptibility to infections and some cancers, as a consequence of immune deficiency. Patients are often infected by intracellular microbes, such as viruses, Pneumocystis carinii, and atypical mycobacteria, all of which are normally combated by T cell–mediated immunity. Many of these microbes are present in the environment, but they do not infect healthy individuals with intact immune systems. Because these infections are seen in immunodeficient individuals, in whom the microbes have an opportunity to establish infection, these types of infections are said to be "opportunistic." Many of the opportunistic infections are caused by viruses, such as cytomegalovirus. AIDS patients show defective cytolytic T lymphocyte (CTL) responses to viruses, even though HIV does not infect CD8+ T cells. It is believed that the defective CTL responses are because CD4+ helper T cells (the main targets of HIV) are required for full CD8+ CTL responses against many viral antigens (see Chapters 5 and 6). AIDS patients are at increased risk for infections by extracellular bacteria, likely because of impaired helper T cell–dependent antibody responses to bacterial antigens. Patients also become susceptible to cancers that are caused by oncogenic viruses. The two most common types of cancers are B cell lymphomas, caused by the Epstein-Barr virus, and a tumor of small blood vessels that is called Kaposi's sarcoma and is

Figure 12–9   The pathogenesis of disease caused by HIV. The stages of HIV disease correlate with a progressive spread of HIV from the initial site of infection to lymphoid tissues throughout the body. The immune response of the host temporarily controls acute infection but does not prevent establishment of chronic infection of cells in lymphoid tissues. Cytokines produced in response to HIV and other microbes serve to enhance HIV production and progression to AIDS.

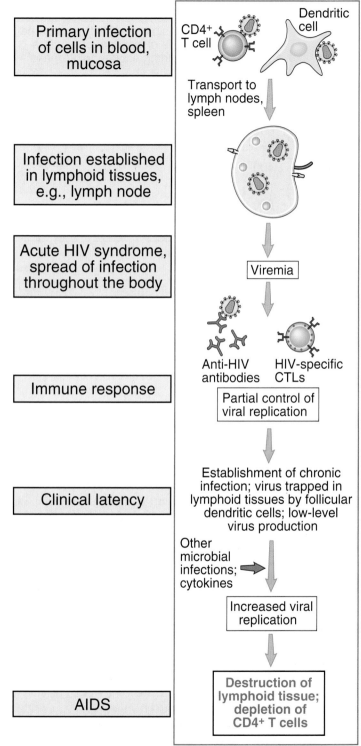

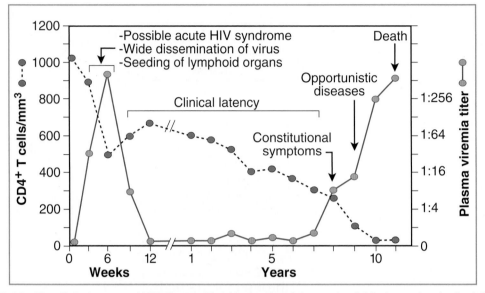

Figure 12–10   The clinical course of HIV disease. Blood-borne virus (plasma viremia) is detected early after infection and may be accompanied by systemic symptoms typical of acute HIV syndrome. The virus spreads to lymphoid organs, but plasma viremia falls to very low levels (only detectable by sensitive reverse transcriptase polymerase chain reaction assays) and stays this way for many years. CD4+ T cell counts steadily decline during this clinical latency period, because of active viral replication and T cell destruction in lymphoid tissues. As the level of CD4+ T cells falls, there is increasing risk of infection and other clinical components of AIDS. (Reproduced with permission from Pantaleo G, C Graziosi, and A Fauci. The immunopathogenesis of human immunodeficiency virus infection. N Engl J Med 328:327-335, 1993.)

caused by a herpesvirus. AIDS patients with advanced disease often suffer from a wasting syndrome with a significant loss of body mass, due to altered metabolism and reduced caloric intake. Some AIDS patients develop dementia, believed to be caused by infection of macrophages (microglia) in the brain.

The immune response to HIV is ineffective in controlling spread of the virus and its pathologic effects. Infected individuals produce antibodies and CTLs against viral antigens, and the responses help to limit the early acute HIV syndrome. But these immune responses usually do not prevent chronic progression of the disease. Antibodies against envelope glycoproteins, such as gp120, may be ineffective because the virus rapidly mutates the region of gp120 that is the target of most antibodies. CTLs are often ineffective in killing infected cells because the virus inhibits the expression of class I MHC molecules by the infected cells. Immune responses to HIV may paradoxically promote spread of the infection. Antibody-coated viral particles may bind to Fc receptors on

macrophages and follicular dendritic cells in lymphoid organs, thus increasing virus entry into these cells and creating additional reservoirs of infection. If CTLs are able to lyse infected cells, this may result in release of viral particles and infection of more cells. And, of course, by infecting and thereby interfering with the function of immune cells, the virus is able to prevent its own eradication.

Therapy and Vaccination Strategies

The current treatment of AIDS is aimed at controlling replication of HIV and the infectious complications of the disease. Cocktails of drugs that block the activity of the viral reverse transcriptase, protease, and integrase enzymes are now being administered early in the course of the infection, with considerable benefit. This treatment, called "highly active antiretroviral therapy (HAART)," is expensive, and its long-term efficacy is not known. The virus is capable of mutations that may render it resistant to these drugs, and the drug treatments do not eradicate reservoirs of latent virus.

The control of HIV worldwide will require the development of effective vaccines. A successful vaccine will likely have to induce an innate immune response, high titers of neutralizing antibodies, a strong T cell response, as well as mucosal immunity. An additional challenge is to be able to protect against all subtypes of HIV. Early efforts focused on gp120 as an immunogen, but these were largely unsuccessful. More recent attempts have involved combinations of DNA immunization and recombinant poxviruses encoding several different HIV proteins. It will take years to judge the effectiveness of new vaccines in clinical trials.

SUMMARY

▶ Immunodeficiency diseases are caused by defects in various components of the immune system and result in increased susceptibility to infections and some cancers. Congenital (primary) immunodeficiency diseases are caused by genetic abnormalities, and acquired (secondary) immunodeficiencies are the result of infections, malnutrition, or treatments for other conditions that adversely affect the cells of the immune system.

▶ Some congenital immunodeficiency diseases are the result of mutations that block the maturation of lymphocytes. Severe combined immunodeficiency (SCID) may be caused by mutations in the cytokine receptor γc chain that reduces the IL-7–driven proliferation of immature lymphocytes, by mutations in enzymes involved in purine metabolism, and by other defects in lymphocyte maturation. Selective B cell maturation defects are seen in X-linked agammaglobulinemia, caused by abnormalities in an enzyme involved in B cell maturation (Btk), and selective T cell maturation defects are seen in the DiGeorge syndrome, in which the thymus does not develop normally.

▶ Some immunodeficiency diseases are caused by defects in lymphocyte activation and functions, despite their normal maturation. The X-linked hyper-IgM syndrome is caused by mutations in CD40 ligand, because of which helper T cell–dependent B cell responses (e.g., Ig heavy chain class switching) and T cell–dependent macrophage activation are defective. The bare lymphocyte syndrome is due to defective expression of class II MHC proteins, resulting in defective maturation and activation of CD4+ T cells.

▶ The acquired immunodeficiency syndrome (AIDS) is caused by the retrovirus human immunodeficiency virus (HIV). HIV infects CD4+ T cells, macrophages, and dendritic cells by using an envelope protein (gp120) to bind to CD4 and chemokine receptors. The viral DNA integrates into the host genome and may be activated to produce infectious virus. Infected cells die during this process of virus replication, and death of cells of the immune system is the principal mechanism by which the virus causes immune deficiency.

▶ The clinical course of HIV infection typically consists of an acute viremia, a period of clinical latency during which there is progressive destruction of CD4+ T cells and dissolution of lymphoid tissues and, ultimately, AIDS, with severe immunodeficiency with opportunistic infections, some cancers, weight loss, and, occasionally, dementia. Treatment of HIV infection is designed to interfere with the life cycle of the virus. Many attempts at vaccine development are ongoing.

⇄ Review Questions

1 What are the most common clinical and pathologic manifestations of immunodeficiency diseases?

2 What are some of the mutations that may block the maturation of T and B lymphocytes?

3 What are some of the mutations that may block the activation or effector functions of CD4+ T cells, and what are the clinical and pathologic consequences of these mutations?

4 How does HIV infect cells and replicate inside infected cells?

5 What are the principal clinical manifestations of HIV infection, and what is the pathogenesis of these manifestations?

Suggested Readings

Chapter 1

Burnet FM. A modification of Jerne's theory of antibody production using the concept of clonal selection. Australian Journal of Science 20:67-69, 1957.

Cyster JG. Chemokines and cell migration in secondary lymphoid organs. Science 286:2098-2102, 1999.

Fu Y-X, and DD Chaplin. Development and maturation of secondary lymphoid tissues. Annual Review of Immunology 17:399-433, 1999.

Jerne NK. The natural-selection theory of antibody formation. Proceedings of the National Academy of Sciences USA 41:849-857, 1955.

Kunkel EJ, and EC Butcher. Chemokines and the tissue-specific migration of lymphocytes. Immunity 16:1-4, 2002.

Chapter 2

Aderem A, and DM Underhill. Mechanisms of phagocytosis in macrophages. Annual Review of Immunology 17:593-623, 1999.

Biron CA, LP Coussens, KB Nguyen, GC Pien, and TP Salazar-Mather. Natural killer cells in antiviral defense: function and regulation by innate cytokines. Annual Review of Immunology 17:189-220, 1999.

Hack CE, LA Aarden, and LG Thijs. Role of cytokines in sepsis. Advances in Immunology 66:101-195, 1997.

Janeway C, and R Medzhitov. Innate immune recognition. Annual Review of Immunology 20:197-216, 2002.

Lieberman N, and O Mandelboim. The role of NK cells in innate immunity. Advances in Experimental Medicine and Biology 479:137-145, 2000.

Takeda K, T Kaisho, and S Akira. Toll-like receptors. Annual Review of Immunology 21:335-376, 2003.

Chapter 3

Guermonprez P, J Valladeau, L Zitvogel, C Théry, and S Amigorena. Antigen presentation and T cell stimulation by dendritic cells. Annual Review of Immunology 20:621-667, 2002.

Klein J, and A Sato. The HLA system. New England Journal of Medicine 343:702-709 and 782-786, 2000.

Kumánovics A, T Takada, and KF Lindahl. Genomic organization of the mammalian MHC. Annual Review of Immunology 21:629-657, 2003.

Rock KL, and AL Goldberg. Degradation of cell proteins and generation of MHC class I–presented peptides. Annual Review of Immunology 17:739-779, 1999.

The MHC Sequencing Consortium. Complete sequence and gene map of a human major histocompatibility complex. Nature 401:921-923, 1999.

Tortorella D, BE Gewurz, MH Furman, DJ Schust, and HL Ploegh. Viral subversion of the immune system. Annual Review of Immunology 18:861-926, 2000.

Chapter 4

Bassing CH, W Swat, and FW Alt. The mechanism and regulation of chromosomal V(D)J recombination. Cell 109(Suppl):S45-S55, 2002.

Bjorkman PJ. MHC restriction in three dimensions: a view of T cell receptor/ligand interactions. Cell 89:167-170, 1997.

Garcia KC, L Teyton, and IA Wilson. Structural basis of T cell recognition. Annual Review of Immunology 17:369-397, 1999.

Muljo SA, and MS Schlissel. Pre-B and pre-T-cell receptors: conservation of strategies in regulating early lymphocyte development. Immunological Review 175:80-93, 2000.

Nemazee D. Receptor selection in B and T lymphocytes. Annual Review of Immunology 18:19-51, 2000.

Niiro H, and EA Clark. Regulation of B-cell fate by antigen-receptor signals. Nature Reviews Immunology 2:945-956, 2002.

Starr TK, SC Jameson, and KA Hogquist. Positive and negative selection of T cells. Annual Review of Immunology 21:139-176, 2003.

Chapter 5

Del Prete G. The concept of type-1 and type-2 helper T cells and their cytokines in humans. International Review of Immunology 16:427-455, 1998.

Germain RN, and I Stefanova. The dynamics of T cell receptor signaling: complex orchestration and the key roles of tempo and cooperation. Annual Review of Immunology 19:467-522, 1999.

Lanzavecchia A, and F Sallusto. Dynamics of T lymphocyte responses: intermediates, effectors, and memory cells. Science 290:92-97, 2000.

Murphy KM, and SL Reiner. The lineage decisions of helper T cells. Nature Reviews Immunology 2:933-944, 2002.

Samelson LE. Signal transduction mediated by the T cell antigen receptor: the role of adapter proteins. Annual Review of Immunology 20:371-394, 2002.

Sharpe AH, and GJ Freeman. The B7-CD28 superfamily. Nature Reviews Immunology 2:116-126, 2002.

Sims TN, and ML Dustin. The immunological synapse: integrins take the stage. Immunological Reviews 186:100-117, 2002.

Chapter 6

Grewal IS, and RA Flavell. CD40 and CD154 in cell-mediated immunity. Annual Review of Immunology 16:111-135, 1998.

Heath WR, and FR Carbone. Cross-presentation in viral immunity and self-tolerance. Nature Reviews Immunology 1:126-134, 2001.

Schaible UE, HL Collins, and SHE Kaufmann. Confrontation between intracellular bacteria and the immune system. Advances in Immunology 71:267-377, 1999.

Von Andrian UH, and CR Mackay. T-cell function and migration. New England Journal of Medicine 343:1020-1034, 2000.

Wong P, and EG Pamer. CD8 T cell responses to infectious pathogens. Annual Review of Immunology 21:29-70, 2003.

Chapter 7

Clark EA, and JA Ledbetter. How B and T cells talk to each other. Nature 367:425-428, 1994.

Fagarasan S, and T Honjo. T-independent immune response: new aspects of B cell biology. Science 290:89-92, 2000.

Fearon DT, and MC Carroll. Regulation of B lymphocyte responses to foreign and self-antigens by the CD19/CD21 complex. Annual Review of Immunology 18:393-422, 2000.

Gold MR, and AL DeFranco. Biochemistry of B lymphocyte activation. Advances in Immunology 55:221-295, 1994.

Honjo T, K Kinoshita, and M Muramatsu. Molecular mechanism of class switch recombination: linkage with somatic hypermutation. Annual Review of Immunology 20:165-196, 2002.

Papavasiliou FN, and DG Schatz. Somatic hypermutation of immunoglobulin genes: merging mechanisms for genetic diversity. Cell 109(Suppl): S35-S44, 2002.

Przylepa J, C Himes, and G Kelsoe. Lymphocyte development and selection in germinal centers. Current Topics in Microbiology and Immunology 229:85-104, 1998.

Chapter 8

Bachmann MF, and RM Zinkernagel. Neutralizing antiviral B cell responses. Annual Review of Immunology 15:235-270, 1997.

Barrington R, M Zhang, M Fischer, and MC Carroll. The role of complement in inflammation and adaptive immunity. Immunological Reviews 180:5-15, 2001.

Corthesy B, and JP Kraehenbuhl. Antibody-mediated protection of mucosal surfaces. Current Topics in Microbiology and Immunology 236:93-111, 1999.

Marshall-Clarke S, D Reen, L Tasker, and J Hassan. Neonatal immunity: how well has it grown up? Immunology Today 21:35-41, 2000.

Ravetch JV, and S Bolland. IgG Fc receptors. Annual Review of Immunology 19:275-290, 2001.

Chapter 9

Anderton SM, and DC Wraith. Selection and fine-tuning of the autoimmune T-cell repertoire. Nature Review Immunology 2:487-498, 2002.

Goodnow CC, JG Cyster, SB Hartley, SE Bell, MP Cooke, JI Healy, S Akkaraju, JC Rathmell, SL Pogue, and KP Shokat. Self-tolerance checkpoints in B lymphocyte development. Advances in Immunology 59:279-368, 1995.

Lenardo M, FK-M Chan, F Hornung, H McFarland, R Siegel, J Wang, and L Zheng. Mature T lymphocyte apoptosis—immune regulation in a dynamic and unpredictable antigenic environment. Annual Review of Immunology 17:221-253, 1999.

Matzinger P. Tolerance, danger, and the extended family. Annual Review of Immunology 12:991-1045, 1994.

Sakaguchi S. Regulatory T cells: key controllers of immunologic self-tolerance. Cell 101:455-458, 2000.

Shevach EM. CD4+ CD25+ suppressor T cells: more questions than answers. Nature Review Immunology 2:389-400, 2002.

Van Parijs L, and AK Abbas. Homeostasis and self-tolerance in the immune system: turning lymphocytes off. Science 280:243-248, 1998.

Von Herrath MG, Harrison LC. Regulatory lymphocytes: Antigen-induced regulatory T cells in autoimmunity. Nature Review Immunology 3:223-232, 2003.

Walker LS, and AK Abbas. The enemy within: keeping self-reactive T cells at bay in the periphery. Nature Review Immunology 2:11-19, 2002.

Chapter 10

Burnet FM. The concept of immunological surveillance. Progress in Experimental Tumor Research 13:1-27, 1970.

Denton MD, CC Magee, and MH Sayegh. Immunosuppressive strategies in transplantation. Lancet 353:1083-1091, 1999.

Gould DS, and H Auchincloss Jr. Direct and indirect recognition: the role of MHC antigens in graft rejection. Immunology Today 20:77-82, 1999.

Pardoll D. Does the immune system see tumors as foreign or self? Annual Review of Immunology 21:807-839, 2003.

Rosenberg SA. A new era for cancer immunotherapy based on the genes that encode tumor antigens. Immunity 10:281-287, 1999.

Salama AD, G Remuzzi, WE Harmon, and MH Sayegh. Challenges to achieving clinical transplantation tolerance. Journal of Clinical Investigation 108:943-948, 2001.

Timmerman JM, and R Levy. Dendritic cell vaccines for cancer immunotherapy. Annual Review of Medicine 50:507-529, 1999.

Van Der Bruggen P, Y Zhang, P Chaux, V Stroobant, C Panichelli, ES Schultz, J Chapiro, BJ Van Den Eynde, F Brasseur, and T Boon. Tumor-specific shared antigenic peptides recognized by human T cells. Immunological Reviews 188:51-64, 2002.

Yee C, and P Greenberg. Modulating T-cell immunity to tumours: new strategies for monitoring T-cell responses. Nature Review Cancer 2:409-419, 2002.

Chapter 11

Costa JJ, PF Weller, and SJ Galli. The cells of the allergic response. Journal of the American Medical Association 278:1815-1822, 1997.

Gould HJ, BJ Sutton, AJ Beavil, RL Beavil, N McCloskey, HA Coker, D Fear, L Smurthwaite. The biology of IgE and the basis of allergic disease. Annual Review of Immunology 21:579-628, 2003.

Kalden JR, FC Breedveld, H Burkhardt, and GR Burmester. Immunological treatment of autoimmune diseases. Advances in Immunology 68:333-418, 1998.

Kay AB. Allergy and allergic diseases. New England Journal of Medicine 30-37, 109-113, 2001.

Kinet J-P. The high affinity IgE receptor: from physiology to pathology. Annual Review of Immunology 17:931-972, 1999.

Kohl J. Anaphylatoxins and infectious and non-infectious inflammatory diseases. Molecular Immunology 38:175-187, 2001.

Metcalfe DD, D Baram, and YA Mekori. Mast cells. Physiologic Reviews 77:1033-1079, 1997.

Naparstek Y, and PH Poltz. The role of autoantibodies in autoimmune diseases. Annual Review of Immunology 11:79-104, 1993.

Ono SJ. Molecular genetics of allergic diseases. Annual Review of Immunology 18:347-366, 2000.

Wardlaw AJ, R Moqbel, and AB Kay. Eosinophils: biology and role in disease. Advances in Immunology 60:151-266, 1995.

Chapter 12

Berger EA, PM Murphy, and JM Farber. Chemokine receptors as HIV-1 coreceptors: roles in viral entry, tropism, and disease. Annual Review of Immunology 17:657-700, 1999.

Blankson JN, D Persaud, and RF Siliciano. The challenge of viral reservoirs in HIV-1 infection. Annual Review of Medicine 53:557-593, 2002.

Buckley RH. Advances in Immunology: Primary immunodeficiency diseases due to defects in lymphocytes. New England Journal of Medicine 343:1313-1324, 2000.

Finzi D, and RF Siliciano. Viral dynamics in HIV-1 infection. Cell 93:665-671, 1998.

Fischer A, and B Malissen. Natural and engineered disorders of lymphocyte development. Science 280:237-243, 1998.

Fisher A, M Cavazzana-Calvo, G DeSaint Basile, JP DeVollartay, JP DiSanto, C Hivroz, F Rieux-Laucant, and F LeDeist. Naturally occurring primary deficiencies of the immune system. Annual Review of Immunology 15:93-124, 1997.

Frankel AD, and JAT Young. HIV-1: fifteen proteins and an RNA. Annual Review of Biochemistry 67:1-25, 1998.

Grossman Z, M Meier-Schellersheim, AE Sousa, RM Victorino, WE Paul. CD4$^+$ T-cell depletion in HIV infection: are we closer to understanding the cause? Nature Medicine 8:319-323, 2002.

Hazenberg MD, D Harmann, H Schuitemaker, and F Miedema. T cell depletion in HIV-1 infection: CD4$^+$ T cells go out of stock. Nature Immunology 1:285-289, 2000.

Ho DD, and Y Huang. The HIV-1 vaccine race. Cell 110:135-138, 2002.

Peterlin BM, Trono D. Hide, shield and strike back: how HIV-infected cells avoid immune eradication. Nature Review Immunology 3:97-107, 2003.

Principal Features of CD Molecules

CD number	Common synonyms	Molecular structure, Family	Main cellular expression	Known or proposed functions
CD1a*	R4	49 kD; class I MHC family; β_2 microglobulin associated	Thymocytes, dendritic cells (including Langerhans cells)	Presentation of nonpeptide (lipid and glycolipid) antigens to some T cells
CD1b	—	45 kD; class I MHC family; β_2 microglobulin associated	Same as CD1a	Same as CD1a
CD1c	—	43 kD; class I MHC family; β_2 microglobulin associated	Thymocytes, dendritic cells (including Langerhans cells), some B cells	Same as CD1a
CD1d	—	43 kD; class I MHC family; β_2 microglobulin associated	Thymocytes, dendritic cells (including Langerhans cells), intestinal epithelial cells	Same as CD1a
CD2	T11; LFA-2; sheep red blood cell receptor	50 kD; Ig superfamily; CD2/CD48/CD58 family	T cells, thymocytes, NK cells	Adhesion molecule (binds CD58); T cell activation; CTL- and NK cell–mediated lysis
CD3γ	T3; Leu-4	25–28 kD; associated with CD3δ and CD3ϵ in TCR complex; Ig superfamily; ITAM in cytoplasmic tail	T cells, thymocytes	Cell surface expression of and signal transduction by the T cell antigen receptor

*The small letters affixed to some CD numbers refer to complex CD molecules that are encoded by multiple genes or that belong to families of structurally related proteins. For instance, CD1a, CD1b, and CD1c are structurally related, but distinct forms of a β_2-microglobulin-associated nonpolymorphic protein.

CD number	Common synonyms	Molecular structure, Family	Main cellular expression	Known or proposed functions
CD3δ	T3; Leu-4	20 kD; associated with CD3δ and CD3ε in TCR complex; Ig superfamily; ITAM in cytoplasmic tail	T cells, thymocytes	Cell surface expression of and signal transduction by the T cell antigen receptor
CD3ε	T3; Leu-4	20 kD; associated with CD3δ and CD3ε in TCR complex; Ig superfamily; ITAM in cytoplasmic tail	T cells, thymocytes	Required for cell surface expression of and signal transduction by the T cell antigen receptor
CD4	T4; Leu-3; L3T4	55 kD; Ig superfamily	Class II MHC–restricted T cells, thymocyte subsets, monocytes, and macrophages	Signaling and adhesion coreceptor in class II MHC–restricted antigen-induced T cell activation (binds to class II MHC molecules); thymocyte development; primary receptor for HIV retroviruses
CD5	T1; Ly-1	67 kD; scavenger receptor family	T cells, thymocytes, B cell subset	Signaling molecule; binds CD72
CD6	T12	100–130 kD; scavenger receptor family	T cells, thymocytes, subset of B cells	Adhesion of developing thymocytes with thymic epithelial cells; role in T cell activation
CD7	—	40 kD	Hematopoietic stem cells, thymocytes, subset of T cells	Signaling
CD8α	T8; Leu-2; Lyt2	34 kD; expressed as homodimer or heterodimer with CD8β; Ig superfamily	Class I MHC–restricted T cells, thymocyte subsets	Signaling and adhesion coreceptor in class I MHC–restricted antigen-induced T cell activation (binds to class I MHC molecules); thymocyte development

CD number	Common synonyms	Molecular structure, Family	Main cellular expression	Known or proposed functions
CD8β	T8; Leu-2; Lyt2	34 kD; expressed as heterodimer with CD8α; Ig superfamily	Same as CD8α	Same as CD8α
CD9	DRAP-27; MRP-1	24 kD; tetraspan (TM4SF) family	Platelets, pre-B and immature B cells, activated and differentiating B cells, activated T cells, eosinophils, basophils, endothelial cells, brain and peripheral nerves, vascular smooth muscle cells, cardiac muscle cells, epithelial cells	Role in platelet activation; cell adhesion and migration
CD10	Common acute lymphoblastic leukemia antigen (CALLA); neutral endopeptidase metalloendo-peptidase; enkephalinase	100 kD	Immature and some mature B cells; lymphoid progenitors, granulocytes	Metalloproteinase
CD11a	LFA-1 α chain; α_L integrin subunit	180 kD; noncovalently linked to CD18 to form LFA-1 integrin	Leukocytes	Cell:cell adhesion; binds to ICAM-1 (CD54), ICAM-2 (CD102), and ICAM-3 (CD50)
CD11b	Mac-1; Mo1; CR3 (iC3b receptor); αM integrin chain	165 kD; noncovalently linked to CD18 to form Mac-1 integrin	Granulocytes, monocytes/ macrophages, NK cells	Phagocytosis of iC3b-coated particles; neutrophil and monocyte adhesion to endothelium (binds CD54) and extracellular matrix proteins
CD11c	p150; CR4 α chain; α_X integrin chain	145 kD; noncovalently linked to CD18 to form p150,95 integrin	Monocytes/ macrophages, granulocytes, NK cells	Similar functions to CD11b; major CD11CD18 integrin on macrophages

CD number	Common synonyms	Molecular structure, Family	Main cellular expression	Known or proposed functions
CDw12[†]	p90–120	90–120 kD	Monocytes, granulocytes, NK cells	Phosphoprotein; no known function
CD13	Aminopeptidase N	150 kD; peptidase M1 family	Monocytes, granulocytes, endothelial cells	Aminopeptidase involved in trimming peptides bound to class II molecules and cleaving MIP-1 chemokine to alter target cell specificity; coronavirus receptor
CD14	Mo2; LPS receptor	53 kD; PI linked	Monocytes, macrophages, granulocytes, soluble form in serum	Binds complex of LPS and LPS-binding protein; required for LPS-induced macrophage activation
CD15	Lewis^x (Le^x)	Trisaccharide (poly-N-acetyllactosamine) present on several membrane glycoproteins and glycolipids	Granulocytes, monocytes	See CD15s
CD15s	Sialyl Lewis X (sLex)	Poly-N-acetyllactosamine; terminal tetrasaccharide on several cell surface glycoproteins	Leukocytes, endothelium	Leukocyte adhesion to endothelial cells; ligand for CD62E, P (selectins)
CD16a	FcγRIIIA	50–70 kD; Ig superfamily	NK cells, macrophages, mast cells	Immune complex–induced cellular activation; antibody-dependent cellular cytotoxicity
CD16b	FcγRIIIB	50 kD; PI linked; Ig superfamily	Neutrophils	Synergy with FcγRII in immune complex–mediated neutrophil activation

[†]Antibodies that have been submitted recently or whose reactivity has not been fully confirmed are said to identify putative CD molecules, indicated with a "w" (for "workshop") designation.

CD number	Common synonyms	Molecular structure, Family	Main cellular expression	Known or proposed functions
CDw17	Lactosylceramide	Lactosyl disaccharide group of the glycosphingolipid lactosylceramide	Monocytes, granulocytes, platelets, subset of B cells	? Phagocytosis of bacteria
CD18	β chain of LFA-1 family; β$_2$ integrin subunit	95 kD; noncovalently linked to CD11a, CD11b, or CD11c to form β$_2$ integrins	Leukocytes	See CD11a, CD11b, CD11c
CD19	B4	95 kD; Ig superfamily	Most B cells	B cell activation; forms a coreceptor complex with CD21 and CD81, which delivers signals that synergize with signals from B cell antigen receptor complex
CD20	B1	35–37 kD; tetraspan (TM4SF) family	Most or all B cells	? Role in B cell activation or regulation; calcium ion channel
CD21	CR2; C3d receptor; B2	145 kD; regulators of complement activation family	Mature B cells, follicular dendritic cells	Receptor for complement fragment C3d; forms a coreceptor complex with CD19 and CD81, which delivers activating signals in B cells; Epstein-Barr virus receptor
CD22	BL-CAM; Lyb8	130–140 kD; ITIM in cytoplasmic tail; Ig superfamily	B cells	Regulation of B cell activation, cross-regulation with CD19
CD23	FcεRIIb; low-affinity IgE receptor	45 kD; C-type lectin	Activated B cells, monocytes, macrophages	Low-affinity Fcε receptor, induced by IL-4; ? regulation of IgE synthesis; ? triggering of monocyte cytokine release

CD number	Common synonyms	Molecular structure, Family	Main cellular expression	Known or proposed functions
CD24	Heat-stable antigen (HSA)	35–45 kD; PI linked	B cells, granulocytes	?
CD25	IL-2 receptor α chain; TAC; p55	55 kD; regulators of complement activation family; noncovalently associates with IL-2Rβ (CD122) and IL-2Rγ (CD132) chains to form high-affinity IL-2 receptor	Activated T and B cells, activated macrophages	Binds IL-2; subunit of IL-2R
CD26	Adenosine deaminase–binding protein; dipeptidyl-peptidase IV	110 kD; type II transmembrane molecule	Activated T and B cells, macrophages, NK cells	Serine peptidase; ? signaling in T cells
CD27	—	Homodimer of 55-kD chains; TNF-R family	Most T cells, medullary thymocytes, memory B cells, NK cells	Binds CD70; mediates costimulatory signals for T and B cell activation; involved in murine T cell development
CD28	Tp44	Homodimer of 44-kD chains; Ig superfamily	T cells (most CD4, some CD8 cells)	T cell receptor for costimulator molecules CD80 (B7-1) and CD86 (B7-2)
CD29	β chain of VLA antigens; β₁ integrin subunit; platelet GPIIa	130 kD; noncovalently linked with CD49a–d chains to form VLA (β₁) integrins	Leukocytes	Leukocyte adhesion to extracellular matrix proteins and endothelium (see CD49)
CD30	Ki-1; Ber-H2 antigen	120 kD; TNF-R family	Activated T and B cells, NK cells, monocytes, Reed-Sternberg cells in Hodgkin's disease	Role in activation-induced cell death of CD8⁺ T cells; binds to CD153 (CD30L) on neutrophils, activated T cells, and macrophages
CD31	PECAM-1	130–140 kD; Ig superfamily	Platelets, monocytes, granulocytes, B cells, endothelial cells	Adhesion molecule involved in the leukocyte diapedesis

CD number	Common synonyms	Molecular structure, Family	Main cellular expression	Known or proposed functions
CD32	FcγRIIA; FcγRIIB; FcγRIIC	40 kD; Ig superfamily; A, B, and C forms; ITIM in cytoplasmic tail of B form, ITAM in cytoplasmic tail of A and C forms	Macrophages, granulocytes, B cells, eosinophils, platelets	Fc receptor for aggregated IgG; binds C-reactive protein; role in phagocytosis, ADCC; acts as inhibitory receptor that terminates activation signals initiated by the B cell antigen receptor
CD33	Sialoadhesin; sialic acid–dependent cytoadhesion molecule	67 kD; Ig superfamily; sialic acid–binding Ig-like lectin family; ITIMs in cytoplasmic tail	Monocytes, myeloid progenitor cells	Binds sialic acid; ? regulation of signaling in myeloid cells
CD34	gp 105–120	116 kD; sialomucin	Precursors of hematopoietic cells, endothelial cells in high endothelial venules	Cell-cell adhesion; binds CD62L (L-selectin)
CD35	CR1; C3b receptor	190–285 kD (four products of polymorphic alleles); regulators of complement activation family	Granulocytes, monocytes, erythrocytes, B cells, follicular dendritic cells	Binds C3b and C4b; promotes phagocytosis of C3b- or C4b-coated particles and immune complexes; regulates complement activation
CD36	Platelet GPIIIb; GPIV	85–90 kD	Platelets, mature monocytes and macrophages, microvascular endothelial cells	Scavenger receptor for oxidized low-density lipoprotein; platelet adhesion; phagocytosis of apoptotic cells
CD37	—	Composed of two or three 40 to 52 kD chains; tetraspan (TM4SF) family	B cells, some T cells and myeloid cells	Forms complexes in membrane with CD53, CD81, CD82, and MHC class II molecules; ? signal transduction

CD number	Common synonyms	Molecular structure, Family	Main cellular expression	Known or proposed functions
CD38	T10	45 kD	Early and activated B cells, plasma cells, activated T cells	Ectoenzyme with NAD glycohydrolase, ADP ribosyl cyclase, and cyclic ADP ribose hydrolase activities
CD39	ENTPD1: ectonucleoside triphosphate diphospho-hydrolase 1	78 kD; ecto-apyrase gene family	Activated B cells, activated NK cells, some T cells, endothelial cells	Ectoenzyme with ADPase and ATPase activities; regulation of platelet aggregation and thrombosis
CD40	—	Homodimer of 44 to 48 kD chains; TNF-R family	B cells, macrophages, dendritic cells, endothelial cells	Binds CD154 (CD40 ligand); role in T cell–dependent B cell, macrophage, dendritic cell, and endothelial cell activation
CD41	Glycoprotein IIb (GPIIb); α_{IIb} integrin chain	Heterodimer of GPIIba (120 kD) and GPIIbb (23 kD); noncovalently linked with GPIIIa (CD61) to form GPIIb/IIIa integrin	Platelets, megakaryocytes	Platelet aggregation and activation; binds fibrinogen, fibronectin (recognizes RGD sequence)
CD42a	Platelet GPIX	22 kD; forms complex with CD42b, c, and d	Platelets, megakaryocytes	Platelet adhesion; binds von Willebrand factor, thrombin
CD42b	Platelet GPIbα	145 kD; disulfide linked with CD42c and forms complex with CD42a and d; mucin	See CD42a	See CD42a
CD42c	Platelet GPIbβ	25 kD; disulfide linked with CD42b and forms complex with CD42a and d	See CD42a	See CD42a
CD42d	Platelet GPV	82 kD; forms complex with CD42a, b, and c	See CD42a	See CD42a

CD number	Common synonyms	Molecular structure, Family	Main cellular expression	Known or proposed functions
CD43	Sialophorin; leukosialin	95–135 kD; sialomucin	Leukocytes (except circulating B cells)	Adhesive and anti-adhesive functions
CD44	Pgp-1; Hermes	80 to >100 kD, highly glycosylated; cartilage link protein family	Leukocytes, erythrocytes	Binds hyaluronan; involved in leukocyte adhesion to endothelial cells and extracellular matrix; leukocyte aggregation
CD45	Leukocyte common antigen (LCA); T200; B220	Multiple isoforms, 180–220 kD (see CD45R); protein tyrosine phosphatase receptor family; fibronectin type III family	Hematopoietic cells	Tyrosine phosphatase; plays critical role in T and B cell antigen receptor–mediated signaling
CD45R	Forms of CD45 with restricted cellular expression	CD45RO: 180 kD CD45RA: 220 kD CD45RB: 190, 205, and 220 kD isoforms	CD45RO: memory T cells, subset of B cells, monocytes, macrophages CD45RA: naive T cells, B cells, monocytes CD45RB: B cells, subset of T cells	See CD45
CD46	Membrane cofactor protein (MCP)	52–58 kD; regulators of complement activation family	Leukocytes, epithelial cells, fibroblasts	Regulation of complement activation
CD47R	Rh-associated protein; integrin-associated protein (IAP); CDw149	45–60 kD; Ig superfamily	Broad	Thrombospondin receptor; adhesion
CD48	BCM1; Blast-1; Hu; Lym3; OX-45	45 kD; PI linked; Ig superfamily; CD2/CD48/CD58 family	Leukocytes	Ligand for CD244; mouse receptor for CD2; ? role in leukocyte adhesion and signaling
CD49a	α_1 integrin subunit	210 kD; noncovalently linked to CD29 to form VLA-1 (β_1 integrin)	Activated T cells, monocytes	Leukocyte adhesion to extracellular matrix; binds collagens, laminin

CD number	Common synonyms	Molecular structure, Family	Main cellular expression	Known or proposed functions
CD49b	α_2 integrin subunit; platelet GPIa	170 kD; noncovalently linked to CD29 to form VLA-2 (β_1 integrin)	Platelets, activated T cells, monocytes, some B cells	Leukocyte adhesion to extracellular matrix; binds collagen, laminin
CD49c	α_3 integrin subunit	Dimer of 130 and 25 kD chains; noncovalently linked to CD29 to form VLA-3 (β_1 integrin)	T cells, some B cells, monocytes	Leukocyte adhesion to extracellular matrix; binds fibronectin, collagens, laminin
CD49d	α_4 integrin subunit	150 kD; noncovalently linked to CD29 to form VLA-4 ($\alpha_4\beta_1$) integrin or to β_7 to form $\alpha_7\beta_7$ integrin	T cells, monocytes, B cells	Leukocyte adhesion to endothelium and extracellular matrix; binds to VCAM-1 and MAdCAM-1; binds fibronectin and collagens
CD49e	α_5 integrin subunit	Heterodimer of 135 and 25 kD chains; noncovalently linked to CD29 to form VLA-5 (β_1 integrin)	T cells, few B cells and monocytes	Adhesion to extracellular matrix; binds fibronectin
CD49f	α_6 integrin subunit	Heterodimer of 125 and 25 kD chains; noncovalently linked to CD29 to form VLA-6 (β_1 integrin)	Platelets, megakaryocytes, activated T cells, monocytes	Adhesion to extracellular matrix; binds fibronectin
CD50	ICAM-3	110–140 kD; Ig superfamily	Leukocytes, some endothelium	Adhesion; binds CD11aCD18
CD51	α_V integrin subunit; vitronectin receptor α chain	Heterodimer of 125 and 24 kD chains; noncovalently associates with CD61 to form vitronectin receptor integrin	Platelets, megakaryocytes	Adhesion: receptor for vitronectin, fibrinogen, von Willebrand factor (binds RGD sequence)
CD52	—	25–29 kD	Thymocytes, lymphocytes, monocytes, macrophages, male genital tract epithelial cells	Function unknown; anti-CD52 antibodies used to treat lymphoid malignant tumors
CD53	OX44	32–42 kD; tetraspan (TM4SF) family	Hematopoietic cells	? Signaling

CD number	Common synonyms	Molecular structure, Family	Main cellular expression	Known or proposed functions
CD54	ICAM-1	75–114 kD; Ig superfamily	Endothelial cells, T cells, B cells, monocytes, endothelial cells (cytokine inducible)	Cell-cell adhesion; ligand for CD11aCD18 (LFA-1) and CD11bCD18 (Mac-1); receptor for rhinovirus
CD55	Decay-accelerating factor (DAF)	55–70 kD; PI linked; regulators of complement activation family	Broad	Regulation of complement activation; binds C3b, C4b
CD56	Leu-19; NKH1	175–220 kD; isoform of neural cell adhesion molecule (N-CAM); Ig superfamily	NK cells, subset of T and B cells, brain	Homotypic adhesion
CD57	HNK-1; Leu-7	Carbohydrate epitope on many cell surface glycoproteins and glycolipids	NK cells, subset of T cells, monocytes	? Adhesion
CD58	Lymphocyte function–associated antigen-3 (LFA-3)	40–70 kD; PI linked or integral membrane protein; CD2/CD48/CD58 family	Broad	Leukocyte adhesion; T cell costimulation; binds CD2
CD59	Membrane inhibitor of reactive lysis (MIRL)	18–20 kD; PI linked; Ly-6 superfamily	Broad	Binds C9; inhibits formation of complement membrane attack complex
CDw60	GD3	120 kD; 9-O-acetylated disialosyl group predominantly found on ganglioside D3	Subset of T cells, platelets, thymic epithelium, activated keratinocytes	Unknown
CD61	β_3 integrin subunit; vitronectin receptor β chain; GPIIIa component of GPIIb/GPIIIa integrin	110 kD; noncovalently linked to CD51 to form vitronectin receptor (integrin); noncovalently linked to CD41 to form GPIIb/GPIIIa (integrin)	Platelets, megakaryocytes, endothelial cells, leukocytes	See CD51, CD41
CD62E	E-selectin; ELAM-1	115 kD; selectin family	Endothelial cells	Leukocyte-endothelial adhesion

CD number	Common synonyms	Molecular structure, Family	Main cellular expression	Known or proposed functions
CD62L	L-selectin; LAM-1; MEL-14	74–95 kD; selectin family	B cells, T cells, monocytes, granulocytes, some NK cells	Leukocyte-endothelial adhesion; homing of naive T cells to peripheral lymph nodes
CD62P	P-selectin; gmp 140; PADGEM	120 kD; selectin family	Platelets, endothelial cells; (present in granules, translocated to cell surface upon activation)	Leukocyte adhesion to endothelium, platelets; binds CD162 (PSGL-1)
CD63	Granulophysin; lysosome-associated membrane protein 3 (LAMP-3)	40–60 kD; tetraspan (TM4SF) family	Activated platelets, endothelial cells, neutrophils, monocytes, macrophages	Unknown
CD64	FcγRI	75 kD; Ig superfamily; noncovalently associated with the common FcRγ chain	Monocytes, macrophages, activated neutrophils	High-affinity Fcγ receptor; role in phagocytosis, ADCC, macrophage activation
CD65	Ceramide-dodecasac-charide; VIM-2	Carbohydrate epitope on ceramide glycolipid	Granulocytes	Unknown
CD66a	NCA-160 biliary glycoprotein (BGP)	140–180 kD; Ig superfamily; carcinoembryonic antigen (CEA) family	Granulocytes, epithelial cells	Unknown; receptor for *Neisseria gonorrhoeae* and *Neisseria meningitidis*
CD66b	CD67; CGM6; NCA-95	95–100 kD; Ig superfamily; carcinoembryonic antigen (CEA) family	Granulocytes	? Role in cell-cell adhesion; ? role in signaling
CD66c	NCA	90 kD; Ig superfamily; carcinoembryonic antigen (CEA) family	Granulocytes, epithelial cells	? Role in cell-cell adhesion; ? regulates integrin activity
CD66d	CGM1	35 kD; Ig superfamily; carcinoembryonic antigen (CEA) family	Granulocytes	? Role in cell-cell adhesion; ? regulates integrin activity

CD number	Common synonyms	Molecular structure, Family	Main cellular expression	Known or proposed functions
CD66e	Carcinoembryonic antigen (CEA)	180–220 kD; Ig superfamily; carcinoembryonic antigen (CEA) family	Colonic and other epithelial cells	? Adhesion; clinical marker of carcinoma burden
CD66f	Pregnancy-specific glycoprotein (PSG)	54–72 kD; Ig superfamily; carcinoembryonic antigen (CEA) family	Placental syncytiotrophoblasts, fetal liver	Unknown
CD68	Macrosialin	110 kD; mucin; lysosome-associated membrane protein (LAMP) family; scavenger receptor family	Monocytes, macrophages, dendritic cells, granulocytes, activated T cells, subset of B cells, intracellular protein, weak surface expression	Unknown
CD69	Activation inducer molecule (AIM)	Homodimer of 28 to 32 kD chains; C-type lectin	Activated leukocytes including T cells, B cells, NK cells, neutrophils, basophils, eosinophils, platelets, Langerhans cells	Signaling in different cell types
CD70	Ki-24	75–170 kD; TNF family	Activated T and B cells, macrophages	Binds CD27; provides costimulatory signals for T and B cell activation
CD71	T9; transferrin receptor	Homodimer of 95-kD chains	Activated T and B cells, macrophages, proliferating cells	Receptor for transferrin; role in iron metabolism, cell growth
CD72	Lyb-2 (mouse)	Homodimer of 39 to 43 kD chains; C-type lectin	B cells	Ligand for CD5; ? role in T cell–B cell interactions
CD73	Ecto-5'-nucleotidase	69–70 kD; PI linked	Subsets of T and B cells, germinal center follicular dendritic cells	Ecto-5'-nucleotidase; signaling in T cells
CD74	Class II MHC invariant (γ) chain; I_i	33–35 and 41 kD isoforms	B cells, monocytes, macrophage, other class II MHC–expressing cells	Associates with and directs intracellular sorting of newly synthesized class II MHC molecules

CD number	Common synonyms	Molecular structure, Family	Main cellular expression	Known or proposed functions
CD75	Lactosamines	Carbohydrate epitope		Unknown
CD75s	—	Carbohydrate epitope; sialoglycan	Mature B cells, subset of T cells	Cell adhesion; binds CD22
CD77	Pk blood group antigen; Burkitt's lymphoma antigen (BLA); ceramide trihexoside (CTH); globotri-aosylceramide (Gb3)	Carbohydrate epitope	Germinal center B cells	Unknown; ? induces apoptosis
CD79a	Igα, MB1	32–33 kD; forms dimer with CD79b; Ig superfamily; ITAM in cytoplasmic tail	Mature B cells	Required for cell surface expression of and signal transduction by the B cell antigen receptor complex
CD79b	Igβ, B29	37–39 kD; forms dimer with CD79a; Ig superfamily; ITAM in cytoplasmic tail	Mature B cells	Required for cell surface expression of and signal transduction by the B cell antigen receptor complex
CD80	B7-1; BB1	60 kD; Ig superfamily	Dendritic cells, activated B cells and macrophages	Costimulator for T lymphocyte activation; ligand for CD28 and CD152 (CTLA-4)
CD81	Target for antiproliferative antigen-1 (TAPA-1)	26 kD; tetraspan (TM4SF) family	Hematopoietic cells, endothelium, epithelial cells	B cell activation; forms a coreceptor complex with CD19 and CD21, which delivers signals that synergize with signals from B cell antigen receptor complex
CD82	4F9; C33; IA4; KAI1; R2	45–90 kD; tetraspan (TM4SF) family	Broad	? Signal transduction

CD number	Common synonyms	Molecular structure, Family	Main cellular expression	Known or proposed functions
CD83	HB15	43 kD; Ig superfamily	Dendritic cells, Langerhans cells, germinal center B cells	Unknown
CD84	—	68–80 kD; Ig superfamily; CD2/CD48/CD58 family	Monocytes, macrophages, subset of T cells, mature B cells, platelets	Unknown
CD85	Ig-like transcript (ILT)/leukocyte Ig-like receptor (LIR)	110 kD; Ig superfamily; killer cell Ig-like receptors (KIR)	NK cells, B cells, plasma cells; monocytes, T cell subset	NK cell inhibitory receptor
CD86	B7-2	80 kD; Ig superfamily	B cells, monocytes, dendritic cells; some T cells	Costimulator for T lymphocyte activation; ligand for CD28 and CD152 (CTLA-4)
CD87	Urokinase plasminogen activator receptor (uPAR)	35–59 kD; PI linked	T cells, NK cells, monocytes, neutrophils, endothelial cells	Receptor for urokinase plasminogen activator; role in inflammatory cell adhesion and migration
CD88	C5a receptor	43 kD; G protein–coupled, 7-membrane–spanning receptor family	Granulocytes, dendritic cells, mast cells	Receptor for C5a complement fragment; role in complement-induced inflammation
CD89	Fcα receptor (FcαR)	45–100 kD; Ig superfamily; noncovalently associated with the common FcR γ chain	Granulocytes, monocytes, macrophages, T cells, NK cells	Binds IgA; mediates IgA-dependent cellular cytotoxicity
CD90	Thy-1	25–35 kD; PI linked; Ig superfamily	Thymocytes, peripheral T cells (mice), neurons (all species)	Marker for T cells; ? role in T cell activation

CD number	Common synonyms	Molecular structure, Family	Main cellular expression	Known or proposed functions
CD91	α2-macroglobulin receptor; low-density lipoprotein receptor–related protein (LRP)	600 kD; LDL receptor family	Macrophages and monocytes	Binds low-density lipoproteins
CD92	CTL1	70 kD	Monocytes, granulocytes, endothelium	Unknown
CDw93	—	110 kD; sialoglycoprotein	Neutrophils, monocytes, endothelial cells	Unknown
CD94	Kp43; KIR	30 kD; C-type lectin; on NK cells, covalently assembles with other C-type lectin molecules (NKG2)	NK cells; subset of CD8+ T cells	CD94/NKG2 complex functions as an NK cell killer inhibitory receptor; binds HLA-E class I MHC molecules
CD95	Fas antigen, APO-1	Homotrimer of 45 kD chains; TNF receptor family	Multiple cell types	Binds Fas ligand; mediates signals leading to activation-induced cell death
CD96	T cell activation increased late expression (TACTILE)	160, 180, 240 kD forms; Ig superfamily; mucin	T cells	Unknown
CD97	BL-KDD/F12	74, 80, 89 kD forms; G protein–coupled receptor family	Broad	Unknown
CD98	4F2; FRP-1	Heterodimer of 40 and 80-kD subunits	Broad	? Amino acid transporter
CD99	E2; MIC2	32 kD	Broad	Unknown
CD100	SEMA4D	120 kD; Ig superfamily; semaphorin	Hematopoietic cells	? Signaling
CD101	P126; V7	Homodimer of 120 kD chains; Ig superfamily	Granulocytes, monocytes, dendritic cells, activated T cells	? Inhibitory signaling in T cells

CD number	Common synonyms	Molecular structure, Family	Main cellular expression	Known or proposed functions
CD102	ICAM-2	55–65 kD; Ig superfamily	Endothelial cells, monocytes, some lymphocytes	Ligand for CD11aCD18 (LFA-1); cell-cell adhesion
CD103	HML-1; α_E integrin subunit	Dimer of 150 and 25 kD subunits; noncovalently linked to β_7 integrin subunit to form $\alpha_E\beta_7$ integrin	Intraepithelial lymphocytes, other cell types	Role in T cell homing to mucosa; binds E-cadherin
CD104	β_4 integrin subunit	205–220 kD; noncovalently linked to CD49f (α_6) integrin subunit to form $\alpha_6\beta_4$ integrin	Thymocytes, epithelial cells	Adhesion; binds laminin
CD105	Endoglin	Homodimer of 90-kD subunits	Endothelial cells, activated macrophages	Binds TGF-β; modulates cellular responses to TGF-β
CD106	Vascular cell adhesion molecule-1 (VCAM-1); INCAM-110	100–110 kD; Ig superfamily	Endothelial cells, macrophages, follicular dendritic cells, marrow stromal cells	Adhesion; receptor for CD49dCD29 (VLA-4) integrin; role in lymphocyte trafficking, activation; role in hematopoiesis
CD107a	Lysosome-associated membrane-protein 1 (LAMP-1)	110–120 kD	Activated platelets, activated T cells, activated endothelium, activated neutrophils	Lysosomal protein translocated to cell surface after activation; ? adhesion
CD107b	Lysosome-associated membrane protein 2 (LAMP-2)	120 kD	Activated platelets, activated T cells, activated endothelium, activated neutrophils	Lysosomal protein translocated to cell surface after activation; ? adhesion
CD108	John-Milton-Hagen (JMH) human blood group antigen	76 kD; PI linked	Erythrocytes, lymphocytes	Unknown
CD109	8A3; E123	170 kD; PI linked	Endothelial cells, activated platelets, activated T lymphocytes	Unknown

CD number	Common synonyms	Molecular structure, Family	Main cellular expression	Known or proposed functions
CD110	MPL; TPO-R; C-MPL	85–92 kD; hematopoietin receptor family	Hematopoietic cells	Thrombopoietin receptor; megakaryocyte differentiation
CD111	PVRL1; PRR1; HevC; nectin-I	75 kD; Ig superfamily; poliovirus receptor family	Hematopoietic cells; epithelial cells; neurons	Adhesion molecule; herpesvirus receptor
CD112	PVR2; HveB; nectin-2	64–72 kD; Ig superfamily; poliovirus receptor family	Hematopoietic cells	Adhesion; herpesvirus receptor
CD114	Granulocyte colony-stimulating factor (G-CSF) receptor	150 kD; Ig superfamily; type I cytokine receptor family	Granulocytes, monocytes, platelets, endothelial cells, hematopoietic cells	Binds and mediates biologic effects of G-CSF
CD115	Macrophage colony-stimulating factor receptor (M-CSFR); CSF-1R	150 kD; Ig superfamily; tyrosine kinase receptor family	Monocytes, macrophages, hematopoietic cells	Binds and mediates biologic effects of M-CSF
CD116	Granulocyte-monocyte colony-stimulating factor receptor (GM-CSFR) α chain	80 kD; interacts with the common β subunit (CDw131) of the GM-CSF, IL-3, and IL-5 receptors; type I cytokine receptor family	Myeloid cells and their hematopoietic precursors	Binds and mediates biologic effects of GM-CSF
CD117	c-Kit, stem cell factor receptor	145 kD; Ig superfamily; tyrosine kinase receptor family	Hematopoietic stem and progenitor cells, tissue mast cells	Binds and mediates biologic effects of c-Kit ligand (stem cell factor)
CD118	Interferon (IFN)-α, β receptor	Type II cytokine receptor family	Broad	Binds and mediates biologic effects of IFN-α/β
CD119	Interferon (IFN)-γ receptor	90–100 kD; type II cytokine receptor family	Macrophages, monocytes, dendritic cells, B cells, T cells, endothelium, epithelial cells	Binds and mediates biologic effects of IFN-γ

CD number	Common synonyms	Molecular structure, Family	Main cellular expression	Known or proposed functions
CD120a	55 kD tumor necrosis factor (TNF) receptor; TNF-RI	Homotrimer of 55 kD chains; TNF-R family	Broad	Binds and mediates most biologic effects of TNF-α and TNF-β
CD120b	75 kD tumor necrosis factor (TNF) receptor; TNF-RII	Homotrimer of 75 kD chains; TNF-R family	Broad	Binds and mediates some biologic effects of TNF-α and TNF-β
CD121a	Type 1 IL-1 receptor	80 kD; Ig superfamily	Broad	Binds and mediates biologic effects of IL-1α and IL-1β
CD121b	Type 2 IL-1 receptor	60–70 kD; Ig superfamily	B cells	Decoy receptor that binds IL-1α and IL-1β but does not mediate biologic effects
CD122	IL-2 receptor β chain	70–75 kD; type I cytokine receptor family; associates with CD25 and CD132 to form high-affinity IL-2R	T cells, B cells, NK cells, monocytes, macrophages	Signaling and binding component of IL-2 and IL-15 receptors; critical for mediating biologic effects of IL-2 and IL-15 on T cells and NK cells
CD123	IL-3 receptor α chain	70 kD; type I cytokine receptor family; associates with the common CD131 signaling chain	Monocytes, macrophages, megakaryocytes, bone hematopoietic precursor cells	Binds IL-3 and in association with CD131, mediates biologic effects of IL-3
CDw124	IL-4 receptor α chain	140 kD; type I cytokine receptor family; associates with CD132 to form functional IL-4 receptor	B cells, T cell, endothelium, hematopoietic precursor cells	Cytokine binding subunit of IL-4 receptor; also subunit of IL-13 receptor
CD125	IL-5 receptor α chain	60 kD; type I cytokine receptor family; associates with CDw131 to form functional IL-5 receptor	Eosinophils, activated B cells, basophils	Binds IL-5 and in association with CDw131 mediates biologic effects of IL-5

CD number	Common synonyms	Molecular structure, Family	Main cellular expression	Known or proposed functions
CD126	IL-6 receptor α chain	80 kD; type I cytokine receptor family; Ig superfamily; associates with CDw130 to form functional IL-6 receptor	Activated B cells, plasma cells, other leukocytes	Binds IL-6 and in association with CDw130 mediates biologic effects of IL-6
CD127	IL-7 receptor α chain	65–70/90 kD; type I cytokine receptor family; associates with CD132 to form functional IL-7 receptor	Lymphocyte precursors in bone marrow, T cells	Binds IL-7 and in association with CD132 mediates biologic effects of IL-7
CDw128a	CXCR1; IL-8 receptor α	58–67; G protein–coupled, 7-membrane–spanning receptor family	Neutrophils, basophils, mast cells, T cell subsets	Binds and mediates biologic effects of IL-8
CDw128b	CXCR2; IL-8 receptor β	G protein–coupled, 7-membrane–spanning receptor family	Neutrophils, mast cells	Binds and mediates biologic effects of IL-8
CD129	Unassigned			
CD130	IL-6 receptor β chain (IL-6Rβ); IL-11 receptor β chain (IL-11Rβ); oncostatin M receptor β chain (OSMRβ); leukemia inhibitory factor receptor β (LIFRβ); gp 130	130–140 kD; Ig superfamily; type I cytokine receptor family; associates with ligand binding chains of IL-6 (CD126), IL-11, oncostatin M, and leukemia inhibitory factor receptors	Broad	Signaling functions of receptors for IL-6, IL-11, oncostatin M, and LIF
CD131	Common β subunit of IL-3 receptor (IL-3R), IL-5 receptor (IL-5R), and granulocyte-monocyte colony-stimulating factor receptor (GM-CSFR)	120–140 kD; Ig superfamily; type I cytokine receptor family; associates with α chains of IL-3R (CD123), IL-5R (CD125), and GM-CSFR (CD116)	Myeloid cells and their progenitors, early B cells	Signaling functions of receptors for IL-3, IL-5, and GM-CSF

CD number	Common synonyms	Molecular structure, Family	Main cellular expression	Known or proposed functions
CD132	Common γ chain (γc) of IL-2 receptor (IL-2R), IL-4 receptor (IL-4R), IL-7 receptor (IL-7R), IL-9 receptor (IL-9R), and interleukin-15 receptor (IL-15R)	65 kD; Ig superfamily; type I cytokine receptor family; associates with other chains of IL-2R (CD25, CD122), IL-4R (CD124), IL-7R (CD127), IL-9R, and IL-15R (IL-15Rα, CD122)	T cells, B cells, NK cells, monocytes, macrophages, neutrophils	Some of the signaling functions of receptors for IL-2, IL-4, IL-7, IL-9, and IL-15
CD133	PROML1; AC133; hematopoietic stem cell antigen	120 kD; pentaspan transmembrane glycoprotein family	Various stem cells	Unknown
CD134	OX40	50 kD; TNF receptor family	Activated T cells	Costimulatory signaling in T cells; binds OX40 ligand
CD135	FMS-like tyrosine kinase 3 (Flt-3); Flk-2; STK-1	130 kD; tyrosine kinase receptor family	Myeloid and B cell progenitor cells	Growth factor receptor involved in hematopoiesis; binds Flt-3
CDw136	Macrophage-stimulating protein receptor (MSP receptor); Ron	Heterodimer of 150-kD and 40-kD chains; tyrosine kinase receptor family	Epithelial cells from various tissues	Role in cell migration and growth; binds incompletely characterized growth factors—macrophage stimulating protein (MSP) and hepatocyte growth factor-like (HGFL)
CDw137	4-1BB, induced by lymphocyte activation (ILA)	85 kD; TNF-receptor family	T lymphocytes, B lymphocytes, monocytes, epithelial cells	Costimulation of T cells; binds an incompletely characterized ligand on B cells and macrophages
CD138	Syndecan-1	Heparan sulfate proteoglycan	Antibody-secreting B cells	Unknown

CD number	Common synonyms	Molecular structure, Family	Main cellular expression	Known or proposed functions
CD139		209, 228 kD	B lymphocytes, monocytes, granulocytes	Unknown
CD140a	Platelet-derived growth factor receptor α (PDGFR α)	180 kD; tyrosine kinase receptor family; associates with β chain of PDGFR	Broad	In association with CD140b, binds and mediates biologic effects of PDGF
CD140b	Platelet-derived growth factor receptor β (PDGFR β)	180 kD; tyrosine kinase receptor family; associates with α chain of PDGFR	Broad	In association with CD140a, binds and mediates biologic effects of PDGF
CD141	Fetomodulin; thrombomodulin (TM)	75 kD, 105 kD; C-type lectin	Endothelium	Regulation of coagulation
CD142	Coagulation factor III; thromboplastin; tissue factor (TF)	Coagulation factor III; thromboplastin; tissue factor (TF)	Epithelial cells and stromal cells in various tissues, activated endothelial cells	Binds factor VIIa to form an enzyme that initiates the blood clotting cascade; regulates factor VIIa serine protease activity
CD143	Angiotensin-converting enzyme (ACE)	170–180 kD	Endothelial cells, epithelial cells, neurons, activated macrophages, some T cells	Peptidyl-dipeptide hydrolase involved in metabolism of vasoactive peptides angiotensin II and bradykinin
CD144	Cadherin-5; VE-cadherin	139, 135 kD; cadherin family	Endothelial cells	Organizes adherent junction in endothelial cells, which control cell-cell adhesion, permeability, and migration
CD146	A32; MCAM, MUC18, Mel-CAM, S-endo	118, 139 kD; Ig superfamily	Endothelium, smooth muscle, subpopulation of activated T cells	? Cell junction adhesion molecule
CD147	5A11; basigin; CE9; HT7; M6; neurothelin; OX-47	55–65 kD; Ig superfamily	Leukocytes, red blood cells, platelets, endothelial cells	? Adhesion

CD number	Common synonyms	Molecular structure, Family	Main cellular expression	Known or proposed functions
CD148	HPTP-η	240–260 kD; protein tyrosine phosphatase	Granulocytes, monocytes, T cells, dendritic cells, platelets, fibroblasts, nerve cells	Unknown
CD150	Signaling lymphocyte activation molecule (SLAM); IPO-3	75–95 kD; Ig superfamily	Thymocytes, activated lymphocytes, dendritic cells, endothelial cells	Regulation of B cell–T cell interactions and proliferative signals in B lymphocytes; binds itself as a self ligand
CD151	PETA-3; SFA-1	32 kD; tetraspan (TM4SF) family	Platelets, megakaryocytes, hematopoietic cells, epithelial cells, endothelium	? Adhesion, platelet aggregation
CD152	Cytotoxic T lymphocyte–associated protein-4 (CTLA-4)	33, 50 kD; Ig superfamily	Activated T lymphocytes	Inhibitory signaling in T cells; binds CD80 (B7-1) and CD86 (B7-2) on antigen-presenting cells
CD153	CD30 ligand (CD30L)	40 kD; TNF family	Activated T cells, resting B cells, granulocytes, thymocytes	Role in activation-induced cell death of CD8+ T cells; binds to CD30
CD154	CD40 ligand (CD40L); T-BAM; TNF-related activation protein (TRAP); gp39	Homotrimer of 32 to 39 kD chains; TNF receptor family	Activated CD4+ T cells	Activates B cells, macrophages, and endothelial cells; ligand for CD40
CD155	Poliovirus receptor	80–90 kD; Ig superfamily	Broad	Unknown function; used by poliovirus to infect cells
CD156a	ADAM8; MS2	69 kD; metalloprotease family; disintegrin family	Neutrophils, monocytes	? Role in leukocyte extravasation
CD156b	ADAM17: tumor necrosis factor α converting enzyme (TACE)	100–120 kD; disintegrin and metalloprotease families	Broad	Proteolysis and release of active forms of TNF and TGFα

CD number	Common synonyms	Molecular structure, Family	Main cellular expression	Known or proposed functions
CD157	BP-3/IF-7; BST-1; Mo5	42–45, 50 kD; PI linked	Granulocytes, monocytes, B and T cell progenitors, bone marrow stromal cells	ADP ribosyl cyclase and cyclic ADP ribose hydrolase activities; ? role in lymphocyte development
CD158	Killer cell Ig-like receptors (KIR); KIR2D, KIR3D	50, 58, 70 kD; Ig superfamily; killer cell Ig-like receptors (KIR); ITIMs or ITAMs in cytoplasmic tail	NK cells, some T cells	Inhibition or activation of NK cells upon binding class I MHC molecules
CD159A	NKG2A; NKG2B; KLRC1: killer cell lectin-like receptor subfamily C	C-type lectin; ITIMs in cytosplasmic tails of NKG2A; NKG2B	NK cells	Inhibition or activation of NK cells
CD160	BY55	Homodimer of 80 kD chains; Ig superfamily; glycosylphosphatidyl-inositol-linked	NK cells, some T cells	Binds to class I or class I–like MHC molecules
CD161	NKR-P1A; KLRB1	Homodimer of 40 kD chains; C-type lectin	NK cells, subset of T cells	Role in NK cell activation
CD162	PSGL-1	Homodimer of 120 kD chains; sialomucin	T cells, monocytes, granulocytes, some B cells	Ligand for selectins (CD62E, CD62P, CD62L); adhesion of leukocytes to endothelium
CD163	GHI/61; M130	130 kD; scavenger receptor cysteine-rich family	Monocytes, macrophages	Unknown
CD164	MUC-24; multiglycosylated core protein 24 (MGC-24v)	80–90 kD; sialomucin	Hematopoietic progenitor cells	? Adhesion of hematopoietic cells to bone marrow stroma
CD165	AD2; gp37	37, 42 kD	Mature lymphocytes, thymocytes, thymic epithelial cells, monocytes, platelets, CNS neurons	? Adhesion between thymocytes and thymic epithelial cells

CD number	Common synonyms	Molecular structure, Family	Main cellular expression	Known or proposed functions
CD166	BEN; DM-GRASP; KG-CAM; SC-1; activated leukocyte cell adhesion molecule (ALCAM)	100–105 kD; Ig superfamily	Activated T cells, activated monocytes, epithelium, neurons, fibroblasts	Binds CD6; unknown function
CD167a	DDR1; trkE; cak; eddr1	62 kD; tyrosine kinase receptor family	Normal and transformed epithelial cells	Binds collagen
CD168	HMMR; IHABP; RHAMM	88, 84, 80 kD	Thymocytes, hematopoietic progenitors, malignant B cells, monocytes	Binds hyaluronan; stimulates cellular motility
CD169	Sialoadhesin; siglec-1	180 kD; Ig superfamily; sialic acid–binding Ig-like lectin (siglec) family	Macrophages	Binds sialylated ligands; cell-cell and cell-matrix adhesion
CD170	Siglec-5; OBBP2, CD33L2	70 kD homodimer; Ig superfamily; sialic acid binding–Ig-like lectin (siglec) family	Neutrophils, monocytes, macrophages	Binds sialylated ligands; cell-cell and cell-matrix adhesion
CD171	L1; L1CAM; N-CAM L1	140–220 kD depending on cell type; Ig superfamily	Neurons, Schwann cells, epithelial cells, CD4+ T cells, myelomonocytic cells	Cell adhesion molecule required for normal neurohistogenesis
CD172a	SIRP, MYD-1, SHPS1, SHPS-1, protein tyrosine phosphatase, nonreceptor type substrate 1	Ig superfamily, signal-regulatory-protein (SIRP) family; ITIM in cytoplasmic tail	Neutrophils, monocytes	Inhibitory receptor
CD173	Blood group H type 2	Carbohydrate epitope	Broad	Blood group antigen
CD174	Lewis y	Carbohydrate epitope	Broad	Blood group antigen
CD175	Tn	Carbohydrate epitope	Broad	Blood group antigen
CD175s	Sialyl-Tn	Carbohydrate epitope	Broad	Blood group antigen

CD number	Common synonyms	Molecular structure, Family	Main cellular expression	Known or proposed functions
CD176	TF	Carbohydrate epitope	Broad	Blood group antigen
CD177	NB1; HNA-2a	64–68 kD	Neutrophils	Unknown
CD178	FasL; CD95L; APO-1; TNFSF6; APT1LG1;	40 kD; forms homotrimers; TNF family	Activated T cells, NK cells, tumor cells, retinal cells, endothelial cells; broadly inducible	Binds CD95 (Fas); induces apoptosis via Fas pathway
CD179a	VpreB; VPREB1; IGVPB; IgΙ	16–18 kD; Ig superfamily	Pro-B and early pre-B cells	Associates noncovalently with CD179b to form surrogate light chain component of pre-B cell receptor required for B cell development
CD179b	IGLL1; lambda5; Igomega; IGVPB; 14.1 chain	22 kD; Ig superfamily	Pro-B and early pre-B cells	Associates noncovalently with CD179a to form surrogate light chain component of pre-B-cell receptor required for B cell development
CD180	LY64; RP105	95–105 kD; Toll-like receptor (TLR) family	B cells, monocytes, dendritic cells	Associates with MD-1 to form RP105/MD-1 complex, which works with TLR-4 in LPS-induced signaling
CD183	CXCR3; GPR9; CKR-L2; IP10-R; Mig-R	40 kD; CXCR chemokine receptor family	T cells, subsets of B cells and NK cells	Cell surface receptor for chemokines, including IP10, Mig, and I-TAC
CD184	CXCR4; fusin; LESTR; NPY3R; HM89; FB22	40 kD; CXCR chemokine receptor family	Broadly expressed on blood and tissue cells	Cell surface receptor for chemokine SDF1; cofactor for T cell–tropic HIV entry into cells

CD number	Common synonyms	Molecular structure, Family	Main cellular expression	Known or proposed functions
CD195	L1; L1CAM; N-CAM L1	40 kD; CCR chemokine receptor family	T cells and macrophages	Cell surface receptor for chemokines MCP-2, MIP-1α, MIP-1β, and RANTES; cofactor for macrophage-tropic HIV entry into cells
CDw197	CCR7; CMKBR7; BLR2; EBI1	40 kD; CCR chemokine receptor family	T cells, dendritic cells	Cell surface receptor for chemokines ELC and SLC
CD200	OX-2	41 or 47 kD; Ig superfamily	B cells, CNS neurons, microglial cells	Unknown
CD201	EPC R; CCCA; CCD41; bA42O4.2	49 kD; CD1 MHC family	Endothelial cells	Binds protein C and mediates endothelial cell activation
CD202b	Tie2; tek	145 kD; Ig superfamily; receptor tyrosine kinase family	Endothelial cells, early hematopoietic cells	Role in vascular maturation and remodeling
CD203c	NPP3; PDNP3; PD-Iβ; B10; gp130RB13-6; ENPP3	270 kD; type II transmembrane molecule; ectonucleotide enzyme family	Basophils, mast cells	Ectoenzyme that cleaves phosphodiester and phosphosulfate bonds, including deoxynucleotides, nucleotide sugars, and NAD
CD204	Macrophage scavenger receptor 1; MSR1	220 kD; scavenger receptor family; collagen-like domain	Myeloid cells	Role in cellular internalization of oxidized low-density lipoproteins and many other molecules
CD205	DEC205; LY75; GP200-MR6	205 kD; mannose receptor family	Dendritic cells, B cells	Putative role in antigen uptake
CD206	Macrophage mannose receptor (MMR); MRC1	162 kD; mannose receptor family; C-type lectin family	Macrophages, immature dendritic cells	Binds high-mannose oligosaccharides on microbes; pattern recognition receptor of innate immune system

CD number	Common synonyms	Molecular structure, Family	Main cellular expression	Known or proposed functions
CD207	Langerin	40 kD; mannose receptor family; C-type lectin family	Langerhans cells	Antigen capture and routing to nonclassical antigen-processing pathway
CD208	Lysosome-associated membrane protein 3; DC-LAMP; TSC403	70–90 kD; lysosome-associated membrane protein (LAMP) family	Dendritic cells	Role in transfer of peptide-MHC class II molecules to the surface of dendritic cells
CD209	Dendritic cell–specific ICAM3-grabbing nonintegrin (DCSIGN)	44 kD; mannose receptor family; C-type lectin	Dendritic cells	Binds ICAM-3 and high-mannose oligosaccharides; cell adhesion receptor mediating dendritic cell migration and T cell activation; HIV receptor
CDw210	IL-10 receptor α; IL10R	90–110 kD; type II cytokine receptor family	Hematopoietic cells	Subunit of IL-10 receptor; associates with IL-10Rβ
CD212	IL-12 receptor β1; IL12Rβ	Type I cytokine receptor superfamily	Hematopoietic cells	Subunit of the IL-12 receptor complex; associates with IL-12Rβ2
CD213a1	IL-13 receptor α1; IL-13Rα1; IL13RA1; IL13RA	65 kD; Ig superfamily	Broad	Subunit of IL-13 and IL-4 receptor complexes
CD213a2	IL-13 receptor α2; IL-13Rα2; IL-13R; IL13BP	56 kD; type I cytokine receptor superfamily	Broad	High-affinity, nonsignaling IL-13 decoy receptor
CDw217	IL-17 receptor; HIL-17R; VDw217; AW538159	120 kD; cytokine receptor	Hematopoietic cells	Binds and mediates biologic effects of IL-17
CD220	Insulin receptor; INSR	135 kD (α) and 90 kD (β) subunits; tyrosine kinase receptor family	Broad	Binds and mediates many biologic effects of insulin

CD number	Common synonyms	Molecular structure, Family	Main cellular expression	Known or proposed functions
CD221	Insulin-like growth factor 1 receptor; IGFR1; JTK13	80 kD (α) and 71 kD (β) subunits; tyrosine kinase receptor family	Broad	Binds insulin and IGF and induces DNA synthesis and differentiation; delivers cell survival signals
CD222	Insulin-like growth factor 2 receptor; IGF2R; IGFIIR; mannose-6 phosphate receptor; M6P-R; CIMPR; CI-MPR	250 kD; lectin	Broad	Internalization of IGF-II; internalization and sorting of lysosomal enzymes and other M6P-containing proteins
CD223	Lymphocyte activation gene 3; LAG3	Ig superfamily; CD4 related	Activated T cells and NK cells	Binds class II MHC; unknown function
CD224	γ Glutamyl transpeptidase; GGT, GGT1; EC2.3.2.2	62–68 kD and 22 kD subunits; ectoenzyme, peptidase family T3	Renal tubular cells, pancreas, epididymis, seminal vesicles, vascular endothelium, macrophages, activated T cells, subset of B cells	Role in γ glutamyl cycle involving the degradation and neosynthesis of glutathione
CD225	Interferon-induced transmembrane protein 1; LEU13	17 kD	Leukocytes, endothelial cells	Component of a multimeric complex involved in the transduction of antiproliferative and homotypic adhesion signals
CD226	DNAM-1; PTA1; TLiSA1	65 kD; Ig superfamily	T cells, NK cells, platelets, monocytes, subset of B cells, thymocytes, activated endothelial cells	Mediates cellular adhesion and activation; ligand unknown
CD227	MUC1; episialin; PUM; PEM; EMA; DF3 antigen; H23 antigen	300–700 kD; mucin	Glandular and ductal epithelial cells, human adenocarcinoma, activated T cells, activated monocytes, activated dendritic cells, some B cells	Cell-cell and cell-matrix adhesion; signal transduction; target for immunotherapy of tumors

CD number	Common synonyms	Molecular structure, Family	Main cellular expression	Known or proposed functions
CD228	Melanotrans-ferrin; melanoma-associated antigen p97; MTF1; MAP97	97 kD; transferrin superfamily	Melanomas	Iron transport functions
CD229	Ly9	100, 120 kD; Ig superfamily; CD2/CD48/CD58 family	B cells, T cells, thymocytes	Putative adhesion functions
CD230	Prion protein (p27–30); CJD, PrP, PRIP, PrPc	27–30 kD; prion family; neuronal sialoglycoprotein	Broad	Cellular protein of unknown function; structural isoform is the transmissible agent causing spongiform encephalopathies
CD231	TM4SF2; A15; TALLA-1; MXS1; CCG-B7; TALLA	150 kD; tetraspan (TM4SF) family	Neurons, neuroblastoma cells, T cell acute lymphoblastic leukemic cells	Unknown
CD232	Plexin C1; PLXN-C1; semaphorin receptor; VESPR	200 kD; plexin family	Neurons	Receptor for virally encoded semaphorins; regulation of cell dissociation and repulsion
CD233	Band 3; erythrocyte membrane protein band 3; AE1; SLC4A1; Diego blood group; EPB3	95–110 kD; anion exchanger family	Erythrocytes, renal tubular epithelial cells	Anion exchanger; attachment site for underlying cytoskeleton
CD234	Fy-glycoprotein; Duffy antigen; duffy antigen receptor for chemokines	35 kD; chemokine receptor family	Erythrocytes; endothelial cells	Bears the Duffy blood group antigens; nonspecific nonsignaling receptor for various chemokines; *Plasmodium vivax* and *Plasmodium knowlesi* receptor

CD number	Common synonyms	Molecular structure, Family	Main cellular expression	Known or proposed functions
CD235a	Glycophorin A; MN; GPA; MNS	31 kD; glycophorin A family; sialoglycoprotein	Erythrocytes	Prevention of red cell aggregation in the circulation; bears the antigenic determinants for the MN and Ss blood groups
CD235b	Glycophorin B; SS; MNS	24 kD; glycophorin A family; sialoglycoprotein	Erythrocytes	Bears the antigenic determinants for the MN and Ss blood groups
CD236	Glycophorin C/D	24 kD; sialoglycoprotein	Erythrocytes	Mutated form of glycophorin D bears Webb and Dutch blood group antigens; *Plasmodium falciparum* receptor
CD236R	Glycophorin C; GYPC; Gerbich blood group	32 kD; sialoglycoprotein	Erythrocytes	Bears the Gerbich blood group antigens; role in maintenance of the erythrocyte shape
CD238	Kell	93 kD; zinc metalloglycoproteins family	Erythrocytes	Bears the Kell blood group antigens
CD239	B cell adhesion molecule; B-CAM; Lutheran blood group; Auberger blood group	78–85 kD; Ig superfamily	Broad	Bears the Lutheran blood group antigens
CD240CE	Rhesus blood group; CcEe antigens; Rh30CE	30 kD	Erythrocytes	Rh Cc and Ee blood group antigens; associates with Rh50, CD47, and glycophorin B to form the Rh antigen; membrane transport function

CD number	Common synonyms	Molecular structure, Family	Main cellular expression	Known or proposed functions
CD240D	Rh30D; Rh protein, D antigen	30 kD	Erythrocytes	Major antigen of the Rh system; associates with Rh50, CD47, and glycophorin B to form the RhD group; membrane transport function
CD241	Rhesus blood group–associated glycoprotein RhAg; RH50A	50 kD	Erythrocytes	Role in transport of Rh antigen to cell surface of red blood cells
CD242	ICAM-4; Landsteiner-Wiener blood group	42 kD; ICAM family	Erythrocytes	Adhesion molecule; binds LFA-1; bears Landsteiner-Wiener blood group antigen
CD243	Multidrug resistance-1; MDR-1; P glycoprotein 1; P-GP, PGY1, ABC20, GP170	1170 kD; ATP-binding cassette (ABC) transporter family; MDR/TAP subfamily	Broad	ATP-dependent efflux pump for xenobiotic hydrophobic compounds (e.g., drugs); transporter in the blood-brain barrier
CD244	2B4; NAIL; p38	70 kD; Ig superfamily; CD2/CD48/CD58 family	NK cells, ~50% of CD8$^+$ T cells, $\gamma\delta$ T cells, subset of CD4$^+$ T cells, monocytes, basophils	High-affinity receptor for CD48; modulates various functions of NK cells
CD245	p220/240; NPAT	220/240 kD	T cells	Cell cycle regulation
CD246	Anaplastic lymphoma kinase; Ki-1	177 kD; tyrosine kinase receptor family; insulin receptor subfamily	Brain, anaplastic lymphomas	Unknown; fusion protein with nucleolar phosphoprotein nucleophosmin (NPM) found in anaplastic lymphomas

CD number	Common synonyms	Molecular structure, Family	Main cellular expression	Known or proposed functions
CD247	Zeta chain; TCRζ	21–23 kD; ITAMs in cytoplasmic tail	T cells, NK cells	Signaling chain of TCR and NK cell–activating receptors

The complete listing of CD molecules is published in Mason D (ed). Leucocyte Typing VII. Oxford University Press, Oxford, 2002.

Current CD molecule information is also available in Shaw S, L Turni, and K Katz (eds). Protein Reviews on the Web: An International WWW Resource/Journal. http://www.ncbi.nlm.nih.gov/prow/

Additional details of the individual CD molecules may be found in Barclay AN, ML Birkeland, MH Brown, AD Beyers, SJ Davis, C Somoza, and AF Williams (eds). The Leukocyte Antigen Facts Book, 2nd ed. Academic Press, New York, 1997.

Abbreviations: ADCC, antibody-dependent cell-mediated cytotoxicity; ADP, adenosine diphosphate; ATP, adenosine triphosphate; CEA, carcinoembryonic antigen; CR1, type 1 complement receptor; CTL, cytolytic T lymphocyte; ELAM, endothelial cell leukocyte adhesion molecule; GMP, granule membrane protein; GP, glycoprotein; HIV, human immunodeficiency virus; ICAM, intercellular adhesion molecule; IFN, interferon; Ig, immunoglobulin; IL, interleukin; kD, kilodalton; ITAM, immunoreceptor tyrosine-based activation motif; ITIM, immunoreceptor tyrosine-based inhibition motif; LAMP, lysosomal membrane-associated glycoprotein; LFA, lymphocyte function-associated antigen; LPS, lipopolysaccharide; MAC, membrane attack complex; MAdCAM, mucosal addressin cell adhesion molecule; MHC, major histocompatibility complex; NAD, nicotinamide adenine dinucleotide; NK, natural killer; PECAM, platelet endothelial cell adhesion molecule; PI, phosphatidylinositol; TAC, T cell activation antigen; TCR, T cell receptor; TGF, transforming growth factor; TNF, tumor necrosis factor; VCAM, vascular cell adhesion molecule; VLA, very late activation.

Glossary

ABO blood group antigens. Glycosphingolipid antigens present on many cell types, including red blood cells and endothelial cells, which differ between different individuals depending on inherited alleles encoding the enzymes required for synthesis of the antigens. The ABO antigens act as alloantigens responsible for blood transfusion reactions and hyperacute rejection of allografts.

Accessory molecule. A lymphocyte cell surface molecule distinct from the antigen receptor complex that mediates adhesive or signaling functions important for activation or migration of the lymphocyte.

Acquired immunodeficiency. A deficiency in the immune system that is acquired after birth, because of infections, malnutrition, and therapies that deplete immune cells, and is not related to a genetic defect.

Acquired immunodeficiency syndrome (AIDS). A disease caused by human immunodeficiency virus (HIV) infection that is characterized by depletion of CD4$^+$ T cells leading to a profound defect in cell-mediated immunity. Clinically, AIDS includes opportunistic infections, malignancies, wasting, and encephalopathy.

Activation phase. A phase of an adaptive immune response that follows the recognition of antigen and is characterized by proliferation of lymphocytes and their differentiation into effector cells.

Active immunity. The form of adaptive immunity that is induced by exposure to a foreign antigen and activation of lymphocytes, in which the immunized individual plays an active role in responding to the antigen. Compare with **passive immunity**.

Acute phase response. The increase in plasma concentrations of several proteins, called acute phase reactants, that occurs as part of the innate immune response to infections. These proteins, including C-reactive protein, fibrinogen, and serum amyloid A protein, are synthesized by the liver in response to inflammatory cytokines, especially IL-6 and TNF.

Acute rejection. A form of graft rejection involving vascular and parenchymal injury mediated by T cells, macrophages, and antibodies, which usually begins after the first week of transplantation. The differentiation of the effector T cells and the production of antibodies that mediate acute rejection occur in response to graft antigens.

Adapter protein. Proteins involved in lymphocyte signal transduction pathways, which serve as bridge molecules or scaffolds for the recruitment of other signaling molecules. Adapter molecules involved in T cell activation include LAT, SLP-76, and Grb-2.

Adaptive immunity. The form of immunity that is mediated by lymphocytes and is stimulated by exposure to infectious agents. In contrast to innate immunity, adaptive immunity is characterized by exquisite specificity for distinct macromolecules, and "memory," which is the ability to respond more vigorously to repeated exposures to the same microbe.

Adhesion molecule. A cell surface molecule whose function is to promote adhesive interactions with other cells or the extracellular matrix. Leukocytes express various types of adhesion molecules, such as selectins and integrins, and these molecules play important roles in cell migration and activation in innate and adaptive immune responses.

Adjuvant. A substance, distinct from antigen, that enhances T cell activation by promoting the accumulation of antigen-presenting cells at a site of antigen exposure and by enhancing the expression of costimulators and cytokines by the antigen-presenting cells.

Affinity. The strength of the binding between a single binding site of a molecule (e.g., an antibody) and a ligand (e.g., an antigen), represented by the dissociation constant (K_d). A smaller K_d indicates a stronger or higher affinity interaction.

Affinity maturation. The process that leads to increased affinity of antibodies for a protein antigen as a humoral response progresses. Affinity maturation is the result of somatic mutation of Ig genes followed by selective survival of the B cells producing the highest affinity antibodies.

Allele. One of different forms of a gene present at a particular chromosomal locus. An individual who is heterozygous at a locus has two different alleles, each on a different chromosome, one inherited from the mother and one from the father. If there are many different alleles for a particular gene in a population, the gene or locus is said to be *polymorphic.* The major histocompatibility locus is extremely polymorphic.

Allelic exclusion. The expression of only one of two inherited alleles encoding immunoglobulin heavy and light chains and T cell receptor β chains. Allelic exclusion occurs when the protein product of one productively recombined antigen receptor locus on one chromosome blocks the rearrangement of the corresponding locus on the other chromosome.

Allergen. An antigen that elicits an immediate hypersensitivity (allergic) reaction. Allergens are proteins, or chemicals bound to proteins, that induce IgE antibody production in atopic individuals.

Allergy. A form of atopy or immediate hypersensitivity disease, often referring to the type of antigen that elicits the disease, such as food allergy, bee sting allergy, and penicillin allergy. All these conditions are related to antigen-induced mast cell or basophil activation.

Alloantigen. A cell or tissue antigen that is present in some members of a species and not others and which is recognized as foreign on an allograft. Alloantigens are the products of polymorphic genes.

Allogeneic graft. An organ or tissue graft from a donor who is of the same species but genetically not identical to the recipient (also called an allograft).

Alloreactive. Reactive to alloantigens; describes T cells or antibodies from one individual that will recognize antigens on cells or tissues of another genetically nonidentical individual.

Altered peptide ligands (APLs). Peptides with altered T cell receptor contact residues that elicit responses different from the responses to the native peptide. APLs may be important in the regulation of T cell activation in physiologic, pathologic, or therapeutic situations.

Alternative pathway of complement activation. An antibody-independent pathway of activation of the complement system that occurs when the C3b protein binds to microbial cell surfaces. The alternative pathway is a component of the innate immune system and mediates inflammatory responses to infection as well as direct lysis of microbes.

Anaphylatoxins. The C5a, C4a, and C3a complement fragments that are generated during complement activation. The anaphylatoxins bind specific cell surface receptors and promote acute inflammation by stimulating neutrophil chemotaxis and by activating mast cells.

Anaphylaxis. An extreme systemic form of immediate hypersensitivity, also called anaphylactic shock, in which mast cell or basophil mediators cause bronchial constriction, massive tissue edema, and cardiovascular collapse.

Anergy. A state of unresponsiveness to antigenic stimulation. Lymphocyte anergy (also called clonal anergy) is the failure of clones of T or B cells to react to antigen, and this may be a mechanism of maintaining immunologic tolerance to self antigens. In clinical practice, anergy refers to a generalized defect in T cell–dependent cutaneous delayed-type hypersensitivity reactions to common antigens.

Antibody. A type of glycoprotein molecule, also called immunoglobulin (Ig), produced by B lymphocytes, that binds antigens, often with a high degree of specificity and high affinity. The basic structural unit of an antibody is composed of two identical heavy chains and two identical light chains. Amino-terminal variable regions of the heavy and light chains form the antigen binding sites, whereas the carboxy-terminal constant regions of the heavy chains functionally interact with other molecules in the immune system. In any individual, there are millions of different antibodies, each with a unique antigen-binding site. Secreted antibodies perform various effector functions, including neutralizing antigens, activating complement, and promoting phagocytosis and destruction of microbes.

Antibody-dependent cell-mediated cytotoxicity (ADCC). A process by which natural killer (NK) cells are targeted to IgG-coated cells, resulting in the lysis of the antibody-coated cells. A specific receptor for the constant region of IgG, called FcγRIII (CD16), is expressed on the NK cell membrane and mediates the binding to the IgG.

Antibody feedback. The down-regulation of antibody production by secreted IgG antibodies that occurs when antigen-antibody complexes simultaneously engage B cell membrane Ig and Fcγ receptors. Under these conditions, the cytoplasmic tails of the Fcγ receptors deliver inhibitory signals to the B cell.

Antibody repertoire. The collection of different antibody specificities expressed in an individual.

Antibody-secreting cells. A B lymphocyte that has undergone differentiation and produces the secretory form of Ig. Antibody-secreting cells are produced in response to antigen and reside in lymphoid follicles in spleen and lymph node, as well as in the bone marrow. Plasma cells are typical antibody-secreting cells.

Antigen. A molecule that binds to an antibody or a T cell antigen receptor (TCR). Antigens that bind to antibodies include all classes of molecules. TCRs only bind peptide fragments of proteins complexed with major histocompatibility molecules; both the peptide ligand and the native protein from which it is derived are called T cell antigens.

Antigen presentation. The display of peptides bound by major histocompatibility molecules on the surface of an antigen-presenting cell, permitting specific recognition by T cell receptors and activation of T cells.

Antigen processing. The intracellular conversion of protein antigens derived from the extracellular space or the cytosol into peptides and loading of these peptides onto major histocompatibility complex molecules for display to T lymphocytes.

Antigen-presenting cell (APC). A cell that displays peptide fragments of protein antigens, in association with major histocompatibility (MHC) molecules on its surface, and activates antigen-specific T cells. In addition to displaying peptide-MHC complexes, APCs must also express costimulatory molecules to optimally activate T lymphocytes.

Antiserum. Serum from an individual previously immunized against an antigen that contains antibody specific for that antigen.

Apoptosis. A process of cell death, which is characterized by DNA cleavage, nuclear condensation and fragmentation, and plasma membrane blebbing, leading to phagocytosis of the cell, without inducing an inflammatory response. This type of cell death is important in lymphocyte development, regulation of lymphocyte responses to foreign antigens, and maintenance of tolerance to self antigens.

Arthus reaction. A localized form of experimental immune complex–mediated vasculitis induced by injecting an antigen subcutaneously into a previously immunized animal or an animal that has been given intravenous antibody specific for the antigen. Circulating antibodies bind to the injected antigen, forming immune complexes that deposit in the walls of small arteries at the injection site, giving rise to a local cutaneous vasculitis with necrosis.

Atopy. The propensity of an individual to produce IgE antibodies in response to various environmental antigens and to develop strong immediate hypersensitivity (allergic) responses. People who have allergies to environmental antigens, such as pollen or house dust, are said to be atopic.

Autoantibody. An antibody specific for a self antigen. Autoantibodies can cause damage to cells and tissues and are produced in excess in many autoimmune diseases such as systemic lupus erythematosus.

Autoimmune disease. A disease caused by a breakdown of self-tolerance such that the adaptive immune system responds to self antigens and mediates cell and tissue damage. Autoimmune diseases can be organ-specific (e.g., thyroiditis or diabetes) or systemic (e.g., systemic lupus erythematosus).

Autoimmunity. The response of the adaptive immune system to self antigens that occurs when mechanisms of self-tolerance fail.

Autologous graft. A tissue or organ graft in which the donor and recipient are the same individual. Autologous bone marrow and skin grafts are commonly performed in clinical medicine.

Avidity. The overall strength of interaction between two molecules, such as an antibody and antigen. The avidity depends on both the affinity and the valency of interactions. Therefore, the avidity of a pentameric IgM antibody, with 10 antigen binding sites, for a multivalent antigen may be much greater than the avidity of a dimeric IgG molecule for the same antigen. Avidity can also be used to describe the strength of cell-cell interactions, which are mediated by many binding interactions between cell surface molecules.

B lymphocyte. The only cell type capable of producing antibody molecules and therefore the central cellular component of humoral immune responses. B lymphocytes, or B cells, develop in the bone marrow, and mature B cells are found mainly in lymphoid follicles in secondary lymphoid tissues, in bone marrow, and in low numbers in the circulation.

B lymphocyte antigen receptor (BCR) complex. A multiprotein complex expressed on the surface of B lymphocytes that recognizes antigen and transduces activating signals. The BCR complex includes membrane Ig, which is responsible for binding antigen, and the associated Igα and Igβ proteins, which initiate signaling events.

Bare lymphocyte syndrome. An immunodeficiency disease characterized by the lack of class II major histocompatibility complex (MHC) molecule expression, leading to defects in antigen presentation and cell-mediated immunity. The disease is caused by mutations in genes encoding factors that regulate class II MHC gene transcription.

Basophil. A type of bone marrow–derived circulating granulocyte with structural and functional similarities to mast cells, including granules containing many of the same inflammatory mediators as mast cells, and expression of a high-affinity Fc receptor for IgE. Basophils that are recruited into tissue sites where antigen is present may contribute to immediate hypersensitivity reactions.

Bone marrow. The central cavity of bone that is the site of generation of all circulating blood cells in the adult, including immature lymphocytes, and the site of B cell maturation.

Bone marrow transplantation. The transplantation of bone marrow stem cells that give rise to all mature blood cells and lymphocytes, performed clinically to treat hematopoietic/lymphopoietic disorders and malignancies; also used in various immunologic experiments in animals.

Bronchial asthma. An inflammatory disease usually caused by repeated immediate hypersensitivity reactions in the lung, leading to intermittent and reversible airway obstruction, chronic bronchial inflammation with eosinophils, and bronchial smooth muscle cell hypertrophy and hyper-reactivity.

C3 convertase. A multiprotein enzyme complex generated by the early steps of complement activation, which cleaves C3, giving rise to two proteolytic products called C3a and C3b.

C5 convertase. A multiprotein enzyme complex generated by C3b binding to C3 convertase, which cleaves C5 and initiates the late steps of complement activation.

Caspases. Intracellular cysteine proteases that cleave substrates at the carboxy-terminal sides of aspartic acid residues and are components of enzymatic cascades that cause apoptotic death of cells. Lymphocyte caspases may be activated by two distinct pathways, one of which is associated with mitochondrial permeability changes in growth factor–deprived cells and the other with signals from death receptors in the plasma membrane.

CD molecules. Cell surface molecules expressed on various cell types in the immune system that are designated by the "cluster of differentiation" or CD *nomenclature*. See Appendix I for a list of CD molecules.

Cell-mediated immunity. The form of adaptive immunity that is mediated by T lymphocytes and serves as the defense mechanism against microbes that survive within phagocytes or infect nonphagocytic cells. Cell-mediated immune responses include CD4+ T cell–mediated activation of macrophages that have phagocytosed microbes and CD8+ cytolytic T lymphocyte killing of infected cells.

Central tolerance. A form of self-tolerance that is induced in generative ("central") lymphoid organs as a consequence of immature self-reactive lymphocytes recognizing self antigens, leading to their death or inactivation. Central tolerance prevents the emergence of lymphocytes with high-affinity receptors for ubiquitous self antigens that are present in the bone marrow or thymus and are likely to be present throughout the body.

Chédiak-Higashi syndrome. A rare autosomal recessive immunodeficiency disease due to a defect in cytoplasmic granules of various cell types that affects the lysosomes of neutrophils and macrophages, as well as the granules of cytolytic T lymphocytes and natural killer cells. Patients show reduced resistance to infections with pyogenic bacteria.

Chemokine receptors. Cell surface receptors for chemokines that transduce signals, which stimulate migration of leukocytes. These receptors are members of the seven transmembrane α-helical, G protein–linked family of receptors.

Chemokines. A large family of structurally homologous, low molecular weight cytokines that stimulate leukocyte movement and regulate the migration of leukocytes from the blood to tissues.

Chemotaxis. Movement of a cell directed by a chemical concentration gradient. The movement of lymphocytes, polymorphonuclear leukocytes, monocytes, and other leukocytes into various tissues is often directed by gradients of chemokines.

Chronic granulomatous disease (CGD). A rare inherited immunodeficiency due to a defect in the gene encoding a component of the phagocyte oxidase enzyme, which is needed for microbial killing by polymorphonuclear leukocytes and macrophages. The disease is characterized by recurrent intracellular bacterial and fungal infections, often accompanied by chronic cell-mediated immune responses and the formation of granulomas.

Chronic rejection. A form of allograft rejection characterized by fibrosis with loss of normal organ structures occurring over a prolonged period of time. In many cases, the major pathologic event in chronic rejection is graft arterial occlusion that occurs due to proliferation of intimal smooth muscle cells and is called graft arteriosclerosis.

Class I MHC molecule. One of two forms of polymorphic, heterodimeric membrane proteins that bind and display peptide fragments of protein antigens on the surface of antigen-presenting cells for recognition by T lymphocytes. Class I MHC molecules display peptides derived from the cytoplasm of the cell.

Class II–associated invariant chain peptide (CLIP). A peptide remnant of the invariant chain that sits in the class II MHC peptide-binding cleft and is removed by the action of the HLA-DM molecule before the cleft becomes accessible to peptides produced from endocytosed protein antigens.

Class II MHC molecule. One of two forms of polymorphic, heterodimeric membrane proteins that bind and display peptide fragments of protein antigens on the surface of antigen-presenting cells for recognition by T lymphocytes. Class II MHC molecules display peptides derived from proteins that are internalized into phagocytic/endocytic vesicles.

Classical pathway of complement activation. The pathway of complement system activation that is initiated by binding of antigen-antibody complexes to the C1 molecule, inducing a proteolytic cascade involving multiple other complement proteins. The classical pathway is an effector arm of the humoral immune system that generates inflammatory mediators, opsonins for phagocytosis of antigens, and lytic complexes that destroy cells.

Clonal ignorance. A form of lymphocyte unresponsiveness in which self antigens are ignored by the immune system, even though lymphocytes specific for those antigens remain viable and functional.

Clonal selection hypothesis. A fundamental tenet of the immune system (no longer a hypothesis) stating that every individual possesses numerous clonally derived lymphocytes, each clone having arisen from a single precursor and being capable of recognizing and responding to a distinct antigenic determinant. When an antigen enters, it selects a specific preexisting clone and activates it.

Collectins. A family of proteins, including mannose-binding lectins, that are characterized by the presence of a collagen-like domain and a lectin (i.e., carbohydrate-binding) domain. Collectins play a role in the innate immune system by acting as microbial pattern recognition receptors, and they may activate the complement system by binding to C1q.

Colony-stimulating factors (CSFs). Cytokines that promote the expansion and differentiation of bone marrow progenitor cells. CSFs are essential for maturation of red blood cells, granulocytes, monocytes, and lymphocytes. Examples of CSFs are granulocyte-monocyte colony-stimulating factor, c-*kit* ligand, and interleukin-3.

Combinatorial diversity. Describes the many different combinations of variable, diversity, and joining segments that are possible as a result of somatic recombination of DNA in the immunoglobulin and T cell receptor loci during B cell or T cell development. This is one mechanism for the generation of large numbers of different antigen receptor genes from a limited number of gene segments.

Complement. A system of serum and cell surface proteins that interact with one another and with other molecules of the immune system to generate important effectors of innate and adaptive immune responses. There are three pathways of complement activation that differ in how they are initiated. The classical pathway is activated by antigen-antibody complexes, the alternative pathway by microbial surfaces, and the lectin pathway by plasma lectins that bind to microbes. Each complement pathway consists of a cascade of proteolytic enzymes that generate inflammatory mediators and opsonins and leads to the formation of a lytic complex that inserts in cell membranes.

Complement receptor, type 2 (CR2). A receptor expressed on B cells and follicular dendritic cells that binds proteolytic fragments of the C3 complement protein, including C3d, C3dg, and iC3b. CR2 functions to stimulate humoral immune responses by enhancing B cell activation by antigen and by promoting the trapping of antigen-antibody complexes in germinal centers. CR2 is also the receptor for Epstein-Barr virus.

Complementarity-determining region (CDR). Short segments of the immunoglobulin and T cell receptor (TCR) proteins in which most of the sequence differences among different antibodies or TCRs are confined and which make contact with antigen. There are three CDRs in the variable domain of each antigen receptor polypeptide chain and six CDRs in an intact Ig or TCR molecule. These "hypervariable" segments assume loop structures that together form a surface that is complementary to the three-dimensional structure of the bound antigen.

Constant (C) region. The portion of immunoglobulin (Ig) or T cell receptor (TCR) polypeptide chains that does not vary in sequence among different clones of B and T cells and is not involved in antigen binding. The C regions are encoded by DNA sequences in the Ig and TCR gene loci that are spatially separate from the sequences that encode the variable (V) regions.

Contact sensitivity. The propensity to develop a T cell–mediated, delayed-type hypersensitivity reaction in the skin on contact with a particular chemical agent. Chemicals that elicit contact sensitivity bind to and modify self proteins or molecules on the surfaces of antigen-presenting cells, which are then recognized by CD4$^+$ or CD8$^+$ T cells.

Coreceptor. A lymphocyte surface receptor that binds to a part of an antigen at the same time as membrane immunoglobulin (Ig) or T cell receptor (TCR) binds the antigen and that delivers signals required for optimal lymphocyte activation. CD4 and CD8 are T cell coreceptors that bind nonpolymorphic regions of a major histocompatibility complex molecule concurrently with the TCR binding to polymorphic residues and the displayed peptide. The type 2 complement receptor (CR2) is a coreceptor on B cells that binds to complement-coated antigens, at the same time that membrane Ig binds an epitope of the antigen.

Costimulator. A molecule on the surface of an antigen-presenting cell that provides a stimulus ("second signal") required for activation of naive T cells, in addition to antigen (the "first signal"). The best defined costimulators are the B7 molecules on professional antigen-presenting cells that bind to the CD28 molecule on T cells.

Crossmatching. A screening test performed to minimize the chance of graft rejection, in which the patient in need of an allograft is tested for the presence of preformed antibodies against donor cell surface antigens (usually major histocompatibility antigens). The test involves mixing the recipient serum with leukocytes from potential donors, adding complement, and examining it to see if cell lysis occurs.

Cross presentation. A mechanism by which a professional antigen-presenting cell (APC) displays the antigens of another cell (e.g., a virus-infected or tumor cell) and activates (or primes) a naive CD8+ cytolytic T lymphocyte. This occurs, for example, when an infected (often damaged) cell is ingested by a professional APC and the microbial antigens are processed and presented in association with major histocompatibility complex molecules, just like any other phagocytosed antigen. The professional APC also provides costimulation for the T cells. Also called **cross-priming.**

Cutaneous immune system. The components of the innate and adaptive immune system found in the skin that function together in a specialized way to detect and respond to antigens that enter through the skin. Components of the cutaneous immune system include keratinocytes, Langerhans cells, intraepithelial lymphocytes, and dermal lymphocytes.

Cyclosporine (Cyclosporin A). An immunosuppressive drug used to prevent allograft rejection, which functions by blocking T cell cytokine gene transcription. Cyclosporine binds to a cytosolic protein called cyclophilin, and cyclosporine-cyclophilin complexes bind to and inhibit the phosphatase calcineurin, thereby inhibiting activation and nuclear translocation of the transcription factor NFAT.

Cytokines. Secreted proteins that function as mediators of immune and inflammatory reactions. In innate immune responses, cytokines are produced by macrophages and NK cells and, in adaptive immune responses, mainly by T lymphocytes.

Cytolytic (or cytotoxic) T lymphocyte (CTL). A type of T lymphocyte whose major effector function is to recognize and kill host cells infected with viruses or other intracellular microbes. CTLs usually express CD8 and recognize microbial peptides displayed by class I major histocompatibility complex molecules. CTL killing of infected cells involves release of cytoplasmic granules whose contents include membrane pore-forming proteins and enzymes.

Defensins. Cysteine-rich peptides produced in epithelia and neutrophil granules, which act as broad-spectrum antibiotics that kill a wide variety of bacteria and fungi.

Delayed-type hypersensitivity (DTH). An immune reaction in which T cell–dependent macrophage activation and inflammation cause tissue injury. A DTH reaction to subcutaneous injection of antigen is often used as an assay for cell-mediated immunity (e.g., the PPD skin test for immunity to *Mycobacterium tuberculosis*).

Dendritic cells. Bone marrow–derived cells, found in epithelia and most organs, morphologically characterized by thin membranous projections. Dendritic cells function as antigen-presenting cells for naive T lymphocytes and are important for initiation of adaptive immune responses to protein antigens.

Desensitization. A method for treating immediate hypersensitivity disease (e.g., allergies) that involves repetitive administration of low doses of an antigen to which individuals are allergic. This process often prevents severe allergic reactions on subsequent environmental exposure to the antigen, but the mechanisms are not well understood.

Determinant. The portion of a macromolecular antigen to which an antibody or T cell receptor binds. For a T cell, a determinant is the peptide portion of a protein antigen that binds to a major histocompatibility complex molecule and is recognized by the T cell receptor. It is synonymous with **epitope.**

Di George syndrome. A T cell deficiency due to a congenital malformation that results in defective development of the thymus, parathyroid glands, and other structures that arise from the third and fourth pharyngeal pouches.

Direct antigen presentation. Presentation of cell surface allogeneic major histocompatibility complex (MHC) molecules by graft antigen-presenting cells to the recipient's T cells, leading to T cell activation, with no requirement for processing. Direct recognition of foreign MHC molecules is a cross-reaction of a normal T cell receptor, which was selected to recognize a self MHC molecule plus foreign peptide, with an allogeneic MHC molecule plus peptide. (Contrasts to "indirect presentation" of alloantigens.)

Diversity. The existence of a large number of lymphocytes with different antigenic specificities in any individual (i.e., the lymphocyte repertoire is large and diverse). Diversity is a fundamental property of the adaptive immune system and is the result of variability in the structures of the antigen-binding sites of lymphocyte receptors for antigens (antibodies and T cell receptors).

Diversity (D) segments. Short coding sequences between the variable (V) and constant (C) gene segments in the immunoglobulin heavy chain and TCR β and δ loci, which, together with J segments, are somatically recombined with V segments during lymphocyte development. The resulting recombined V-D-J DNA codes for the antigen receptor V region.

DM. See **HLA-DM.**

DNA vaccine. A method for vaccination in which an individual is inoculated with a bacterial plasmid containing a complementary DNA encoding a protein antigen. DNA vaccines presumably work because professional antigen-presenting cells are transfected *in vivo* by the plasmid and express immunogenic peptides that elicit specific responses. Furthermore, the plasmid DNA includes unmethylated CpG nucleotides (typical of bacterial DNA) that act as adjuvants.

Double-negative thymocyte. A subset of developing T cells in the thymus that express neither CD4 nor CD8. Most double-negative thymocytes are at an early developmental stage and do not express antigen receptors. They will later express both CD4 and CD8 during the intermediate "double-positive" stage before further maturation to single-positive T cells expressing only CD4 or only CD8.

Double-positive thymocyte. A subset of developing T cells in the thymus at an intermediate developmental stage, which express both CD4 and CD8. Double-positive thymocytes also express T cell receptors and are subject to selection processes, the survivors of which mature to single-positive T cells expressing only CD4 or only CD8.

Effector cells. The cells that perform effector functions during an immune response, such as secreting cytokines (e.g., helper T cells), killing microbes (e.g., macrophages, neutrophils, and eosinophils), killing microbe-infected host cells (e.g., CTLs), or secreting antibodies (e.g., differentiated B cells).

Effector phase. The phase of an immune response, following the recognition and activation phases, in which a microbe or toxin is destroyed or inactivated. For example, in a humoral immune response, the effector phase may be characterized by antibody-dependent complement activation and phagocytosis of bacteria opsonized with antibody and/or complement.

Endosome. An intracellular membrane-bound vesicle into which extracellular proteins are internalized during antigen processing. Endosomes have an acidic pH and contain proteolytic enzymes that degrade proteins into peptides that bind to class II major histocompatibility complex (MHC) molecules. A subset of class II MHC-rich endosomes, called MIIC, plays a special role in antigen processing and presentation by the class II pathway.

Endotoxin. A component of the cell wall of gram-negative bacteria, also called lipopolysaccharide, which is released from dying bacteria and which stimulates many innate immune responses, including the secretion of cytokines and induction of microbicidal activities of macrophages and the expression of adhesion molecules for leukocytes on endothelium. Endotoxin contains both lipid components and carbohydrate (polysaccharide) moieties.

Endotoxin shock. See **Septic shock.**

Envelope glycoprotein (Env). A membrane glycoprotein encoded by a retrovirus that is expressed on the plasma membrane of infected cells and on the host cell–derived membrane coat of viral particles. Env proteins are often required for viral infectivity. The Env proteins of human immunodeficiency virus include gp41 and gp120, which bind to CD4 and chemokine receptors on human T cells and mediate fusion of the viral and T cell membranes.

Enzyme-linked immunosorbent assay (ELISA). A method for quantifying an antigen immobilized on a solid surface using a specific antibody with a covalently coupled enzyme. The amount of antibody that binds the antigen is proportional to the amount of antigen present and is determined by spectrophotometrically measuring the conversion of a clear substrate to a colored product by the coupled enzyme.

Eosinophil. A bone marrow–derived granulocyte that is abundant in the inflammatory infiltrates of immediate hypersensitivity late phase reactions and that contributes to many of the pathologic processes in allergic diseases. Eosinophils are important in defense against extracellular parasites, such as helminths.

Epitope. The specific portion of a macromolecular antigen to which an antibody binds. In the case of a protein antigen recognized by a T cell, an epitope is the peptide portion that binds to a major histocompatibility complex molecule for recognition by the T cell receptor. It is synonymous with **determinant.**

Epstein-Barr virus (EBV). A double-stranded DNA virus of the herpesvirus family that is the etiologic agent of infectious mononucleosis and is associated with some

B cell malignancies and nasopharyngeal carcinoma. EBV infects B lymphocytes and some epithelial cells by specifically binding to the complement receptor type 2 (CR2 or CD21).

F(ab')₂ fragment. A proteolytic fragment of an IgG molecule that includes two complete light chains but only the variable domain, first constant domain, and hinge region of the two heavy chains. F(ab')₂ fragments retain the entire bivalent antigen-binding region of an intact IgG but cannot bind complement or IgG Fc receptors. They are used in research and therapeutic applications when antigen binding is desired without antibody effector functions.

Fab fragment. A proteolytic fragment of an IgG antibody molecule that includes one complete light chain paired with one heavy chain fragment containing the variable domain and only the first constant domain. A Fab fragment retains the ability to bind an antigen but cannot interact with IgG Fc receptors on cells, nor with complement. Therefore, Fab preparations are used in research and therapeutic applications when antigen binding is desired without activation of effector functions. (A Fab' fragment retains the hinge region of the heavy chain.)

Fas. A member of the tumor necrosis factor receptor family, which is expressed on the surface of T cells and many other cell types and which initiates a signaling cascade leading to the apoptotic death of the cell. The death pathway is initiated when Fas binds to Fas ligand expressed on activated T cells. Fas-mediated killing of T cells, called activation-induced cell death, is important for the maintenance of self-tolerance. Mutations in the Fas gene cause systemic autoimmune disease in mice and humans. Also called CD95.

Fas ligand. A membrane protein that is a member of the tumor necrosis factor family of proteins, which is expressed on activated T cells. Fas ligand binds to Fas, thereby stimulating a signaling pathway leading to apoptotic death of the Fas-expressing cell. Mutations in the Fas ligand gene like mutations in Fas cause systemic autoimmune disease in mice.

Fc (fragment crystalline). A proteolytic fragment of antibody that contains only the disulfide linked carboxy-terminal regions of the two heavy chains. The Fc region mediates effector functions by binding to cell surface receptors of phagocytes and NK cells or the C1 complement protein. (Fc fragments are so named because they tend to crystallize out of solution.)

Fc receptor (FcR). A cell surface receptor specific for the carboxy-terminal constant region of an Ig molecule. Fc receptors are typically multichain protein complexes that include Ig-binding components and signaling components. There are several types of Fc receptors, including those specific for different IgG isotypes, IgE, and IgA. Fc receptors mediate many of the effector functions of antibodies, including phagocytosis of antibody-coated (opsonized) microbes, antigen-induced activation of mast cells, and activation of natural killer cells.

FcεRI. A high-affinity receptor for the carboxy-terminal constant region of IgE molecules, which is expressed on mast cells and basophils. FcεRI molecules on mast cells are usually occupied by IgE, and antigen-induced crosslinking of these IgE-FcεRI complexes activates the mast cell and initiates immediate hypersensitivity reactions.

Fcγ receptor (FcγR). A specific cell surface receptor for the carboxy-terminal constant region of IgG molecules. There are several different types of Fcγ receptors, including the high-affinity FcγRI that mediates phagocytosis by macrophages and neutrophils, the low-affinity FcγRIIb that transduces inhibitory signals in B cells, and the low-affinity FcγRIIIB that mediates targeting and activation of natural killer cells.

Flow cytometry. A method of analysis of the phenotype of cell populations requiring a specialized instrument (flow cytometer) that can detect fluorescence on individual cells in a suspension and thereby determine the number of cells expressing the molecule to which a fluorescent probe binds. Suspensions of cells are incubated with fluorescently labeled antibodies or other probes, and the amount of probe bound by each cell in the population is measured by passing the cells one at a time through a fluorimeter with a laser-generated incident beam.

Fluorescence-activated cell sorter (FACS). An adaptation of the flow cytometer that is used for the purification of cells from a mixed population depending on which and how much fluorescent probe the cells bind. Cells are first stained with fluorescently labeled probe, such as an antibody specific for a surface antigen of a cell population. The cells are then passed one at a time through a fluorimeter with a laser-generated incident beam and are differentially deflected by electromagnetic fields whose strength and direction are varied according to the measured intensity of the fluorescence signal.

Follicle. See Lymphoid follicle.

Follicular dendritic cells. Cells found in lymphoid follicles that express complement receptors, Fc receptors, and CD40 ligand and have long cytoplasmic processes that form a meshwork that is integral to the architecture of the lymphoid follicles. Follicular dendritic cells display antigens on their surface for recognition by B cells and are involved in the activation and selection of B cells expressing high-affinity membrane Ig during the process of affinity maturation.

G proteins. Proteins that bind guanyl nucleotides and act as exchange molecules, catalyzing the replacement of bound GDP by GTP. G proteins with bound GTP can activate a variety of cellular enzymes in different signaling cascades. Trimeric GTP-binding proteins are associated with the cytoplasmic portions of many cell surface receptors, such as chemokine receptors. Other small soluble G proteins, such as Ras and Raf, are recruited into signaling pathways by adapter proteins.

Generative lymphoid organs. Organs where lymphocytes develop from immature precursors. The bone marrow and thymus are the major generative lymphoid organs where B cells and T cells develop, respectively.

Germinal center. A central, light-staining region within a lymphoid follicle in spleen, lymph node, or mucosal lymphoid tissue that forms during T cell–dependent humoral immune responses and is the site of B cell affinity maturation.

Glomerulonephritis. Inflammation of the renal glomeruli, often initiated by immunopathologic mechanisms, such as deposition of circulating antigen-antibody complexes in the glomerular basement membrane or binding of antibodies to antigens expressed in the glomerulus. The antibodies can activate complement and phagocytes, and the resulting inflammatory response can lead to renal failure.

Graft. A tissue or organ that is removed from one site and is placed in another site, usually in a different individual.

Graft arteriosclerosis. Occlusion of graft arteries due to proliferation of intimal smooth muscle cells. This process is evident within 6 months to 1 year after transplantation and is responsible for chronic rejection of vascularized organ grafts. The mechanism is likely to be a result of a chronic immune response to vessel wall alloantigens. It is also called accelerated arteriosclerosis.

Graft rejection. A specific immune response to an organ or tissue graft that leads to inflammation, damage, and possibly graft failure.

Graft-versus-host disease. A disease occurring in bone marrow transplant recipients that is caused by the reaction of mature T cells in the marrow graft against alloantigens on host cells. The disease most often affects skin, liver, and intestines.

Granulocyte colony-stimulating factor (G-CSF). A cytokine made by activated T cells, macrophages, and endothelial cells at sites of infection that acts on bone marrow to increase production of and mobilize neutrophils to replace those consumed in inflammatory reactions.

Granulocyte-monocyte colony-stimulating factor (GM-CSF). A cytokine made by activated T cells, macrophages, endothelial cells, and bone marrow stromal fibroblasts that acts on progenitors in the bone marrow to increase production of neutrophils and monocytes.

Granuloma. A nodule of inflammatory tissue composed of clusters of activated macrophages and T lymphocytes, often with associated necrosis and fibrosis. Granulomatous inflammation is a form of chronic delayed-type hypersensitivity, often in response to persistent microbes, such as *Mycobacterium tuberculosis* and some fungi, or in response to particulate antigens that are not readily phagocytosed.

Granzyme. A serine protease enzyme found in the granules of cytolytic T lymphocytes and natural killer cells that is released by exocytosis, enters target cells, mainly through perforin-created "holes," and proteolytically cleaves and activates caspases, which in turn cleave several substrates and induce target cell apoptosis.

H-2 molecule. A major histocompatibility complex (MHC) molecule in the mouse. The mouse MHC was originally called the H-2 locus.

Haplotype. The set of major histocompatibility complex alleles inherited from one parent and therefore on one chromosome.

Hapten. A small chemical that can bind to an antibody but must be attached to a macromolecule (carrier) to stimulate an adaptive immune response specific for that chemical. For example, immunization with dinitrophenol (DNP) alone does not stimulate an anti-DNP antibody response, but immunization with the DNP hapten attached to a protein does stimulate anti-DNP antibody production.

Heavy chain. See **Immunoglobulin heavy chain.**

Heavy chain class (isotype) switching. The process by which a B lymphocyte changes the isotype of the antibodies it produces, from IgM to IgG, IgE, or IgA, without changing the specificity of the antibody. Heavy chain class switching is regulated by helper T cell cytokines and CD40 ligand and involves recombination of heavy chain VDJ segments with downstream constant region gene segments.

Helminth. A parasitic worm. Helminthic infections often elicit T_H2 responses with eosinophil-rich inflammatory infiltrates and IgE production.

Helper T lymphocytes. The functional subset of T lymphocytes whose main effector functions are to activate macrophages in cell-mediated immune responses and promote B cell antibody production in humoral immune responses. These effector functions are mediated by secreted cytokines and by T cell CD40 ligand binding to macrophage or B cell CD40. Most helper T cells express the CD4 molecule.

Hematopoiesis. The development of mature blood cells, including erythrocytes, leukocytes, and platelets, from pluripotential stem cells in the bone marrow and fetal liver. Hematopoiesis is regulated by several different cytokines produced by bone marrow stromal cells, T cells, and other cell types.

High endothelial venule (HEV). Specialized venules that are the sites of lymphocyte extravasation from the blood into the stroma of a peripheral lymph node or mucosal lymphoid tissues. HEVs are lined by plump endothelial cells that protrude into the vessel lumen and express unique adhesion molecules involved in binding naive T cells.

Hinge region. A region of immunoglobulin heavy chains between the first two constant domains that can assume multiple conformations, thereby imparting a flexibility in the orientation of the two antigen-binding sites. Because of the hinge region, an antibody molecule can simultaneously bind two epitopes that are anywhere within reach of one another.

Histamine. A vasoactive amine, stored in the granules of mast cells, that is one of the important mediators of immediate hypersensitivity. Histamine binds to specific receptors in various tissues and causes increased vascular permeability and contraction of bronchial and intestinal smooth muscle.

HLA. See Human leukocyte antigen.

HLA-DM (also called DM). A peptide exchange molecule that plays a critical role in the class II major histocompatibility complex (MHC) pathway of antigen presentation. HLA-DM is found in the specialized MIIC endosomal compartment and facilitates the removal of the invariant chain-derived CLIP peptide and the binding of other peptides to class II MHC molecules. HLA-DM is encoded by a gene in the MHC and is structurally similar to class II MHC molecules, but it is not polymorphic. Called H-2M in the mouse.

Homeostasis. In the adaptive immune system, the maintenance of a constant number and diverse repertoire of lymphocytes, despite the emergence of new lymphocytes and tremendous expansions of individual clones that may occur during responses to microbial antigens. Homeostasis is achieved by regulated pathways of lymphocyte death and inactivation.

Homing of lymphocytes. The directed migration of subsets of circulating lymphocytes into particular tissue sites. Lymphocyte homing is regulated by the selective expression of adhesion molecules, called homing receptors, on the lymphocytes and the tissue-specific expression of endothelial ligands for these homing receptors, called addressins, in different vascular beds. For example, some T lymphocytes preferentially home to intestinal lymphoid tissue (e.g., Peyer's patches), and this is regulated by binding of the $\alpha 4\beta 1$ integrin on the T cells to the MAdCAM ("mucosal addressin cell adhesion molecule") addressin on Peyer's patch endothelium.

Homing receptor. Adhesion molecules expressed on the surface of lymphocytes that are responsible for the different pathways of lymphocyte recirculation and tissue homing. Homing receptors bind to ligands (called addressins) expressed on endothelial cells in particular vascular beds.

Human immunodeficiency virus (HIV). The etiologic agent of acquired immunodeficiency disease (AIDS). HIV is a retrovirus that infects a variety of cell types, including CD4-expressing helper T cells, macrophages, and dendritic cells, and causes a chronic progressive destruction of the immune system.

Human leukocyte antigens (HLA). Major histocompatibility complex (MHC) molecules expressed on the surface of human cells. Human MHC molecules were first identified as alloantigens on the surface of white blood cells (leukocytes) that bound serum antibodies from individuals previously exposed to other individuals' cells (e.g., mothers or transfusion recipients).

Humanized antibody. A monoclonal antibody encoded by a recombinant hybrid gene and composed of the antigen-binding sites from a murine monoclonal antibody and the constant region of a human antibody. Humanized antibodies are less likely than mouse monoclonal antibodies to induce an anti-antibody response in humans; they are used clinically in the treatment of tumors and transplant rejection.

Humoral immunity. The type of adaptive immune response mediated by antibodies that are produced by B lymphocytes. Humoral immunity is the principal defense mechanism against extracellular microbes and their toxins.

Hybridoma. A cell line derived by cell fusion, or somatic cell hybridization, between a normal lymphocyte and an immortalized lymphocyte tumor line. B cell hybridomas, created by fusion of normal B cells of defined antigen specificity with a myeloma cell line, are used to produce monoclonal antibodies. T cell hybridomas, created by fusion of a normal T cell of defined specificity with a T cell tumor line, are commonly used in research.

Hyperacute rejection. A form of allograft or xenograft rejection that begins within minutes to hours after transplantation and is characterized by thrombotic occlusion of the graft vessels. Hyperacute rejection is mediated by preexisting antibodies in the host circulation that bind to donor endothelial antigens such as blood group antigens or major histocompatibility complex (MHC) molecules.

Hypersensitivity diseases. Disorders caused by immune responses. Hypersensitivity diseases include autoimmune diseases, in which immune responses are directed against self antigens, and diseases that result from uncontrolled or excessive responses against foreign antigens, such as microbes and allergens. The tissue damage that occurs in hypersensitivity diseases is the result of the same effector mechanisms used by the immune system to protect against microbes.

Hypervariable region. Short segments of about 10 amino acid residues within the variable regions of antibody or T cell receptor (TCR) proteins, which form loop structures that contact antigen. There are three hypervariable regions, also called **complementarity-determining regions,** in each antibody heavy chain and light chain and in each TCR α and β chain. Most of the variability between different antibodies or TCRs is located within these regions.

Idiotope. A unique determinant on an antibody or T cell receptor molecule, usually formed by one or more of the hypervariable regions. Idiotopes may be recognized as "foreign" in an individual because they are usually present in quantities too low to induce self-tolerance.

Idiotype. The unique structures present in the antigen-binding regions of the antibodies or T cell receptors produced by a single clone of lymphocytes. A theory, called the network hypothesis, postulates that a network of complementary interactions involving idiotypes and anti-idiotypes reach a steady state at which the immune system is at homeostasis and that antigen perturbs this steady state. The importance of such a network has not been established.

Igα and Igβ. Proteins that are required for surface expression and signaling functions of membrane immunoglobulin (Ig) on B cells. Igα and Igβ pairs are disulfide-linked to one another and noncovalently associated with the cytoplasmic tail of membrane Ig, forming the B cell receptor complex. The cytoplasmic domains of Igα and Igβ contain immunoreceptor tyrosine-based activation motifs (ITAMs) that are involved in early signaling events during antigen-induced B cell activation.

Immature B lymphocyte. A membrane IgM^+, IgD^- B cell, recently derived from marrow precursors, that does not proliferate or differentiate in response to antigens but rather may undergo apoptotic death or become functionally unresponsive. Immature B cells that are specific for self antigens present in the bone marrow are negatively selected by encounter with these antigens and do not complete their maturation.

Immediate hypersensitivity. The type of immune reaction responsible for allergic diseases and dependent on IgE plus antigen-mediated stimulation of tissue mast cells and basophils. The mast cells and basophils release mediators that cause increased vascular permeability, vasodilation, bronchial and visceral smooth muscle contraction, and inflammation.

Immune complex. A complex of one or more antibody molecules with bound antigen. Because each antibody molecule has a minimum of two antigen-binding sites and many antigens contain multiple epitopes, immune complexes can vary greatly in size. Immune complexes activate effector mechanisms of humoral immunity, such as the classical complement pathway and Fc receptor-mediated phagocyte activation. Deposition of circulating immune complexes in blood vessel walls, renal glomeruli, and joint synovia can lead to inflammation and disease.

Immune complex disease. An inflammatory disease caused by deposition of antigen-antibody complexes in blood vessel walls resulting in local complement activation and phagocyte recruitment. Immune complexes may form because of overproduction of antibodies to microbial antigens or because of autoantibody production in the setting of an autoimmune disease such as systemic lupus erythematosus. Immune complex deposition in arteries, kidney glomeruli, and joint synovia may cause vasculitis, glomerulonephritis, and arthritis, respectively.

Immune privileged site. A site in the body that is inaccessible to, or actively suppresses, immune responses. The anterior chamber of the eye, the testes, and the brain are examples of immune privileged sites.

Immune response. A collective and coordinated response to the introduction of foreign substances in an individual mediated by the cells and molecules of the immune system.

Immune surveillance. The concept that a physiologic function of the immune system is to recognize and destroy clones of transformed cells before they grow into tumors and to kill tumors after they are formed. This term is sometimes used in a general sense to describe the function of T lymphocytes in detecting and destroying any cell, not necessarily a tumor cell, that is expressing a foreign antigen (e.g., if it is infected with an intracellular microbe).

Immune system. The molecules, cells, tissues, and organs that collectively function to provide immunity, or protection, against infectious pathogens.

Immunodominant epitope. The portion of an antigen that is recognized by the majority of the lymphocytes specific for that antigen. For T cells, immunodominant epitopes correspond to the peptides generated within antigen-presenting cells that bind most avidly to MHC molecules and are most likely to stimulate T cells.

Immunofluorescence. A technique in which a molecule is detected using an antibody labeled with a fluorescent probe. For example, in immunofluorescence microscopy, cells that express a particular surface antigen can be stained with a fluorescein-conjugated antibody specific for the antigen and then visualized under a fluorescent microscope.

Immunogen. An antigen that induces an immune response. Not all antigens are immunogens. For example, small molecular weight compounds (haptens) may not stimulate an immune response unless they are linked to macromolecules.

Immunoglobulin. Synonymous with antibody (see **Antibody**).

Immunoglobulin (Ig) domain. A three-dimensional globular structural motif found in many proteins in the immune system, including immunoglobulins, T cell receptors, and major histocompatibility complex molecules. Ig domains are about 110 amino acid residues in length, include an internal disulfide bond, and contain two layers of β-pleated sheet, each layer composed of three to five strands of antiparallel polypeptide chain.

Immunoglobulin (Ig) superfamily. A large family of proteins that contain a globular structural motif called an immunoglobulin (Ig) domain, or Ig fold, originally described in antibodies. Many proteins of importance in the immune system are members of this superfamily, including antibodies, T cell receptors, major histocompatibility complex molecules, CD4, and CD8.

Immunoglobulin (Ig) heavy chain. One of two types of polypeptide chains that compose an antibody molecule. The basic structural unit of an antibody includes two identical, disulfide-linked heavy chains and two identical light chains. Each heavy chain is composed of a variable (V) Ig domain and three or four constant (C) Ig domains. The different antibody isotypes, including IgM, IgD, IgG, IgA, and IgE, are distinguished by structural differences in their heavy chain constant regions. The heavy chain constant regions also mediate effector functions, such as complement activation and engagement of phagocytes.

Immunoglobulin (Ig) light chain. One of two types of polypeptide chains that compose an antibody molecule. The basic structural unit of an antibody includes two identical light chains, each disulfide-linked to one of two identical heavy chains. Each light chain is composed of one variable (V) Ig domain and one constant (C) Ig domain. There are two light chain isotypes, called κ and λ, both functionally identical. About 60% of human antibodies have κ light chains and 40% have λ light chains.

Immunohistochemistry. A technique used to detect the presence of an antigen in histologic tissue sections using an enzyme-coupled antibody that is specific for the antigen. The enzyme converts a colorless substrate to a colored insoluble substance that precipitates at the site where the antibody, and thus the antigen, is localized. The position of the colored precipitate, and therefore the antigen, in the tissue section is observed by conventional light microscopy. Immunohistochemistry is a routine technique in diagnostic pathology and in various fields of research.

Immunoperoxidase. A common immunohistochemical technique in which a horseradish peroxidase–coupled antibody is used to identify the presence of an antigen in a tissue section. The peroxidase enzyme converts a colorless substrate to an insoluble brown product that is observable by light microscopy.

Immunoprecipitation. A technique for the isolation of a molecule from a solution by binding it to an antibody and then rendering the antigen-antibody complex insoluble, either by precipitation with a second anti-antibody or by coupling the first antibody to an insoluble particle or bead.

Immunoreceptor tyrosine-based activation motif (ITAM). A conserved motif composed of two copies of the sequence tyrosine-X-X-leucine (where X is an unspecified amino acid) found in the cytoplasmic tails of various membrane proteins in the immune system that are involved in signal transduction. ITAMs are present in the ζ and CD3 proteins of the T cell receptor complex, in the Igα and Igβ proteins in the B cell receptor complex, and in signaling subunits of several Ig receptors. When these receptors bind their ligands, the tyrosine residues of the ITAMs become phosphorylated, forming docking sites for other molecules involved in propagating cell-activating signal transduction pathways.

Immunoreceptor tyrosine-based inhibition motif (ITIM). A 6-amino acid (isoleucine-X-tyrosine-X-X-leucine) motif found in the cytoplasmic tails of various inhibitory receptors in the immune system, including FcγRIIB on B cells, and the killer inhibitory receptor on natural killer cells. When these receptors bind their ligands, the ITIMs become phosphorylated on their tyrosine residues, forming a docking site for protein tyrosine phosphatases, which in turn function to inhibit other signal transduction pathways.

Immunosuppression. Inhibition of one or more components of the adaptive or innate immune systems, owing to an underlying disease or intentionally induced by drugs for the purpose of preventing or treating graft rejection or autoimmune disease. A commonly used immunosuppressive drug is cyclosporine, which blocks T cell cytokine production.

Immunotherapy. The treatment of a disease using therapeutic agents that promote immune responses. Cancer immunotherapy, for example, involves promoting active immune responses to tumor antigens or administering antitumor antibodies or T cells to establish passive immunity.

Immunotoxins. Reagents that may be used in the treatment of cancer that consist of covalent conjugates of a potent cellular toxin, such as ricin or diphtheria toxin, with antibodies specific for antigens expressed on the surface of tumor cells. It is hoped that such reagents can specifically target and kill tumor cells without damaging normal cells, but safe and effective immunotoxins have yet to be developed.

Inbred mouse strain. A strain of mice created by repetitive mating of siblings, characterized by homozygosity at every genetic locus. Every mouse of an inbred strain is genetically identical (syngeneic) to every other mouse of the same strain.

Indirect antigen presentation. In transplantation immunology, a pathway of presentation of donor (allogeneic) major histocompatibility complex (MHC) molecules by recipient antigen-presenting cells (APCs) involving the same mechanisms used to present microbial proteins. The allogeneic MHC proteins are processed by recipient professional APCs, and peptides derived from the allogeneic MHC molecules are presented, in association with recipient (self) MHC molecules, to host T cells. This is in contrast to direct antigen presentation, which involves recipient T cell recognition of unprocessed allogeneic MHC molecules on the surface of graft cells.

Inflammation. A complex reaction of the innate immune system in vascularized tissues that involves accumulation and activation of leukocytes and plasma proteins at a site of infection, toxin exposure, or cell injury. Inflammation is initiated by changes in blood vessels that promote leukocyte recruitment. Local adaptive immune responses can promote inflammation. While inflammation serves a protective function in controlling infections and promoting tissue repair, it can also cause tissue damage and disease.

Inflammatory bowel disease (IBD). A group of disorders, including ulcerative colitis and Crohn's disease, characterized by chronic inflammation in the gastrointestinal tract. The etiology of IBD is not known, but there is evidence that immune mechanisms may be involved.

Gene knockout mice lacking IL-2, IL-10, or the T cell receptor α chain develop IBD.

Innate immunity. Protection against infections that relies on mechanisms that exist before infection, are capable of rapid responses to microbes, and react in essentially the same way to repeat infections. The innate immune system includes epithelial barriers; phagocytic cells (neutrophils, macrophages); natural killer cells; the complement system; and cytokines, largely made by mononuclear phagocytes, that regulate and coordinate many of the activities of the cells of innate immunity.

Insulin-dependent diabetes mellitus (IDDM). A disease characterized by a lack of insulin, which leads to various metabolic and vascular abnormalities. The insulin deficiency results from destruction of the insulin-producing β cells of the islets of Langerhans in the pancreas, usually a result of T cell–mediated autoimmunity.

Integrins. Heterodimeric cell surface proteins whose major functions are to mediate adhesion of leukocytes to other leukocytes, endothelial cells, and extracellular matrix proteins. Integrins are important for T cell interactions with antigen-presenting cells and for migration of leukocytes from blood into tissues. The ligand-binding affinity of the integrins can be regulated by various stimuli, and the cytoplasmic domains of integrins bind to the cytoskeleton. There are two subfamilies of integrins, and the members of each family express a conserved β chain (β1, or CD18, and β2, or CD29) associated with different α chains. VLA-4 is a β1 integrin expressed on T cells, and LFA-1 is a β2 integrin expressed on T cells and phagocytes.

Interferon-γ (IFN-γ). A cytokine produced by T lymphocytes and natural killer cells whose principal function is to activate macrophages in both innate immune responses and adaptive cell-mediated immune responses. (In the past, IFN-γ was also called immune or type II interferon.)

Interleukin. Another name for a cytokine, originally used to describe a cytokine made by leukocytes, that acts on leukocytes. It is now generally used with a numerical suffix to designate a structurally defined cytokine regardless of source or target.

Interleukin-1 (IL-1). A cytokine produced mainly by activated mononuclear phagocytes whose principal function is to mediate host inflammatory responses in innate immunity. There are two forms of IL-1 (α and β) that bind to the same receptors and have identical biologic effects, including induction of endothelial cell adhesion molecules, stimulation of chemokine production by endothelial cells and macrophages, stimulation of synthesis of acute-phase reactants by the liver, and fever.

Interleukin-10 (IL-10). A cytokine produced by activated macrophages and some helper T cells whose major function is to inhibit activated macrophages and therefore maintain homeostatic control of innate and cell-mediated immune reactions.

Interleukin-12 (IL-12). A cytokine produced by mononuclear phagocytes and dendritic cells that serves as a mediator of the innate immune response to intracellular microbes and is a key inducer of cell-mediated immune responses to these microbes. IL-12 activates natural killer (NK) cells, promotes interferon-γ production by NK cells and T cells, enhances cytolytic activity of NK cells and cytolytic T lymphocytes, and promotes the development of T_H1 cells.

Interleukin-15 (IL-15). A cytokine produced by mononuclear phagocytes and other cells in response to viral infections whose principal function is to stimulate the proliferation of natural killer cells. It is structurally similar to interleukin-2.

Interleukin-18 (IL-18). A cytokine produced by macrophages in response to LPS and other microbial products, which functions together with IL-12 as an inducer of cell-mediated immunity. IL-18 synergizes with interleukin-12 in stimulating the production of IFN-γ by natural killer cells and T cells. IL-18 is structurally homologous to, but is functionally very different from, IL-1.

Interleukin-2 (IL-2). A cytokine produced by antigen-activated T cells that acts in an autocrine manner to stimulate T cell proliferation and also potentiates apoptotic cell death of antigen-activated T cells. Thus, IL-2 is required for both the induction and regulation of T cell–mediated immune responses. IL-2 also stimulates proliferation and differentiation of natural killer cells and B cells.

Interleukin-3 (IL-3). A cytokine produced by CD4$^+$ T cells that promotes the expansion of immature marrow progenitors of all blood cells. IL-3 is also known as multilineage colony-stimulating factor (multi-CSF).

Interleukin-4 (IL-4). A cytokine produced mainly by the T_H2 subset of CD4$^+$ helper T cells whose functions include inducing differentiation of T_H2 cells from naive CD4$^+$ precursors, stimulation of IgE production by B cells, and suppression of interferon-γ–dependent macrophage functions.

Interleukin-5 (IL-5). A cytokine produced by CD4$^+$ T_H2 cells and activated mast cells, which stimulates the growth and differentiation of eosinophils and activates mature eosinophils.

Interleukin-6 (IL-6). A cytokine produced by many cell types including activated mononuclear phagocytes, endothelial cells, and fibroblasts, which functions in both innate and adaptive immunity. IL-6 stimulates the synthesis of acute phase proteins by hepatocytes and stimulates the growth of antibody-producing B lymphocytes.

Interleukin-7 (IL-7). A cytokine secreted by bone marrow stromal cells that stimulates survival and expansion of immature precursors of B and T lymphocytes.

Intracellular bacterium. A bacterium that survives and replicates within cells, usually in phagolysosomes. The principal defense against intracellular bacteria, such as *Mycobacterium tuberculosis*, is cell-mediated immunity.

Intraepidermal lymphocyte. T lymphocytes found within the epidermal layer of the skin. In the mouse, most of the intraepidermal T cells express the $\gamma\delta$ form of T cell receptor. (See **Intraepithelial T lymphocytes.**)

Intraepithelial T lymphocytes. T lymphocytes that are present in the epidermis of the skin and in mucosal epithelia that typically express a very limited diversity of antigen receptors. Some of these lymphocytes may recognize microbial products, such as glycolipids, associated with nonpolymorphic class I major histocompatibility complex–like molecules. Intraepithelial T lymphocytes may be considered effector cells of innate immunity and function in host defense by secreting cytokines and activating phagocytes and by killing infected cells.

Invariant chain (I$_i$). A nonpolymorphic protein that binds to newly synthesized class II major histocompatibility complex (MHC) molecules in the endoplasmic reticulum (ER). The invariant chain prevents loading of the class II MHC peptide-binding cleft with peptides present in the ER, leaving such peptides to bind to class I molecules. The invariant chain also promotes folding and assembly of class II molecules and directs newly formed class II molecules to the specialized endosomal MIIC compartment where peptide loading takes place.

Isotype. A type of antibody determined by which of five different forms of heavy chain are present. Antibody isotypes include IgM, IgD, IgG, IgA, and IgE, and each isotype performs a different set of effector functions. Additional structural variations characterize distinct subtypes of IgG and IgA.

J chain. A protein produced in mature B cells that binds to secreted forms of IgM and IgA molecules and brings together five or two of these molecules, respectively. (Not to be confused with the J segment of antigen-receptor genes.)

Joining (J) segments. Short coding sequences, between the variable (V) and constant (C) gene segments in all the immunoglobulin and T cell receptor loci, which together with D segments are somatically recombined with V segments during lymphocyte development. The resulting recombined V(D)J DNA codes for antigen receptor V regions.

Junctional diversity. The diversity in the antibody and T cell receptor repertoires that is attributed to the random addition or the removal of nucleotide sequences at junctions between V, D, and J gene segments.

Killer inhibitory receptor (KIRs). Receptors on natural killer cells that recognize self class I MHC molecules and deliver inhibitory signals that prevent activation of NK cell cytolytic mechanisms. These receptors ensure that NK cells do not kill normal host cells, which express class I MHC molecules, while permitting lysis of virus-infected cells in which class I MHC expression is suppressed. Several classes of inhibitory receptors have been described, including immunoglobulin superfamily members, heterodimers of CD94 and a lectin and Ly49. All of these receptors contain cytoplasmic tails with immunoreceptor tyrosine inhibition motifs (ITIMs) that are involved in initiating inhibitory signal pathways.

Kinase (protein kinase). An enzyme that adds phosphate groups to the side chains of certain amino acid residues of proteins. Protein kinases in lymphocytes, such as Lck, are involved in signal transduction and the activation of transcription factors. Most protein kinases are specific for tyrosine residues.

Knockout mice. Mice with a targeted disruption of one or more genes, created by homologous recombination techniques. Knockout mice lacking functional genes encoding cytokines, cell surface receptors, signaling molecules, and transcription factors have provided extensive information about the roles of these molecules in the immune system.

Langerhans cell. Immature dendritic cells found as a continuous meshwork in the epidermal layer of the skin, whose major function is to trap and transport protein antigens to draining lymph nodes. During their migration to the lymph nodes, Langerhans cells mature into lymph node dendritic cells that can efficiently process and present antigen to naive T cells.

Large granular lymphocyte (LGL). Another name for a natural killer (NK) cell based on the morphologic appearance of this cell type in the blood.

Late phase reaction. A component of the immediate hypersensitivity reaction that ensues several hours after mast cell and basophil degranulation and is characterized by an inflammatory infiltrate of eosinophils, basophils, neutrophils, and lymphocytes. Repeated bouts of late phase reactions can cause tissue damage.

Lck. An Src family nonreceptor tyrosine kinase that noncovalently associates with the cytoplasmic tails of CD4 and CD8 molecules in T cells and is involved in the early signaling events of antigen-induced T cell activation. Lck mediates tyrosine phosphorylation of the cytoplasmic tails of CD3 and ζ proteins of the T cell receptor complex.

Lectin pathway of complement activation. A pathway of complement activation triggered, in the absence of antibody, by the binding of microbial polysaccharides to circulating lectins like plasma mannose-binding lectin (MBL). MBL is structurally similar to C1q and activates the C1r-C1s enzyme complex (like C1q) or activates another serine esterase, called mannose-binding protein–associated serine esterase. The remaining steps of the lectin pathway, beginning with cleavage of C4, are the same as the classical pathway.

Leishmania. An obligate intracellular protozoan parasite that infects macrophages and can cause a chronic inflammatory disease involving many tissues. *Leishmania* infection in mice has served as a model system for the study of the effector functions of several cytokines and the helper T cell subsets that produce them. T_H1 responses to *Leishmania major* and associated interferon-γ production control infection, whereas T_H2 responses with IL-4 production lead to disseminated lethal disease.

Leukemia. A malignancy of bone marrow precursors of blood cells. Large numbers of leukemic cells usually occupy the bone marrow and often circulate in the blood stream. Lymphocytic leukemias are derived from B or T cell precursors, myelogenous leukemias are derived from granulocyte or monocyte precursors, and erythroid leukemias are derived from red blood cell precursors.

Leukocyte adhesion deficiency (LAD). A rare group of immunodeficiency diseases caused by defective expression of leukocyte adhesion molecules required for tissue recruitment of phagocytes and lymphocytes. LAD I is due to mutations in the gene encoding the CD18 protein, which is part of β_2 integrins. LAD II is caused by mutations in a gene that encodes an enzyme involved in the synthesis of leukocyte ligands for endothelial selectins.

Leukotrienes. A class of arachidonic acid–derived lipid inflammatory mediators produced by the lipoxygenase pathway in many cell types. Mast cells make abundant leukotriene C_4 (LTC_4) and its degradation products LTD_4 and LTE_4, which bind to specific receptors on smooth muscle cells and cause prolonged bronchoconstriction. Leukotrienes contribute to the pathology of bronchial asthma. Collectively, LTC_4, LTD_4, and LTE_4 constitute what was once called "slow-reacting substance of anaphylaxis."

Lipopolysaccharide (LPS). Synonymous with **endotoxin.**

Lymph node. Small nodular, encapsulated aggregates of lymphocyte-rich tissue situated along lymphatic channels throughout the body, where adaptive immune responses to lymph-borne antigens are initiated.

Lymphatic system. A system of vessels throughout the body that collects tissue fluid called lymph, originally derived from the blood, and returns it, via the thoracic duct, to the circulation. Lymph nodes are interspersed along these vessels and trap and retain antigens present in the lymph.

Lymphocyte. A cell type found in the blood, lymphoid tissues, and virtually all organs, that expresses receptors for antigens and mediates immune responses. Lymphocytes include B and T cells (the cells of adaptive immunity and natural killer (NK) cells (mediators of some innate immune responses).

Lymphoid follicle. A B cell–rich region of a peripheral lymphoid organ, such as a lymph node or the spleen, that is the site of antigen-induced B cell proliferation and differentiation. In T cell–dependent B cell responses to protein antigens, a germinal center forms within the follicles.

Lymphokine. An old name for cytokines produced by T lymphocytes. It is now known that the same cytokines may be produced by other cell types.

Lymphokine activated killer (LAK) cell. Natural killer cells with enhanced cytolytic activity for tumor cells as a result of exposure to high doses of interleukin-2. LAK cells generated *in vitro* have been adoptively transferred back into cancer patients to treat their tumors.

Lymphoma. A malignant tumor of B or T lymphocytes, arising in and spreading between lymphoid tissues. Lymphomas often express phenotypic characteristics of the normal lymphocytes from which they were derived.

Lymphotoxin (LT, TNF-β). A cytokine produced by T cells, which is homologous to, and binds to the same receptors as, tumor necrosis factor (TNF). Like TNF, LT has proinflammatory effects, including endothelial and neutrophil activation. LT is also critical for the normal development of lymphoid organs.

Lysosome. A membrane-bound, acidic organelle abundant in phagocytic cells, which contains proteolytic enzymes that degrade proteins derived mainly from the extracellular environment. Lysosomes are involved in the class II major histocompatibility complex (MHC) pathway of antigen processing.

Macrophage. A tissue-based phagocytic cell derived from blood monocytes, which plays important roles in innate and adaptive immune responses. Macrophages are activated by microbial products, such as endotoxin, by molecules such as CD40 ligand, and by T cell cytokines such as interferon-γ. Activated macrophages phagocytose and kill microorganisms, secrete proinflammatory cytokines, and present antigens to helper T cells. Macrophages may assume different morphologic forms in different tissues, including the microglia of the central nervous system, Kupffer cells in the liver, alveolar macrophages in the lung, and osteoclasts in bone.

Major histocompatibility complex (MHC). A large genetic locus (on human chromosome 6 and mouse chromosome 17) that includes the highly polymorphic genes encoding the peptide-binding molecules recognized by T lymphocytes. The MHC locus also includes genes encoding cytokines, molecules involved in antigen processing, and complement proteins.

Major histocompatibility complex (MHC) molecule. A heterodimeric membrane protein encoded in the major histocompatibility complex (MHC) locus that serves as a peptide display molecule for recognition by T lymphocytes. Two structurally distinct types of MHC molecules exist. Class I MHC molecules are present on nucleated cells, bind peptides derived from cytosolic proteins, and are recognized by CD8+ T cells. Class II MHC molecules are restricted largely to professional antigen-presenting cells, macrophages, and B lymphocytes, bind peptides derived from endocytosed proteins, and are recognized by CD4+ T cells.

Mannose receptor. A carbohydrate-binding receptor (lectin) expressed by macrophages that binds mannose and fucose residues on microbial cell walls and mediates phagocytosis of the organisms.

Marginal zone. A peripheral region of splenic lymphoid follicles that contains macrophages that are particularly efficient at trapping polysaccharide antigens. Such antigens may either persist for prolonged periods on the surfaces of marginal zone macrophages, where they are recognized by specific B cells, or they may be transported into follicles.

Mast cell. The major effector cell of immediate hypersensitivity (allergic) reactions. Mast cells are derived from bone marrow precursors, reside in tissues adjacent to blood vessels, express a high-affinity Fc receptor for IgE, and contain numerous mediator-filled granules. Antigen-induced cross-linking of IgE bound to the mast cell Fc receptors causes release of their granule contents as well as synthesis and secretion of other mediators, and this leads to the immediate hypersensitivity reaction.

Maturation of lymphocytes. The process by which pluripotent bone marrow precursor cells develop into mature antigen receptor expressing naive B or T lymphocytes that populate peripheral lymphoid tissues. This process takes place in the specialized environments of the bone marrow (for B cells) and the thymus (for T cells).

Mature B cell. IgM and IgD expressing functionally competent naive B cells that represent the final stage of B cell maturation in the bone marrow and that populate peripheral lymphoid organs.

Membrane attack complex (MAC). A lytic complex of the terminal components of the complement cascade, including multiple copies of C9, which forms in the membranes of target cells on which complement is activated. The MAC causes lethal ionic and osmotic changes of cells.

Memory. The ability of the adaptive immune system to mount more rapid, larger, and more effective responses to repeat encounters with the same antigen.

Memory lymphocytes. B or T lymphocytes that mediate rapid and enhanced (i.e., memory) responses to second and subsequent exposures to antigens. Memory B and T cells are produced by antigen stimulation of naive lymphocytes and survive in a functionally quiescent state for many years after the antigen is eliminated.

MHC restriction. The characteristic of T lymphocytes that they recognize a foreign peptide antigen only when it is bound to a particular allelic form of a major histocompatibility complex molecule.

β_2-Microglobulin. The light chain of a class I major histocompatibility (MHC) molecule. β_2-Microglobulin is an extracellular protein encoded by a nonpolymorphic gene outside the MHC complex and is structurally homologous to an Ig domain and is invariant among all class I molecules.

Migration of lymphocyte. The movement of lymphocytes from the blood stream into tissues.

Mitogen-activated protein (MAP) kinase cascade. A signal transduction cascade initiated by the active form of the Ras protein and involving the sequential activation of three serine/threonine kinases, the last one being the MAP kinase. MAP kinase, in turn, phosphorylates and activates other enzymes or transcription factors. The MAP kinase pathway is one of several signal pathways activated by antigen binding to the T cell receptor.

Mixed leukocyte reaction (MLR). An *in vitro* reaction of alloreactive T cells from one individual against major histocompatibility complex antigens on blood cells from another individual. The MLR involves proliferation of and cytokine secretion by both CD4$^+$ and CD8$^+$ T cells and is used as a screening test to assess the compatibility of a potential graft recipient with a potential donor.

Molecular mimicry. A postulated mechanism of autoimmunity, which is triggered by infection with a microbe that contains antigens that cross-react with self antigens, so that immune responses to the microbe result in reactions against self tissues.

Monoclonal antibody. An antibody that is specific for one antigen and is produced by a B cell hybridoma (a cell line derived by the fusion of a single normal B cell and an immortal B cell tumor line). Monoclonal antibodies are widely employed in research and clinical diagnosis and therapy.

Monocyte. A type of bone marrow–derived circulating blood cell that is the precursor of tissue macrophages. Monocytes are actively recruited into inflammatory sites, where they differentiate into macrophages.

Monocyte colony-stimulating factor (M-CSF). A cytokine made by activated T cells, macrophages, endothelial cells, and bone marrow stromal fibroblasts that stimulates the production of monocytes from bone marrow precursor cells.

Monokines. An old name for cytokines produced by mononuclear phagocytes. It is now known that the same cytokines are produced by many cell types.

Mononuclear phagocytes. Cells with a common bone marrow lineage whose primary function is phagocytosis. These cells function as antigen-presenting cells in the recognition and activation phases of adaptive immune responses and as effector cells in innate and adaptive immunity. Mononuclear phagocytes circulate in the blood in an incompletely differentiated form called monocytes, and once they settle in tissues they mature into cells called macrophages.

Mucosal immune system. A part of the immune system that responds to and protects against microbes that enter the body through mucosal surfaces, such as the gastrointestinal and respiratory tracts. The mucosal immune system is composed of collections of lymphocytes and antigen-presenting cells in the epithelia and lamina propria of mucosal surfaces. The mucosal immune system includes intraepithelial lymphocytes, mainly T cells, and organized collections of lymphocytes, often rich in B cells, below mucosal epithelia, such as Peyer's patches in the gut or tonsils in the pharynx.

Mucosal immunity. The form of protective immunity that acts at mucosal surfaces of the gastrointestinal and respiratory tracts to prevent colonization by ingested and inhaled microbes. The secretion of IgA antibody is an important component of mucosal immunity.

Multiple myeloma. A malignant tumor of antibody-producing B cells that often secretes an immunoglobulin or part of an immunoglobulin molecule. The monoclonal antibodies produced by multiple myelomas were critical for the early biochemical analyses of antibody structure.

Multivalency. The presence of multiple identical copies of an epitope on a single antigen molecule, cell surface, or particle. Multivalent antigens, such as bacterial capsular polysaccharides, are often capable of activating B lymphocytes independent of helper T cells.

Mycobacteria. A genus of bacteria, many species of which can survive within phagocytes and cause disease. The principal host defense against mycobacteria, such as *Mycobacterium tuberculosis*, is cell-mediated immunity.

Naive lymphocyte. A mature B or T lymphocyte that has not previously encountered antigen nor is the progeny of an antigen-stimulated mature lymphocyte. When naive lymphocytes are stimulated by antigen, they differentiate into effector lymphocytes, such as antibody-secreting B cells or effector T lymphocytes. Naive lymphocytes have surface markers and recirculation patterns that are distinct from those of previously activated lymphocytes.

Natural antibodies. IgM antibodies, largely produced by B-1 cells, specific for bacteria that are common in the environment. Normal individuals contain natural antibodies without any evidence of infection, and these antibodies serve as a preformed defense mechanism against microbes that succeed in penetrating epithelial barriers. Some of these antibodies cross-react with ABO blood group antigens and are responsible for transfusion reactions.

Natural killer (NK) cells. A subset of bone marrow–derived lymphocytes, distinct from B and T cells, that function in innate immune responses to kill microbe-infected cells and to activate phagocytes by secreting interferon-γ. NK cells do not express clonally distributed antigen receptors like immunoglobulin or T cell receptors, and their activation is regulated by a combination of cell surface stimulatory and inhibitory receptors, the latter recognizing self MHC molecules.

Negative selection. The process by which developing lymphocytes that express antigen receptors specific for self antigens are eliminated, thereby contributing to the maintenance of self-tolerance. Negative selection of developing T lymphocytes (thymocytes) is best understood and involves high-avidity binding of an immature T cell to self MHC molecules with bound self peptides on thymic antigen-presenting cells, leading to apoptotic death of the T cell.

Neonatal immunity. Passive humoral immunity to infections in mammals in the first months of life, prior to full development of the immune system. Neonatal immunity is mediated by maternally produced antibodies, which are transported across the placenta into the fetal circulation before birth or are derived from ingested milk and transported across the gut epithelium.

Neutrophil. The most abundant circulating white blood cell, also called a **polymorphonuclear leukocyte (PMN),** which is recruited to inflammatory sites and is capable of phagocytosing and enzymatically digesting microbes.

Nitric oxide. A biologic effector molecule with a broad range of activities that, in macrophages, functions as a potent microbicidal agent that kills ingested organisms. Production of nitric oxide (NO) is dependent on an enzyme called NO synthase, which converts L-arginine into NO. Macrophages express an inducible form of NO synthase on activation by various microbial or cytokine stimuli.

N-nucleotides. The name given to nucleotides randomly added to the junctions between V, D, and J gene segments in immunoglobulin or T cell receptor (TCR) genes during lymphocyte development. The addition of up to 20 of these nucleotides, which is mediated by the enzyme terminal deoxyribonucleotidyl transferase, contributes to the diversity of the antibody and TCR repertoires.

Nuclear factor of activated T cells (NFAT). A transcription factor required for the expression of IL-2, IL-4, TNF, and other cytokine genes. There are four different NFATs, each encoded by a separate gene; NFAT1 and NFAT4 are found in T cells. Cytoplasmic NFAT is activated by Ca^{2+}-calmodulin–dependent, calcineurin-mediated dephosphorylation that permits NFAT to translocate into the nucleus and bind to consensus-binding sequences in the regulatory regions of IL-2, IL-4, and other cytokine genes, usually in association with other transcription factors, such as AP-1.

Nuclear factor κB (NF-κB). A family of transcription factors composed of homodimers or heterodimers of proteins homologous to the c-Rel protein. NF-κB proteins are important in the transcription of many genes in both innate and adaptive immune responses.

Oncofetal antigen. Proteins that are expressed at high levels on some types of cancer cells and in normal developing (fetal) but not adult tissues. Antibodies specific for these proteins are often used in histopathologic identification of tumors or to follow the progression of tumor growth in patients. Carcinoembryonic antigen (CEA, CD66) and α-fetoprotein (AFP) are two oncofetal antigens that are commonly expressed by certain carcinomas.

Opsonin. A macromolecule that becomes attached to the surface of a microbe that can be recognized by surface receptors of neutrophils and macrophages and that increases the efficiency of phagocytosis of the microbe. Opsonins include IgG antibodies, which are recognized by Fcγ receptors on phagocytes, and fragments of complement proteins, which are recognized by the type 1 complement receptor (CR1, CD35) and by the leukocyte integrin Mac-1.

Opsonization. The process of attaching opsonins, such as IgG or complement fragments, to microbial surfaces to target the microbes for phagocytosis.

Oral tolerance. The suppression of systemic humoral and cell-mediated immune responses to an antigen after the oral administration of that antigen, due to anergy of antigen-specific T cells or the production of immunosuppressive cytokines such as transforming growth factor-β. Oral tolerance is a possible mechanism for preventing immune responses to food antigens and to bacteria that normally reside as commensals in the intestinal lumen.

Passive immunity. The form of immunity to an antigen that is established in one individual by transfer of antibodies or lymphocytes from another individual who is immune to that antigen. The recipient of such a transfer can become immune to the antigen without ever having been exposed to or having responded to the antigen. An example of passive immunity is the transfer of human sera containing antibodies specific for certain microbial toxins or snake venoms to a previously unimmunized individual.

Pathogenicity. The ability of a microorganism to cause disease. Multiple mechanisms may contribute to pathogenicity, including production of toxins, the stimulation of host inflammatory responses, and the perturbation of host cell metabolism.

Pattern recognition receptors. Receptors of the innate immune system that recognize frequently encountered structures called "molecular patterns" produced by microorganisms and that facilitate innate immune responses against the microorganisms. Examples of pattern recognition receptors of phagocytes include CD14 and Toll-like receptors, which bind bacterial endotoxin, and the mannose receptor, which binds microbial glycoproteins or glycolipids with terminal mannose residues.

Pentraxins. A family of plasma proteins that contain five identical globular subunits; includes the acute phase reactant C-reactive protein.

Peptide-binding cleft. The portion of a major histocompatibility complex (MHC) molecule that binds peptides for display to T cells. The cleft is composed of paired α-helices resting upon a floor made up of an eight-stranded β-pleated sheet. The polymorphic residues, which are the amino acids that vary among different MHC alleles, are located in and around this cleft.

Perforin. A pore-forming protein, homologous to the C9 complement protein, that is present as a monomer in the granules of cytolytic T lymphocytes (CTLs) and natural killer (NK) cells. When perforin monomers are released from granules of activated CTLs or NK cells, they undergo polymerization in the lipid bilayer of the target cell plasma membrane, forming a large aqueous channel. This pore can serve as a channel for influx of enzymes derived from the CTL granules.

Periarteriolar lymphoid sheath (PALS). A cuff of lymphocytes surrounding small arterioles in the spleen, which contains mainly T lymphocytes, about two thirds of which are CD4$^+$ and one third of which are CD8$^+$.

Peripheral lymphoid organs/tissues. Organized collections of lymphocytes and accessory cells, including the spleen, lymph node, and mucosa-associated lymphoid tissues, where adaptive immune responses are initiated.

Peripheral tolerance. Physiologic unresponsiveness to self antigens that are present in peripheral tissues and usually not in the generative lymphoid organs. Peripheral tolerance is induced by the recognition of the antigens without adequate levels of the costimulators that are required for lymphocyte activation or by persistent and repeated stimulation by these self antigens.

Peyer's patches. Organized lymphoid tissues in the lamina propria of the small intestine where immune responses to ingested antigens may be initiated. Peyer's patches are composed mostly of B cells, with smaller numbers of T cells and antigen-presenting cells, all arranged in follicles similar to those found in lymph nodes, often with germinal centers.

Phagocytosis. The process by which certain cells of the innate immune system, including macrophages and neutrophils, engulf large particles (>0.5 μm in diameter) such as intact microbes. The cell surrounds the particle with extensions of its plasma membrane by an energy- and cytoskeleton-dependent process, leading to formation of an intracellular vesicle called a phagosome, which contains the ingested particle.

Phagosome. A membrane-bound intracellular vesicle that contains microbes or particulate material from the extracellular environment. Phagosomes are formed during the process of phagocytosis and fuse with other vesicular structures such as lysosomes, leading to the enzymatic degradation of the ingested material.

Phosphatase (protein phosphatase). An enzyme that removes phosphate groups from the side chains of certain amino acid residues of proteins. Protein phosphatases in lymphocytes, such as CD45 or calcineurin, regulate the activity of various signal transduction molecules and transcription factors. Some protein phosphatases may be specific for phosphotyrosine residues and others for phosphoserine and phosphothreonine residues.

Phospholipase C (PLCγ1). An enzyme that catalyzes the hydrolysis of the plasma membrane phospholipid phosphatidylinositol 4,5-bisphosphate (PIP$_2$), generating two signaling molecules, inositol 1,4,5-trisphosphate (IP_3) and diacylglycerol (DAG). PLCγ1 becomes activated in lymphocytes by antigen binding to the antigen receptor.

Phytohemagglutinin (PHA). A polymeric carbohydrate-binding protein, or lectin, produced by plants, that crosslinks human T cell surface molecules, including the T cell receptor, thereby inducing activation and agglutination of T cells. Because PHA activates all T cells, regardless of antigen specificity, it is called a **polyclonal activator.** In clinical medicine, PHA is used to assess if a patient's T cells are functional or to induce T cell mitosis for the purpose of producing chromosomal spreads for karyotyping.

Plasma cell. A terminally differentiated antibody-secreting B lymphocyte with a characteristic histologic appearance, including oval shape, eccentric nucleus, and a perinuclear halo.

Pluripotent stem cell. An undifferentiated bone marrow cell that divides continuously and gives rise to additional stem cells and to cells of multiple different lineages. A hematopoietic stem cell in the bone marrow will give rise to cells of lymphoid, myeloid, and erythrocytic lineages.

Polyclonal activators. Agents that are capable of activating many clones of lymphocytes, regardless of their antigen specificities. Examples of polyclonal activators include anti-IgM antibodies for B cells and anti-CD3 antibodies and phytohemagglutinin for T cells.

Poly-Ig receptor. An Fc receptor expressed by mucosal epithelial cells that mediates the transport of IgA and IgM through the epithelial cells into the intestinal lumen. (Also called secretory component.)

Polymorphism. The existence of two or more alternative forms, or variants, of a particular gene, which are present at stable frequencies in a population. Each common variant of a polymorphic gene is called an **allele,** and one individual may carry two different alleles of a gene, each inherited from a different parent. The major histocompatibility complex genes are the most polymorphic genes in the mammalian genome.

Polymorphonuclear leukocyte (PMN). A phagocytic cell, also called a **neutrophil,** characterized by a segmented multilobed nucleus and cytoplasmic granules filled with degradative enzymes. PMNs are the most abundant type of circulating white blood cells and are the major cell type mediating acute inflammatory responses to bacterial infections.

Polyvalency. See Multivalency.

Positive selection. The process by which developing T cells in the thymus (thymocytes) whose antigen receptors bind to self major histocompatibility complex (MHC) molecules are rescued from programmed cell death while thymocytes whose receptors do not recognize self MHC molecules die by default. Positive selection ensures that mature T cells are self MHC restricted and that CD8$^+$ T cells are specific for complexes of peptides with class I MHC molecules and CD4$^+$ T cells for complexes of peptides with class II MHC molecules.

Pre-B cell. A developing B cell present only in hematopoietic tissues at a maturational stage characterized by expression of cytoplasmic immunoglobulin (Ig) μ heavy chains but not Ig light chains. Pre-B cell receptors composed of μ chains and surrogate light chains deliver signals that stimulate further maturation of the pre-B cell into an immature B cell.

Pre-B cell receptor. A receptor expressed on maturing B lymphocytes at the pre-B cell stage composed of an immunoglobulin (Ig) μ heavy chain and an invariant surrogate light chain. The surrogate light chain is composed of two proteins, including the λ5 protein that is homologous to λ light chain C domain and the V pre-B protein that is homologous to a V domain. The pre-B cell receptor associates with the Igα and Igβ signal transduction proteins to form the pre-B cell receptor complex. Pre-B cell receptors are required for stimulating the proliferation and continued maturation of the developing B cell. It is not known if the pre-B cell receptor binds a specific ligand.

Pre-T cell. A developing T lymphocyte in the thymus at a maturational stage characterized by expression of the T cell receptor (TCR) β chain, but not the α chain, nor CD4 or CD8. In pre-T cells, the TCR β chain is found on the cell surface as part of the pre-T cell receptor.

Pre-T cell receptor. A receptor expressed on the surface of pre-T cells, composed of the T cell receptor (TCR) β chain and an invariant pre-Tα protein. This receptor associates with the CD3 and ζ molecules, forming the pre-T cell receptor complex. The function of this complex is similar to that of the pre-B cell receptor in B cell development, namely, the delivery of signals that stimulate further proliferation, antigen receptor gene rearrangements, and maturation. It is not known if the pre-T cell receptor binds a specific ligand.

Primary immune response. An adaptive immune response that occurs after the first exposure of an individual to a foreign antigen. Primary responses are characterized by relatively slow kinetics and small magnitude, compared with responses after a second or subsequent exposure.

Primary immunodeficiency. A genetic defect that results in a deficiency in some component of the innate or adaptive immune systems, leading to an increased susceptibility to infections that is frequently manifested early in infancy and childhood but is sometimes clinically detected later in life.

Pro-B cell. A developing B cell in the bone marrow that is the earliest cell committed to the B lymphocyte lineage. Pro-B cells do not produce immunoglobulin, but they can be distinguished from other immature cells by the expression of B-lineage–restricted surface molecules such as CD19 and CD10.

Professional antigen-presenting cells. Antigen-presenting cells for T lymphocytes that are capable of displaying peptides bound to major histocompatibility complex molecules and expressing costimulators. The most important professional APCs for initiating primary T cell responses are dendritic cells.

Programmed cell death. A pathway of cell death by apoptosis, which occurs in lymphocytes deprived of necessary survival stimuli, such as growth factors or costimulators. Programmed cell death, also called "death by neglect," is characterized by release of mitochondrial cytochrome *c* into the cytoplasm, activation of caspase-9, and initiation of the apoptotic pathway.

Prostaglandins. A class of lipid inflammatory mediators derived from arachidonic acid in many cell types via the cyclooxygenase pathway. Activated mast cells make prostaglandin D_2 (PGD$_2$), which binds to receptors on smooth muscle cells and acts as a vasodilator and as a bronchoconstrictor. PGD$_2$ also promotes neutrophil chemotaxis and accumulation at inflammatory sites.

Pro-T cell. A developing T cell in the thymic cortex that is a recent arrival from the bone marrow and does not express T cell receptors, CD3, or ζ chains, nor CD4 or CD8 molecules. Pro-T cells are also called double-negative thymocytes.

Proteasome. A large multiprotein enzyme complex with a broad range of proteolytic activity, which is found in the cytoplasm of most cells and which generates from cytosolic proteins the peptides that bind to class I major histocompatibility complex molecules. Proteins are targeted for proteasomal degradation by covalent linkage of ubiquitin molecules.

Protein kinase C (PKC). Any of several isoforms of an enzyme that mediates the phosphorylation of serine and threonine residues in many different protein substrates and thereby serves to propagate various signal transduction pathways leading to transcription factor activation. In T and B lymphocytes, PKC is activated by diacylglycerol, which is generated in response to antigen receptor ligation.

Protein tyrosine kinase (PTK). See Kinase.

Protozoa. Complex single-celled eukaryotic organisms, many of which are human parasites and cause diseases.

Examples of pathogenic protozoa include *Entamoeba histolytica*, causing amebic dysentery; *Plasmodium*, causing malaria; and *Leishmania* causing leishmaniasis. Protozoa stimulate both innate and adaptive immune responses.

Provirus. A DNA copy of the genome of a retrovirus, which is integrated into the host cell genome, and from which viral genes are transcribed and the viral genome is reproduced. Human immunodeficiency virus (HIV) proviruses can remain inactive for long periods of time and thereby represent a latent form of HIV infection that is not accessible to immune defense.

Purified antigen (subunit) vaccine. Vaccines composed of purified antigens or subunits of microbes. Examples of this type of vaccine include diphtheria and tetanus toxoids, *Pneumococcus* and *Haemophilus influenzae* polysaccharide vaccines, and purified polypeptide vaccines against hepatitis B and influenza virus. Purified antigen vaccines may stimulate antibody and helper T cell responses, but they do not generate cytolytic T lymphocyte responses.

Pyogenic bacteria. Bacteria, such as the gram-positive staphylococci and streptococci, that induce inflammatory responses rich in polymorphonuclear leukocytes (giving rise to pus). Antibody responses to these bacteria greatly enhance the efficacy of innate immune effector mechanisms to clear infections.

Radioimmunoassay (RIA). A highly sensitive and specific immunologic method for quantifying the concentration of an antigen in a solution, which relies on a radioactively labeled antibody specific for the antigen. Usually, two antibodies specific for the antigen are employed. The first antibody is unlabeled but attached to a solid support where it binds and immobilizes the antigen whose concentration is being determined. The amount of the second, labeled antibody that binds to the immobilized antigen, determined by radioactive-decay detectors, is proportional to the concentration of antigen in the test solution.

Reactive oxygen intermediates (ROIs). Highly reactive metabolites of oxygen, including superoxide anion, hydroxyl radical, and hydrogen peroxide, which are produced by activated phagocytes. ROIs are used by the phagocytes to form oxyhalides that damage ingested bacteria. ROIs may also be released from the cells and promote inflammatory responses or cause tissue damage.

Receptor editing. A process by which some immature B cells that recognize self antigens in the bone marrow may be induced to change their immunoglobulin (Ig) specificities. Receptor editing involves reactivation of the RAG genes, additional light chain V-J recombinations, and production of a new Ig light chain, allowing the cell to express a different antigen receptor that is not self-reactive.

Recirculation of lymphocytes. The continuous movement of lymphocytes via the blood stream and lymphatics, between lymph nodes or spleen, and, if activated, to peripheral inflammatory sites.

Recognition phase. The initial phase of an adaptive immune response during which antigen-specific lymphocytes bind to antigens. The recognition phase usually occurs in the specialized environment of secondary lymphoid tissues, such as lymph nodes or spleen, where both antigens and naive lymphocytes are most likely to be colocalized.

Recombination activating gene 1 and 2 (RAG-1 and RAG-2). The genes encoding RAG-1 and RAG-2 proteins, which are the lymphocyte-specific components of the V(D)J recombinase and are critical for DNA recombination events that form functional immunoglobulin and T cell receptor genes. The RAG proteins are expressed in developing B and T cells and bind to recombination recognition sequences, which consist of a highly conserved stretch of seven nucleotides, called the hepatamer, located adjacent to the V, D, or J coding sequence, followed by a spacer of exactly 12 or 23 nonconserved nucleotides, followed by a highly conserved stretch of 9 nucleotides, called the nonamer. Therefore, RAG proteins are required for expression of the antigen receptors and for the maturation of B and T lymphocytes.

Red pulp. An anatomic and functional compartment of the spleen composed of vascular sinusoids, scattered among which are large numbers of macrophages, dendritic cells, sparse lymphocytes, and plasma cells. Red pulp macrophages clear the blood of microbes, other foreign particles, and damaged red blood cells.

Repertoire. The complete collection of antigen receptors, and therefore antigen specificities, expressed by all the B and T lymphocytes of an individual.

Regulatory T cells. A population of T cells that regulate the activation or effector functions of other T cells and may be necessary to maintain tolerance to self antigens. Regulatory T cells express CD4+ and CD25.

Reverse transcriptase. An enzyme encoded by retroviruses, such as human immunodeficiency virus, which synthesizes a DNA copy of the viral genome from the RNA template of the virus. Purified reverse transcriptase is used widely in molecular biology research for purposes of cloning complementary DNAs encoding a gene of interest from messenger RNA. Reverse transcriptase inhibitors are used as drugs to treat HIV-1 infection.

Rheumatoid arthritis. An autoimmune disease characterized primarily by inflammatory damage to joints and sometimes inflammation of blood vessels, lungs, and other tissues. CD4+ T cells, activated B lymphocytes, and plasma cells are found in the inflamed joint lining (synovium), and numerous proinflammatory cytokines, including interleukin-1 and tumor necrosis factor, are present in the synovial (joint) fluid.

Scavenger receptors. A family of cell surface receptors expressed on macrophages, originally defined as receptors that mediate endocytosis of oxidized or acetylated low density lipoprotein particles but that also bind and mediate phagocytosis of a variety of microbes.

SCID mouse. A mouse strain in which B and T cells are absent because of an early block in maturation from bone marrow precursors. SCID mice carry a mutation in a component of the enzyme DNA-dependent protein kinase, which is required for double-stranded DNA break repair. Deficiency of this enzyme results in abnormal joining of immunoglobulin and T cell receptor gene segments during recombination, and therefore a failure to express antigen receptors.

Secondary immune response. An adaptive immune response that occurs on second exposure to an antigen. A secondary response is characterized by more rapid kinetics and greater magnitude relative to the primary immune response that occurs on first exposure.

Secretory component. The proteolytically cleaved portion of the extracellular domain of the poly-Ig receptor, which remains bound to IgA molecules secreted into the intestinal lumen.

Selectin. Any one of three separate but closely related carbohydrate-binding proteins that mediate adhesion of leukocytes to endothelial cells. Each of the selectin molecules is a single-chain transmembrane glycoprotein with a similar modular structure, including an extracellular calcium-dependent lectin domain. The selectins include L-selectin (CD62L) expressed on leukocytes, P-selectin (CD62P) expressed on platelets and activated endothelium, and E-selectin (CD62E) expressed on activated endothelium.

Self major histocompatibility complex (MHC) restriction. The limitation (or restriction) of antigens that can be recognized by an individual's T cells to complexes of peptides bound to MHC molecules that were present in the thymus during T cell maturation (i.e., self MHC molecules). The T cell repertoire is self MHC restricted as a result of the process of positive selection.

Self-tolerance. Unresponsiveness of the adaptive immune system to self antigens, largely as a result of inactivation or death of self-reactive lymphocytes induced by exposure to those self antigens. Self-tolerance is a cardinal feature of the normal immune system, and failure of self-tolerance leads to autoimmune diseases.

Septic shock. An often lethal complication of severe gram-negative bacterial infection with spread to the blood stream (sepsis), which is characterized by vascular collapse, disseminated intravascular coagulation, and metabolic disturbances. This syndrome is due to effects of bacterial lipopolysaccharide (LPS) and cytokines, including tumor necrosis factor, interleukin-12 (IL-12), and IL-1. Septic shock is also called **endotoxin shock.**

Seroconversion. The production of detectable antibodies in the serum specific for a microorganism, during the course of an infection or in response to an immunization.

Serology. The study of blood (serum) antibodies and their reactions with antigens. The term *serology* is often used to refer to the diagnosis of infectious diseases by detection of microbe-specific antibodies in the serum.

Serotype. An antigenically distinct subset of a species of an infectious organism that is distinguished from other subsets by serologic (i.e., serum antibody) tests. Humoral immune responses to one serotype of microbes (e.g., influenza virus) may not be protective against another serotype.

Serum. The cell-free fluid that remains when blood or plasma forms a clot. Blood antibodies are found in the serum fraction.

Serum sickness. A disease caused by injection of large doses of a protein antigen into the blood, characterized by the deposition of antigen-antibody (immune) complexes in blood vessel walls, especially in kidneys and joints. The immune complex deposition leads to complement activation and leukocyte recruitment, causing glomerulonephritis and arthritis. Serum sickness was originally described as a disorder that occurred in patients receiving injections of horse serum containing antitoxin antibodies to prevent diphtheria; these patients made antibodies against horse proteins and immune complexes composed of these antibodies and the injected antigens.

Severe combined immunodeficiencies (SCID). Immunodeficiency diseases in which both B and T lymphocytes do not develop or do not function properly; therefore, both humoral immunity and cell-mediated immunity are impaired. Children with SCID usually present with infections during the first year of life and succumb to these infections unless the immunodeficiency is treated. There are several different genetic causes of SCID.

Signal transducer and activator of transcription (STAT). A member of a family of proteins that function as signaling molecules and transcription factors in response to cytokines binding to type I and type II cytokine receptors. The STATs are present as inactive monomers in the cytoplasm of cells and are recruited to the cytoplasmic tails of cross-linked cytokine receptors where they are tyrosine-phosphorylated by Janus kinases. The phosphorylated STAT proteins dimerize and move to the nucleus, where they bind to specific sequences in the promoter regions of various genes and stimulate their transcription. Different STATs are activated by different cytokines.

Single-positive thymocyte. A maturing T cell precursor in the thymus that expresses CD4 or CD8 molecules but not both. Single positive thymocytes are found mainly in the medulla and have matured from the double-positive stage during which thymocytes express both CD4 and CD8 molecules.

Smallpox. A disease caused by variola virus. Smallpox was the first infectious disease shown to be preventable by vaccination, and the first disease to be completely eradicated by a worldwide vaccination program.

Somatic hypermutation. High-frequency point mutations in immunoglobulin heavy and light chains that occur in germinal center B cells. Mutations that lead to increased affinity of antibodies for antigen impart a selective survival advantage to the B cells producing those antibodies, leading to affinity maturation of a humoral immune response.

Somatic recombination. The process of DNA recombination by which the genes encoding the variable regions of antigen receptors are formed during lymphocyte development. A relatively limited set of inherited, or germline, DNA sequences that are initially separated from one another are brought together by enzymatic deletion of intervening sequences and re-ligation. This process occurs only in developing B and T lymphocytes.

Specificity. A cardinal feature of the adaptive immune system, referring to the ability of immune responses to distinguish between distinct antigens or small parts of macromolecular antigens. This fine specificity is attributed to lymphocyte antigen receptors that may bind to one molecule but not to another with only minor structural differences from the first.

Spleen. A peripheral lymphoid organ located in the left upper quadrant of the abdomen. The spleen is the major site for adaptive immune responses to blood-borne antigens. The red pulp of the spleen is composed of blood-filled vascular sinusoids lined by phagocytes that ingest opsonized microbes and damaged red blood cells. The white pulp of the spleen contains lymphocytes and lymphoid follicles.

Stem cell. An undifferentiated cell that divides continuously and gives rise to additional stem cells and to cells of multiple different lineages. For example, all blood cells arise from a common hematopoietic stem cell in the bone marrow.

Superantigen. Proteins that bind to and activate all the T cells in an individual that express a particular set or family of Vβ T cell receptor (TCR) genes. Superantigens are presented to T cells by binding to nonpolymorphic regions of class II major histocompatibility complex molecules on antigen-presenting cells, and they interact with conserved regions of TCR Vβ domains. Several staphylococcal enterotoxins are superantigens. Their importance lies in their ability to activate many T cells, resulting in large amounts of cytokine production and a clinical syndrome called **toxic shock syndrome** that is similar to septic shock.

Suppressor T cell. T cells that block the activation and functions of other effector T lymphocytes. Some suppressor cells may function by producing cytokines that inhibit immune responses.

Surrogate light chain. A complex of two nonvariable proteins that associate with immunoglobulin μ heavy chains in pre-B cells to form the pre-B cell receptor. The two surrogate light chain proteins include V pre-B protein, which is homologous to a light chain V domain, and λ5, which is covalently attached to the μ heavy chain by a disulfide bond.

Switch recombination. The molecular mechanism underlying immunoglobulin heavy chain class, or isotype, switching, in which a rearranged VDJ gene segment in an antibody-producing B cell recombines with a downstream C gene and the intervening C genes are deleted. DNA recombination events in switch recombination are triggered by CD40 ligation and cytokines and involve nucleotide sequences called switch regions, located in the introns at the 5' end of each C_H locus.

Syngeneic. Genetically identical. All animals of an inbred strain or monozygotic twins are syngeneic.

Syngeneic graft. A graft from a donor who is genetically identical to the recipient. Syngeneic grafts are not rejected.

Systemic lupus erythematosus (SLE). A chronic systemic autoimmune disease that affects predominantly women and is characterized by rashes, arthritis, glomerulonephritis, hemolytic anemia, thrombocytopenia, and central nervous system involvement. Many different autoantibodies are found in SLE patients, particularly anti-DNA antibodies. Many of the manifestations of SLE are due to formation of immune complexes composed of autoantibodies and their antigens and deposition of these complexes in small blood vessels in various tissues. The underlying mechanism for the breakdown of self-tolerance in SLE is not understood.

γδ T cell. A subset of T cells that express a form of antigen receptor (TCR) that is distinct from the more common αβ TCR found on CD4$^+$ and CD8$^+$ T cells. These T cells are abundant in epithelia. They recognize lipids and other nonprotein antigens of microbes.

T cell receptor (TCR). The clonally distributed antigen receptor on CD4$^+$ and CD8$^+$ T lymphocytes that recognizes complexes of foreign peptides bound to self major histocompatibility complex molecules on the surface of antigen-presenting cells. The most common form of TCR is composed of a heterodimer of two disulfide-linked transmembrane polypeptide chains, designated α and β, each containing one amino-terminal Ig-like variable (V) domain, one Ig-like constant (C) domain, a hydrophobic transmembrane region, and a short cytoplasmic region. (Another less common type of TCR, composed of γ and δ chains, is found on a small subset of T cells and recognizes different forms of antigen.)

T cell receptor (TCR) complex. A multiprotein plasma membrane complex on T lymphocytes composed of the highly variable, antigen-binding TCR heterodimer and the invariant signaling proteins CD3 γ, δ, and ε and the ζ chain.

T lymphocyte. The cell type that mediates cell-mediated immune responses in the adaptive immune system. T lymphocytes mature in the thymus, circulate in the blood, populate secondary lymphoid tissues, and are recruited to peripheral sites of antigen exposure. They express antigen receptors (T cell receptors) that recognize peptide fragments of foreign proteins bound to self major histocompatibility complex molecules. Functional subsets of T lymphocytes include CD4$^+$ helper T cells and CD8$^+$ cytolytic T lymphocytes.

T-dependent antigen. An antigen that requires both B cells and helper T cells to stimulate an antibody response. T-dependent antigens are all protein antigens that contain some epitopes recognized by T cells and other epitopes recognized by B cells. The helper T cells produce cytokines and cell surface molecules that stimulate B cell growth and differentiation into antibody-secreting cells. Humoral immune responses to T-dependent antigens are characterized by isotype switching, affinity maturation, and memory.

T_H1 cells. A functional subset of helper T cells that secretes a particular set of cytokines, including interferon-γ, and whose principal function is to stimulate phagocyte-mediated defense against infections, especially with intracellular microbes.

T_H2 cells. A functional subset of helper T cells that secretes a particular set of cytokines, including IL-4 and IL-5, and whose principal functions are to stimulate IgE and eosinophil/mast cell-mediated immune reactions and to down-regulate T_H1 responses.

Thymocyte. A precursor of a mature T lymphocyte present in the thymus.

Thymus. A bilobed organ situated in the anterior mediastinum, which is the site of maturation of T lymphocytes from bone marrow–derived precursors. The thymus is divided into an outer cortex and an inner medulla and contains epithelial cells, macrophages, dendritic cells, and numerous T cell precursors (thymocytes) at various stages of maturation.

T-independent antigen. Nonprotein antigens, such as polysaccharides and lipids, that can stimulate antibody responses without a requirement for antigen-specific helper T lymphocytes. T-independent antigens usually contain multiple identical epitopes that can cross-link antigen receptors of B cells and thereby activate the cells. Humoral immune responses to T-independent antigens show relatively little heavy chain isotype switching or affinity maturation, two processes that require signals from helper T cells.

Tissue typing. The determination of the particular MHC alleles expressed by an individual for the purposes of matching allograft donors and recipients. Tissue typing, also called HLA typing, is usually done by testing whether sera known to be reactive with certain MHC gene products mediate complement-dependent lysis of an individual's lymphocytes. Polymerase chain reaction (PCR) techniques are now also used to determine if an individual carries a particular MHC allele.

Tolerogen. An antigen that induces immunologic tolerance, in contrast to an immunogen, which induces an immune response. Many antigens can be either tolerogens or immunogens, depending on how they are administered. Tolerogenic forms of antigens include large doses of the proteins administered without adjuvants, altered peptide ligands, and orally administered antigens.

Toll-like receptors. Cell surface receptors on phagocytes and other cell types that act as pattern recognition receptors important in the innate immune response to lipopolysaccharides and other microbial products. Toll-like receptors share structural homology and signal transduction pathways with the type I interleukin-1 receptor.

Toxic shock syndrome. An acute illness characterized by shock, skin exfoliation, conjunctivitis, and diarrhea, associated with tampon use and caused by a *Staphylococcus aureus* superantigen.

Transforming growth factor-β (TGF-β). A cytokine produced by activated T cells, mononuclear phagocytes, and other cells, whose principal actions are to inhibit the proliferation and differentiation of T cells, to inhibit the activation of macrophages, and to counteract the effects of proinflammatory cytokines.

Transfusion. Transplantation of circulating blood cells, platelets, or plasma from one individual to another. Transfusions are performed to treat blood loss due to hemorrhage or to treat a deficiency in one or more blood cell types due to inadequate production or excess destruction.

Transfusion reactions. An immunologic reaction against transfused blood products, usually mediated by preformed antibodies in the recipient that bind to donor blood cell antigens, such as ABO blood group antigens or histocompatibility antigens. Transfusion reactions can lead to intravascular lysis of red blood cells and, in severe cases, kidney damage, fever, shock, and disseminated intravascular coagulation.

Transgenic mouse. A mouse that expresses an exogenous gene that has been introduced into the genome by injection of a DNA sequence into the pronuclei of fertilized mouse eggs. Transgenes insert randomly at chromosomal breakpoints and are subsequently inherited as simple mendelian traits. By designing transgenes with tissue-specific regulatory sequences, mice can be produced that express a particular gene only in certain tissues. Transgenic mice are used extensively in immunology research to study the functions of various cytokines, cell surface molecules, and intracellular signaling molecules.

Transporter associated with antigen processing (TAP). An ATP-dependent peptide transporter that mediates the active transport of peptides from the cytosol to the site of assembly of class I major histocompatibility complex (MHC) molecules inside the endoplasmic reticulum. TAP is a heterodimeric molecule composed of TAP-1 and TAP-2 polypeptides, both encoded by genes in the MHC. Because peptides are required for stable assembly of class I MHC molecules, TAP-deficient animals express very few cell surface class I MHC molecules, resulting in diminished development and activation of $CD8^+$ T cells.

Tumor immunity. Protection against the development of tumors mediated by the immune system. Strong immune responses are induced by tumors that express immunogenetic antigens (e.g., tumors that are caused by oncogenic viruses and therefore express viral antigens).

Tumor necrosis factor (TNF-α). A cytokine produced mainly by activated mononuclear phagocytes that functions to stimulate the recruitment of neutrophils and monocytes to sites of infection and to activate these cells to eradicate microbes. TNF stimulates vascular endothelial cells to express adhesion molecules and induces macrophages and endothelial cells to secrete chemokines.

In severe infections, TNF is produced in large amounts and has systemic effects, including induction of fever, synthesis of acute-phase proteins by the liver, and cachexia. When very large amounts of TNF are produced, it can cause intravascular thrombosis and shock (the clinical syndrome of septic shock).

Tumor-infiltrating lymphocytes (TILs). Lymphocytes isolated from the inflammatory infiltrates present in and around surgical resection samples of solid tumors, which are enriched for tumor-specific cytolytic T lymphocytes and natural killer cells. In an experimental mode of cancer treatment, TILs isolated from patients with tumors are expanded *in vitro* by culture with high concentrations of interleukin-2 and are then transferred back into the patients.

Tumor-specific transplantation antigen (TSTA). An antigen expressed on experimental animal tumor cells that can be detected by induction of immunologic rejection of tumor transplants. TSTAs were originally defined on chemically induced rodent sarcomas and were shown to stimulate cytolytic T lymphocyte–mediated tumor transplant rejection of transplanted tumors.

Two-signal hypothesis. A now proven hypothesis that states that the activation of lymphocytes requires two distinct signals, the first being antigen and the second either microbial products or components of innate immune responses to microbes. The requirement for antigen (so-called signal 1) ensures that the ensuing immune response is specific. The requirement for additional stimuli triggered by microbes or innate immune reactions (signal 2) ensures that immune responses are induced when they are needed (i.e., against microbes and other noxious substances) and not against harmless substances, including self antigens. Signal 2 is often referred to as costimulation.

Type I interferons (IFN-α, IFN-β). A family of cytokines, including several structurally related interferon-α (IFN-α) proteins and a single IFN-β protein, all of which have potent antiviral actions. The major source of IFN-α is mononuclear phagocytes, and IFN-β is produced by many cells, including fibroblasts. Both IFN-α and IFN-β bind to the same cell surface receptor and induce similar biologic responses. Type I IFNs inhibit viral replication, increase the lytic potential of natural killer cells, increase expression of class I major histocompatibility complex molecules on virus-infected cells, and stimulate the development of T_H1 cells, especially in humans.

Urticaria. Localized transient swelling and redness of the skin due to leakage of fluid and plasma proteins from small vessels into the dermis during an immediate hypersensitivity reaction.

V gene segments. A DNA sequence that encodes the variable domain of an immunoglobulin heavy chain or light chain or a T cell receptor α, β, γ, or δ chain. Each antigen receptor locus contains many different V gene segments, any one of which may recombine with downstream D or J segments during lymphocyte maturation to form functional antigen receptor genes.

V(D)J recombinase. A collection of enzymes that together mediate the somatic recombination events that form functional antigen receptor genes in developing B and T lymphocytes. Some of the enzymes, such as RAG-1 and RAG-2, are found only in developing lymphocytes, and others are DNA repair enzymes found in most cell types.

Vaccine. A preparation of microbial antigen, often combined with adjuvants, that is administered to individuals to induce protective immunity against microbial infections. The antigen may be in the form of live but avirulent microorganisms, killed microorganisms, or purified macromolecular components of microorganisms.

Variable region. The extracellular amino-terminal region of an immunoglobulin heavy or light chain or a T cell receptor α, β, γ, or δ chain that contains variable amino acid sequences that differ between every clone of lymphocytes and that are responsible for specificity for antigen. The antigen-binding variable sequences are localized to hypervariable segments.

Virus. A primitive obligate intracellular parasitic organism or infectious particle that consists of a simple nucleic acid genome packaged in a protein capsid, sometimes surrounded by a lipid envelope. There are many pathogenic animal viruses that cause a wide range of diseases. Humoral immune responses to viruses can be effective in blocking infection of cells, and natural killer cells and cytolytic T lymphocytes are necessary to kill already infected cells.

Western blot. An immunologic technique to determine the presence of a protein in a biologic sample. The method involves separation of proteins in the sample by electrophoresis, transfer of the protein array from the electrophoresis gel to a support membrane by capillary action (blotting), and finally detection of the protein by binding of an enzymatically or radioactively labeled antibody specific for that protein.

Wheal and flare reaction. Local swelling and redness in the skin at a site of an immediate hypersensitivity reaction. The wheal reflects increased vascular permeability and the flare results from increased local blood flow, both changes resulting from mediators, such as histamine, released from activated dermal mast cells.

White pulp. The part of the spleen that is composed predominantly of lymphocytes, arranged in periarteriolar lymphoid sheaths (PALS) and follicles. The remainder of the spleen contains vascular sinusoids lined with phagocytic cells and filled with blood, called the **red pulp.**

Wiskott-Aldrich syndrome. An X-linked disease characterized by eczema, thrombocytopenia (reduced blood platelets), and immunodeficiency manifested as susceptibility to bacterial infections. The defective gene encodes a cytosolic protein involved in signaling cascades and regulation of the actin cytoskeleton.

Xenoantigen. An antigen on a graft from another species.

Xenogeneic graft. An organ or tissue graft derived from a different species than the recipient. Transplantation of xenogeneic grafts (e.g., from pig) to human is not yet practical because of special problems related to immunologic rejection.

X-linked agammaglobulinemia. An immunodeficiency disease, also called Bruton's agammaglobulinemia, characterized by a block in early B cell maturation and an absence of serum immunoglobulin. Patients suffer from pyogenic bacterial infections. The disease is caused by mutations or deletions in the gene encoding B cell tyrosine kinase (Btk), an enzyme involved in signal transduction in developing B cells.

X-linked hyper-IgM syndrome. A rare immunodeficiency disease caused by mutations in the CD40 ligand gene and characterized by a failure of B cell heavy chain isotype switching and cell-mediated immunity. Patients suffer from both pyogenic bacterial and intracellular microbial infections.

Zeta-associated protein of 70 kD (ZAP-70). An Src family cytoplasmic protein tyrosine kinase that is critical for early signaling steps in antigen-induced T cell activation. ZAP-70 binds to phosphorylated tyrosines in the cytoplasmic tails of the ζ chain of the T cell antigen-receptor complex and, in turn, phosphorylates adapter proteins that recruit other components of the signaling cascade.

ζ chain. A transmembrane protein expressed in T cells as part of the T cell receptor complex, which contains immunoreceptor tyrosine-based activation motifs in its cytoplasmic portion and which binds the ZAP-70 protein tyrosine kinase during T cell activation.

Clinical Cases

This appendix includes five clinical cases illustrating various diseases involving the immune system. These cases are not meant to teach clinical skills but rather to show how the basic science of immunology contributes to our understanding of human diseases. Each case illustrates typical ways a disease manifests, what tests are used in diagnosis, and common modes of treatment. The appendix was compiled with the assistance of Dr. Richard Mitchell, Department of Pathology, Brigham and Women's Hospital, Boston, Massachusetts, and Dr. James Faix, Department of Pathology, Stanford University School of Medicine, Palo Alto, California.

Case 1: Lymphoma

E.B. was a 38-year-old chemical engineer who had been well all of his life. One morning, he noticed a lump in his left groin while showering. It was not tender, and the overlying skin appeared normal. After a few weeks, he began to worry about it because it did not "go away," and he finally made an appointment with a doctor after 2 months. On physical examination, the physician noted a subcutaneous firm, movable nodule, about 3 cm in diameter in the left inguinal region. The doctor asked E.B. if he had recently noticed any infections of his left foot or leg (which E.B. hadn't). The doctor also found some slightly enlarged lymph nodes in E.B.'s right neck. Otherwise, the physical examination was normal. The doctor explained that the nodule was probably a lymph node that was enlarged due to a reaction to some infection. However, he advised E.B. to see a surgeon who would remove the lymph node so that a pathologist could examine it to be sure that it was not malignant.

The lymph node was removed, and histologic examination revealed an expansion of the node by follicular structures composed of monotonous collections of enlarged, activated ("lymphoblastoid") cells (Fig. A-1). Immunohistochemistry revealed that these cells expressed B cell surface molecules. Also, polymerase chain reaction (PCR) analysis of DNA from the lymph node showed a clonal rearrangement of the immunoglobulin heavy chain gene. On this basis, the diagnosis of follicular lymphoma was made.

1. Why does the presence of a clonal rearrangement of immunoglobulin heavy chain genes in the lymph node indicate a neoplasm rather than a response to an infection?

E.B. was treated with chemotherapy. The lymphadenopathy in his neck (which was due to his lymphoma) regressed but, unfortunately, a new enlarged lymph node appeared in his left cervical area about a year later. This lymph node was removed, and it showed follicular lymphoma, with the same histologic features of the original.

2. If one developed an anti-idiotypic antibody against the surface immunoglobulin present on E.B.'s original lymphoma cells, it might not recognize the cells responsible for his recurrence. Why not?

The oncologist caring for E.B. is now planning to administer chemotherapy and radiation to kill all the tumor cells, followed by bone marrow transplantation.

3. Why would it be necessary to perform the bone marrow transplantation, and what will be the status of the patient's immune system after the recommended treatment?

Answers to Questions for Case 1

1. In an infection, many different clones of lymphocytes are activated. More than one clone may be specific for the same microbial antigen, and different clones may be responding to different antigens produced by the microbe. Furthermore, even in a lymph node draining a site of infection, there are many clones of normal B cells not specific for the microbe. Because each clone of B

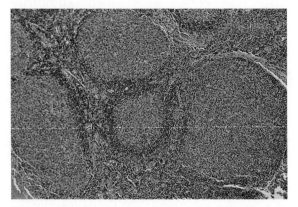

Figure A-1   Lymph node biopsy with follicular lymphoma. The microscopic appearance of the patient's inguinal lymph node is shown. The follicular structures are abnormal, composed of a monotonous collection of neoplastic cells. In contrast, a lymph node with reactive hyperplasia would have follicles with germinal center formation, containing a heterogeneous mixture of cells.

cells has a unique rearrangement of its immunoglobulin heavy and light chain genes (see Chapter 4, pages 79-80), the analysis of heavy chain genes in the polyclonal mixture of B cells in a lymph node draining a site of infection reveals many different (polyclonal) rearrangements. In contrast, B cell lymphomas arise from a single cell with a unique immunoglobulin heavy chain rearrangement, and after the tumor has grown for some time it represents the majority of cells in the lymph node. Therefore, analysis of heavy chain genes in a lymph node with a B cell lymphoma reveals a single dominant heavy chain rearrangement. The PCR is often used for analysis of clonality of B cell tumors. In this method, specific sequences of the tumor DNA are amplified by the use of complementary DNA primers and a DNA polymerase. The size of the amplified products is analyzed by gel electrophoresis. Two primers are typically used, one corresponding to a consensus sequence common to most V segments, the other to a sequence common to most J segments. The length of the amplified PCR product is determined by the unique sequences generated during VDJ joining in each clone of B cells. With a normal population of B cells, many PCR products of different sizes are generated, and these appear as a smear on the gel. In the case of lymphoma, all the B cells have the same VDJ rearrangement and the PCR product is of one size, appearing as a single band on the gel.

2. An anti-idiotypic antibody would recognize the portions of the immunoglobulin that are unique to the original

tumor, that is, the hypervariable portions of the antigen receptors of this clone of B cells. During their lives, the immunoglobulin genes of B cells often undergo extensive somatic mutations; in humoral immune responses to protein antigens, this process accounts for affinity maturation (see Chapter 7, pages 136-140). Somatic mutations of the Ig genes may occur in the tumor cells also, resulting in the appearance of B cells that express a new Ig that is not recognized by the anti-idiotypic antibody.

3. The chemotherapy and radiation treatment, which kills the tumor cells, also destroys the normal hematopoietic cells in the bone marrow. This would be lethal because the patient would not be able to produce red blood cells for oxygen transport, leukocytes for immunity, and platelets to control bleeding. By injecting hematopoietic stem cells from another donor, hematopoiesis can be restored. The stem cells may be administered in the form of whole bone marrow or stem cells purified from the peripheral blood of a donor. Sometimes, the patient's own marrow is harvested before the chemotherapy and irradiation, treated *in vitro* to destroy tumor cells specifically, and then transplanted back into the patient after the antitumor treatments. Early after bone marrow transplantation, patients often show considerable immune deficiencies. Because B and T lymphocyte progenitors arise from bone marrow stem cells, bone marrow transplantation can lead to reconstitution of the patient's adaptive immune system over time.

Case 2: Heart Transplant Complicated by Allograft Rejection

C.M., a computer software salesman, was 48 years old when he came to his primary care physician because of fatigue and shortness of breath. He had not seen a doctor on a regular basis prior to this visit and felt well up until 1 year ago when he began experiencing difficulty climbing stairs or playing basketball with his children. Over the past 6 months he had trouble breathing when he lay down in bed. He did not remember ever experiencing significant chest pain and had no family history of heart disease. He did recall that about 18 months ago he had to take 2 days off from work because of a severe flulike illness.

On examination, he had a pulse of 105, a respiratory rate of 32, and a blood pressure of 100/60 mm Hg and was afebrile. His doctor heard rales (evidence of abnormal fluid accumulation) in the bases of both lungs. His feet and ankles were swollen. A chest x-ray showed pulmonary edema and pleural effusions and a significantly enlarged left ventricle. C.M. was admitted to the cardiology service of the University Hospital. On the basis of further tests, including coronary angiography and echocardiography, a diagnosis of dilated cardiomyopathy was made. The doctors explained to the patient that his heart muscle had been damaged. The cause may have been an episode of inflammation as a complication of a viral infection some time ago, but they could not be sure. The only lifesaving treatment for his condition would be to receive a heart transplant.

A panel-reactive antibody (PRA) test was performed on C.M.'s serum to determine whether he had been previously sensitized to alloantigens. This test showed the patient had no circulating antibodies against HLA antigens, and no further immunologic testing was performed. Two weeks later in a nearby city, a donor heart was removed from a victim of a construction-site accident. The donor had the same ABO blood type as C.M. The transplant surgery, performed 4 hours after the donor heart was removed, went well, and the allograft was functioning properly postoperatively.

1. What problems might arise if the patient and the heart donor have different blood types, or if the patient has high levels of anti-HLA antibodies?

C.M. was placed on immunosuppressive therapy the day after transplantation, which included daily doses of cyclosporine, mycophenolic acid, and prednisone. Endomyocardial biopsies were performed 1 week after surgery and showed no evidence of myocardial injury or inflammatory cells. He was sent home 10 days after surgery, and within a month he was able to do light exercise without problems. Routinely scheduled endomyocardial biopsies performed within the first 3 months after transplantation were normal, but a biopsy performed 14 weeks after surgery showed the presence of numerous lymphocytes within the myocardium and a few apoptotic muscle fibers (Fig. A-2). The findings were interpreted as evidence of acute allograft rejection.

2. What was the patient's immune system responding to, and what were the effector mechanisms in the acute rejection episode?

C.M.'s serum creatinine level, an indicator of renal function, was high (2.2 mg/dL; normal < 1.5 mg/dL). His doctors therefore did not want to increase his cyclosporine dose because this drug can be toxic to the kidneys. He was given three additional doses of a steroid drug over 18 hours, and a repeat endomyocardial biopsy 1 week later showed only a few scattered macrophages and a small focus of healing tissue. C.M. went home feeling well, and he was able to live a relatively normal life, taking cyclosporine, mycophenolic acid, and prednisone daily.

3. What is the goal of the immunosuppressive drug therapy?

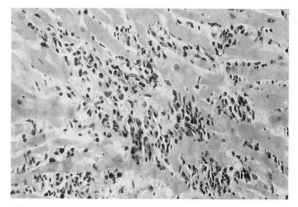

Figure A-2 Endomyocardial biopsy showing acute cellular rejection. The heart muscle is infiltrated by lymphocytes, and necrotic muscle fibers are present. (Courtesy of Dr. Richard Mitchell, Department of Pathology, Brigham and Women's Hospital, Boston, MA.)

Coronary angiograms performed yearly since the transplant showed a gradual narrowing of the lumens of the coronary arteries. In the sixth year after transplantation, C.M. began experiencing some shortness of breath after mild exercise and showed some left ventricular dilatation on radiographic examination. An intravascular ultrasound examination demonstrated significant thickening of the walls and narrowing of the lumen of the coronary arteries (Fig. A-3). An endomyocardial biopsy showed areas of ischemic necrosis. C.M. and his physicians are now considering the possibility of a second cardiac transplant.

4. What process has led to failure of the graft after 6 years?

Answers to Questions for Case 2

1. If the patient and the heart donor had different blood types, or if the patient had high levels of anti-HLA antibodies, a form of rejection called hyperacute rejection might occur after transplantation (see Chapter 10, pages 188-189). Individuals with type A, B, or O blood group have circulating IgM antibodies against the antigens they do not possess (B, A, or both, respectively). People who have received previous blood transfusions, transplants, or were once pregnant may have circulating anti-HLA antibodies. Blood group antigens and HLA antigens are present on endothelial cells. Preformed antibodies, already present in the recipient at the time of transplantation, can bind to these antigens on graft endothelial cells, causing complement activation,

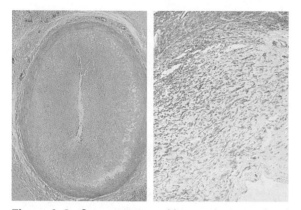

Figure A–3   Coronary artery with transplant-associated arteriosclerosis. This histologic section was taken from a coronary artery of a cardiac allograft that was removed from a patient 5 years after transplantation because of graft failure. The lumen is markedly narrowed by the presence of intimal smooth muscle cells. (Courtesy of Dr. Richard Mitchell, Department of Pathology, Brigham and Women's Hospital, Boston, MA.)

leukocyte recruitment, and thrombosis. As a result, the graft blood supply becomes impaired and the organ can rapidly undergo ischemic necrosis. The panel reactive antibody test is typically performed to determine whether a patient needing a transplant has preexisting antibodies specific for HLA antigens from a random collection of individuals. The test is performed by mixing the patient's serum with a panel of lymphocytes from various donors, adding anti-immunoglobulin antibody (to amplify the reaction) and complement, and examining if the lymphocytes are lysed. The results are expressed as the percentage of donor cells from a panel of donors with which a potential graft recipient's serum reacts. The higher the PRA, the greater the chance that the recipient will reject a graft.

2. In the acute rejection episode, the patient's immune system is responding to alloantigens in the graft (see Chapter 10, pages 185-188). These antigens are likely to include donor MHC molecules encoded by alleles not shared by the recipient, as well as unshared allelic variants of other proteins (minor histocompatibility antigens). These alloantigens may be expressed on the graft endothelial cells, leukocytes, and parenchymal cells within the donor heart. The effector mechanisms in the acute rejection episode include both cell-mediated and humoral immune responses. Recipient CD4+ T cells secrete cytokines that promote macrophage activation and inflammation, which causes myocyte or endothelial

cell injury and dysfunction, and CD8+ cytolytic T lymphocytes directly kill graft cells. Recipient antibodies, produced in response to the graft antigens, bind to graft cells, leading to complement activation and leukocyte recruitment.

3. The goal of the immunosuppressive drug therapy is to impair the recipient's immune response to alloantigens present in the graft, thereby preventing rejection. The drugs work by blocking T cell activation (cyclosporine), lymphocyte proliferation (mycophenolic acid), and inflammatory cytokine production (prednisone). An attempt is made to preserve some immune function to combat infections.

4. The graft has failed as a result of chronic rejection manifested as a thickening of the walls and narrowing of the lumens of the graft arteries (see Chapter 10, pages 188-189). This vascular change, called graft arteriosclerosis, or transplant-associated arteriosclerosis, leads to ischemic damage to the heart and is the most frequent cause of chronic graft failure. It may be caused by a chronic delayed-type hypersensitivity reaction against vessel wall alloantigens, resulting in cytokine-stimulated smooth muscle cell migration into the intima and proliferation of the smooth muscle cells.

Case 3: Allergic Asthma

I.E. was a 10-year-old girl who was brought to her pediatrician's office in November because of frequent coughing for the past 2 days, wheezing, and a feeling of tightness in her chest. Her symptoms had been especially severe at night. In addition to her routine checkups, she had visited the doctor in the past for occasional ear and upper respiratory tract infections but had not previously experienced wheezing or chest tightness. She had eczema, but otherwise, she was in good health and was developmentally normal. Her immunizations were up to date. She lived at home with her mother, father, and two sisters, ages 12 and 4, and a pet cat. Both her parents smoked cigarettes, her father suffered from hay fever, and her older sister had a history of sinus infections in the past.

At the time of her examination, I.E. had a temperature of 37° C (98.6° F), blood pressure of 105/65 mm Hg, and a respiratory rate of 28 breaths per minute. She did not appear short of breath. There were no signs of ear infection or pharyngitis. Auscultation of the chest revealed diffuse wheezing in both lungs without signs of congestive heart failure (rales). There was no evidence of pneumonia. The doctor made a presumptive diagnosis of bronchospasm and referred I.E. to a pediatric allergist-immunologist who was associated with his physicians' group. In the meantime, the patient was given a prescription for a short-acting β₂-adrenergic agonist bronchodilator inhaler, and the child was instructed to administer it every 6 hours to relieve symptoms. This drug binds to β₂-adrenergic receptors on bronchial smooth muscle cells and causes them to relax, resulting in dilatation of the bronchioles.

1. Asthma is an example of "atopy." What are the different ways in which "atopy" may manifest clinically?

One week later, I.E. was seen by the allergist. He auscultated her lungs and confirmed the presence of wheezing. I.E. was instructed to blow into a flowmeter, and the doctor determined that her peak expiratory flow rate was 65% of normal, indicating airway obstruction. The doctor then administered a nebulized bronchodilator, and 10 minutes later performed the test again. The repeat flow rate was 85% of normal, indicating reversibility of the airway obstruction. Blood was drawn and sent for total and differential blood cell count and IgE levels. In addition, a skin test was performed to determine hypersensitivity to various antigens and showed a positive result for cat dander and house dust (Fig. A-4). The patient was instructed to begin using an inhaled corticosteroid and to use her bronchodilator only as needed for respiratory symptoms. She was asked to make a return appointment 2 weeks later for re-evaluation and discussion of blood test results.

2. What is the immunologic basis for a "positive" skin test?

When I.E. returned to the allergist's office, laboratory tests revealed that she had a serum IgE level of 1200 IU/mL

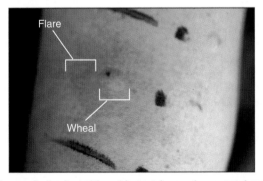

Figure A–4 **A positive skin test for environmental antigens.** Small doses of the antigens are injected intradermally. If mast cells are present with bound IgE specific for the test antigen, the antigen will crosslink the Fc receptors to which the IgE is bound. This induces degranulation of the mast cells and the release of mediators that cause the wheal and flare reaction.

(normal range: 0–180) and a total white blood cell count of 7000 /mm³ with 3% eosinophils (normal < 0.5%). When she returned to the allergist's office a week later, her physical examination was significantly improved, with no audible wheezing. I.E.'s peak expiratory airflow had improved to 90% of predicted. The family was told that I.E. had reversible airway obstruction, possibly triggered by a viral illness and possibly related to cat and dust allergies. The doctor advised the cat should either be given to a friend or at least kept out of I.E.'s bedroom. The mother was told that smoking in the house was probably contributing to I.E.'s symptoms. The doctor recommended that I.E. continue to use the short-acting inhaler for acute episodes of wheezing or shortness of breath. I.E. was asked to return in 3 months, sooner if she used the inhaler more than twice per month.

3. What is the mechanism for the increased IgE levels seen in patients who suffer from allergic symptoms?

The family cat was given to a neighbor, and I.E. did well on the therapy for about 6 months, only experiencing mild wheezing a few times. The next spring, she began to have more frequent episodes of coughing and wheezing. During a soccer game one Saturday, she became very short of breath, and her parents brought her to the emergency department of the local hospital. After confirming that she was experiencing marked upper airway constriction, the emergency department physician treated her with a nebulized β₂-agonist bronchodilator and an oral corticosteroid. After 6 hours, her symptoms resolved, and she was sent home. I.E. was brought to her allergist the next week, who changed her maintenance medication to a different inhaled corticosteroid. She has subsequently been well, with occasional mild "attacks" that are cleared by the bronchodilator inhaler.

4. What are the therapeutic approaches to allergic asthma?

Answers to Questions for Case 3

1. "Atopic" reactions to essentially harmless antigens are mediated by IgE on mast cells but may present in a variety of ways (see Chapter 11, pages 198-200). The symptoms usually reflect the site of entry of the allergen. Hay fever (allergic rhinitis) and asthma are usually responses to inhaled allergens, whereas urticaria and eczema more commonly occur with skin exposure. Although food allergies may cause gastrointestinal symptoms in small children, in adults they usually also provoke systemic urticaria. The most dramatic presentation of allergies to insect venom, foods, or drugs is anaphylaxis, an allergic reaction in which there is systemic

vasodilatation, increased vascular permeability, and bronchoconstriction. This may lead to asphyxia and cardiovascular collapse.

2. Immediate release of histamine from triggered mast cells produces a central "wheal" of edema (due to leakage of plasma) and the surrounding "flare" of vascular congestion (due to vessel dilation). However, it is the subsequent "late phase reaction," characterized by cellular inflammation, that is more characteristic of the damage to tissue affected by allergic diseases. (See Chapter 11, pages 197-198). The allergy skin test should not be confused with the skin test used to assess prior sensitization to certain infectious agents such as *Mycobacterium tuberculosis*. A positive tuberculosis skin test is an example of a delayed-type hypersensitivity (DTH) reaction, mediated by antigen-stimulated helper T cells, which release cytokines such as interferon-γ, leading to macrophage activation and inflammation. (See Chapter 6, pages 112-115).

3. For unknown reasons, these patients mount helper T cell responses of the T_H2 type to a variety of essentially harmless protein antigens, and the T_H2 cells produce IL-4 and IL-5. IL-4 induces IgE synthesis by B cells, and IL-5 promotes eosinophil production and activation (see Chapter 5, pages 95-99 and Chapter 11, pages 194-197). Because atopy appears to run in families, some inherited abnormality in immune regulation (probably multigenic) may be involved. Attention has been focused especially on genes on chromosome 5q (associated with IgE class switching, eosinophil growth, and the β_2-adrenergic receptor) and on 11q (associated with the IgE receptor).

4. A major therapeutic approach for allergies is prevention by avoidance of precipitating allergens, if known. Although therapy has previously been focused on treating the symptoms of bronchoconstriction by elevating intracellular cyclic adenosine monophosphate (cAMP) levels (β_2-adrenergic agents and inhibitors of cAMP degradation), the balance of therapy has shifted to anti-inflammatory agents in recent years. These include corticosteroids (which block cytokine release) and cromolyn (which may inhibit release of mast cell mediators). Newer approaches include receptor antagonists for lipid mediators and inhibitors of leukocyte adhesion.

Case 4: Systemic Lupus Erythematosus (SLE)

N.Z. was a 25-year-old unmarried woman who presented to her primary care physician 2 years ago with the complaints of joint pains involving her wrists, fingers, and ankles. When seen in the office, N.Z. had normal body temperature, heart rate, blood pressure, and respiratory rate. There was a noticeable red rash on her cheeks, most marked around her nose, and on questioning she said the redness got worse after being out in the sun for 1 or 2 hours. The joints of her fingers and her wrists were swollen and tender. The remainder of the physical examination was unremarkable.

Her doctor took a blood sample for various tests. Her hematocrit was 35% (normal 37% to 48%). The total white blood cell count was 9800/mm^3 (within normal range) with a normal differential count. The erythrocyte sedimentation rate was 40 mm/hr (normal 1–20). Her serum antinuclear antibody (ANA) test was positive at 1:256 dilution (normally, negative at 1:8 dilution). Other laboratory findings were unremarkable. Based on these findings, a diagnosis of systemic lupus erythematosus was made. N.Z. was treated with oral prednisone, a corticosteroid, and her joint pain subsided.

1. What is the significance of the positive result for the ANA test?

Three months later, N.Z. began feeling unusually tired and thought that she had the "flu." For about a week she had noticed that her ankles were swollen, and she had difficulty putting on her shoes. She returned to her primary care physician. Her ankles and feet showed severe edema (swollen as a result of extra fluid in the tissue). Her abdomen appeared slightly distended and had a mild shifting dullness on percussion (a sign of an abnormally high amount of fluid in the peritoneal cavity). Her physician ordered several laboratory tests. Her ANA test result was still positive, with a titer of 1:256, and her erythrocyte sedimentation rate was 120 mm/hr. Serum albumin was 0.8 g/dL (normal 3.5–5.0). Measurement of serum complement proteins revealed a C3 of 42 mg/dL (normal 80–180) and a C4 of 5 mg/dL (normal 15–45). Urinalysis showed 4+ proteinuria, red blood cells and white blood cells, and numerous hyaline and granular casts. A 24-hour urine sample contained 4 g of protein.

2. What is the likely reason for the decreased complement levels and the abnormalities in blood and urinary proteins?

Because of the abnormal urinalysis, the doctor recommended that a renal biopsy be taken. This was performed a week later in the outpatient surgery department of the community hospital next door to the doctor's office. The biopsy specimen was examined by routine histologic methods, immunofluorescence, and electron microscopy (Fig. A-5).

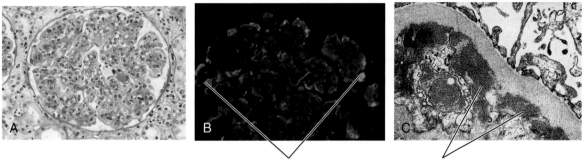

Granular deposits of immunoglobulin
and complement in the basement membrane

Figure A–5 Glomerulonephritis with immune complex deposition in systemic lupus erythematosus. A. A light micrograph of a renal biopsy specimen in which there is neutrophilic infiltration in a glomerulus. B. An immunofluorescence micrograph showing granular deposits of IgG along the basement membrane. (In this technique, called immunofluorescence microscopy, a frozen section of the kidney is incubated with a fluorescein-conjugated antibody against IgG and the site of deposition of the IgG is defined by determining where the fluorescence is located.) C. An electron micrograph of the same tissue revealing immune complex deposition. (Courtesy of Dr. Helmut Rennke, Department of Pathology, Brigham and Women's Hospital, Boston, MA.)

3. What is the explanation for the pathology seen in the kidney?

The physician made the diagnosis of proliferative lupus nephritis and treated N.Z. with a higher dose of prednisone than she was taking previously. The proteinuria and edema subsided over a 2-week period, and serum C3 levels returned to normal. Her corticosteroid dose was tapered down to a lower amount. Over the next few years, she has had intermittent flare-ups of her disease, with joint aches, tissue swelling, and laboratory tests indicating depressed C3 levels and proteinuria. These have been effectively treated with corticosteroids, and she has been able to lead an active life.

4. Some autoimmune diseases are thought to be caused by lymphocytes specific for microbes that are activated by an infection and that cross-react with self antigens. Why is this not likely to be a valid explanation for how SLE develops?

Answers to Questions for Case 4

1. A positive antinuclear antibody test reveals the presence of serum antibodies that bind to components of cellular nuclei. The test is performed by placing different dilutions of the patent's serum on top of a monolayer of human cells on a glass slide. A second fluorescently labeled anti-immunoglobulin is then added, and the cells are examined with a fluorescent microscope to detect if any serum antibodies bound to the nuclei. The ANA titer is the maximum dilution of the serum that still produces detectable nuclear staining. Patients with SLE often have antinuclear antibodies, which may be specific for histones, other nuclear proteins, or double-stranded DNA. These are autoantibodies, and their production is evidence of autoimmunity. Autoantibodies may be produced against red blood cell membrane proteins and many other self antigens.

2. Some of the autoantibodies form circulating immune complexes by binding to antigens in the blood. When these immune complexes deposit in the basement membranes of vessel walls, they may activate the classical pathway of complement, leading to depletion of complement proteins because of consumption. Inflammation caused by the immune complexes in the kidney leads to leakage of protein and red blood cells into the urine. The loss of protein in the urine results in reduced plasma albumin, reduction of osmotic pressure of the plasma, and fluid loss into the tissues, leading to edema of the feet and abdominal distention.

3. The kidney pathology is the result of the deposition of circulating immune complexes in the basement membranes of renal glomeruli. These deposits can be seen by immunofluorescence and electron microscopy. The immune complexes activate complement, and leukocytes are recruited by complement by-products (C3a, C5a) and by binding of leukocyte Fc receptors to the antibodies in the complexes. These leukocytes are activated, and they produce reactive oxygen intermediates and lysosomal enzymes that damage the glomerular

basement membrane. These findings are characteristic of immune complex–mediated tissue injury, and complexes may deposit in joints and small blood vessels anywhere in the body as well as in the kidney. SLE is a prototype of an immune complex disease (see Chapter 11, pages 201-204).

4. The autoantibodies in SLE patients are specific for a wide range of structurally unrelated self antigens. It is therefore unlikely that this represents a cross-reaction with one or a few microbial antigens (so-called molecular mimicry) but rather implicates a fundamental dysregulation of the mechanisms of self-tolerance that affects many different clones of lymphocytes (see Chapter 9, pages 166-176).

Case 5: HIV Infection and Acquired Immunodeficiency Syndrome (AIDS)

J.C. was a 28-year-old carpenter's assistant with a history of HIV infection who came to the emergency department of his local hospital complaining of difficulty in breathing and chills. The patient had a history of intravenous heroin abuse, with an admission to the same hospital 7 years earlier because of a drug overdose. At that time he had tested positive for both anti-HIV and anti-hepatitis B virus antibodies by enzyme-linked immunosorbent assay (ELISA). On discharge from the hospital, he was referred to an HIV clinic, where Western blot testing confirmed the presence of anti-HIV antibodies. A reverse transcriptase PCR test for viral RNA in the blood revealed 15,000 copies/mL of viral genome. His CD4$^+$ T cell count was 800/mm^3 (normal 500 to 1500/mm^3). There was no evidence of opportunistic infections at that time.

1. What major risk factor did this patient have for acquiring HIV infection? What are other risk factors for HIV infection?

J.C. began taking HIV medications including two nucleoside reverse transcriptase inhibitors and one viral protease inhibitor. He also attended a drug abuse rehabilitation program (and has not used illegal drugs since the time of his overdose). He became steadily employed and acquired health insurance benefits. After a year of his triple-drug therapy, J.C.'s CD4$^+$ T cell count remained about 800/mm^3 and a viral load test indicated less than 100 copies/mL. However, over the next 5 years, his CD4$^+$ T cell count gradually declined to 300/mm^3. He assured his doctors that he rarely missed a dose of his medication, which was changed to different reverse transcriptase inhibitors three times, and a different protease inhibitor once, in an attempt to stop the decline in his CD4$^+$ count. He felt well and was able to work

regularly, with the only symptoms being multiple enlarged lymph nodes. He was started on antibiotic prophylaxis for *Pneumocystis carinii* pneumonia 3 years after his initial diagnosis.

2. What caused the gradual decline in the CD4$^+$ T cell count?

After 6 years from the time of initial diagnosis, J.C. began to lose weight. At a clinic visit 6 months ago, he complained of a sore throat and had white plaque lesions in his mouth. Flow cytometry indicated his CD4$^+$ count was 64/mm^3 (Fig. A-6), and the viral load was more than 500,000 copies/mL.

3. What is the likely reason that the anti-HIV drugs given to this patient became ineffective after some time?

In the emergency department, the patient had a temperature of 39° C (102.2° F), blood pressure of 160/55 mm Hg, and shallow respirations at a rate of 40 breaths per minute. He had lost 10 kg of weight since his last clinic visit. Several red skin nodules were present on the patient's chest and arms. A chest radiograph showed a diffuse pneumonia. Intravenous antibiotics were administered for presumed *Pneumocystis carinii* pneumonia, and the patient was admitted to the infectious disease service.

That night, a sputum sample was collected, and the following day skin biopsy specimens were taken from his chest. The sputum sample was stained for microorganisms and revealed numerous *Pneumocystis carinii*. The skin biopsy specimens showed Kaposi's sarcoma. Despite intensive care, the patient's pneumonia progressed and he died 3 days later.

4. Why are AIDS patients at high risk for developing opportunistic infections such as *Pneumocystis carinii* pneumonia and malignancies such as Kaposi's sarcoma?

Answers to Questions for Case 5

1. Intravenous drug use is the major risk factor for HIV infection in this patient. Shared needles among drug addicts transmit blood-borne viral particles from one infected individual to other persons. Other major risk factors for HIV infection include sexual intercourse with an infected individual, transfusion of contaminated blood products, and birth from an infected mother. (See Chapter 12, page 220.)

2. After initial infection, the HIV rapidly enters various types of cells in the body, including CD4$^+$ T lymphocytes, mononuclear phagocytes, and others. Once in an

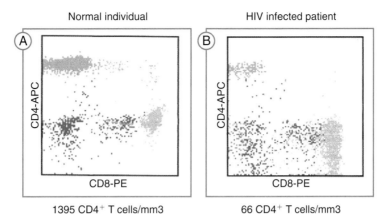

Figure A–6   Flow cytometry analysis of HIV-infected patient's CD4⁺ and CD8⁺ T cells. A suspension of the patient's white blood cells was incubated with monoclonal antibodies specific for CD4 and CD8. The anti-CD4 antibody was labeled with the fluorochrome allophycocyanin (APC), and the anti-CD8 antibody was labeled with the fluorochrome phycoerythrin (PE). These two fluorochromes emit light of different colors when excited by the appropriate wavelengths. The cell suspensions were analyzed in a flow cytometer, which can enumerate the number of cells stained by each of the differently labeled antibodies. In this way the number of CD4⁺ and CD8⁺ T cells can be determined. Shown here are two-color plots of a control blood sample (A) and that of the patient (B). The CD4⁺ T cells are shown in orange (*upper left quadrant*), and the CD8⁺ T cells are shown in green (*lower right quadrant*). (These are not the colors of light emitted by the APC and PE fluorochromes.)

intracellular location, the virus is safe from antibody neutralization. The gradual decline in CD4⁺ T cells in this patient was caused by repetitive cycles of HIV infection and death of CD4⁺ T cells in lymphoid organs. The symptoms of AIDS do not usually occur until the blood count of CD4⁺ T cells is below 200/mm³, reflecting a severe depletion of T cells in the lymphoid organs. (See Chapter 12, pages 220-222.)

3. HIV has a very high mutation rate. Mutations in the reverse transcriptase gene that render the enzyme resistant to nucleoside inhibitors occur frequently in treated patients. Resistance to protease inhibitors may come about by similar mechanisms.

4. The deficiencies in T cell–mediated immunity in AIDS patients lead to impaired immunity to viruses, fungi, and protozoans, which are easily controlled by normal immune system. *Pneumocystis carinii* is a parasite with features of both fungi and protozoans and it is usually eradicated by the action of activated CD4⁺ T cells. Many of the malignancies that are frequent in AIDS patients are associated with oncogenic viruses. For example, Kaposi's sarcoma is associated with human herpesvirus 6 infection. Many of the lymphomas that occur in AIDS patients are associated with the Epstein-Barr virus, and many of the skin and cervical carcinomas that occur in AIDS patients are associated with human papillomavirus.

Index

Note: Page numbers followed by the letter f refer to figures.